Sociology for Social Workers and Probation Officers

How does a social work student make the connection between sociological knowledge and day-to-day social work?

Sociology for Social Workers and Probation Officers provides an introduction to sociological ideas and research and places them firmly into the context of actual social work practice. It encourages readers to develop critical awareness and reach their own judgements about the usefulness and implications of holding certain conceptual positions, and shows how social work can be better informed and improved by doing so.

Fully revised and updated throughout, this second edition examines sociology in relation to key areas of social work and probation practice, and includes one new chapter. Areas covered are:

- family
- childhood
- youth
- community
- care and caring
- health and illness
- crime and deviance.

Essential reading for all social work and probation studies students, this text looks beyond individual and psychological explanations and solutions to develop a sociological knowledge base for social work practice.

Viviene E. Cree is Professor of Social Work Studies at the University of Edinburgh, UK. She is the editor of *Social Work: A Reader* and *Becoming a Social Worker* and co-author of *Social Work: Voices from the Inside*, all published by Routledge. She is also co-author of *Social Work: Making a Difference* and co-editor of the series Social Work in Practice, published jointly by BASW and the Policy Press.

Student Social Work

This exciting new textbook series is ideal for all students studying to be qualified social workers, whether at undergraduate or Masters level. Covering key elements of the social work curriculum, the books are accessible, interactive and thought provoking.

New titles

Human Growth and Development
John Sudbery

Mental Health Social Work in Context
Nick Gould

Social Work and Social Policy
An introduction
Jonathan Dickens

Social Work Placements
Mark Doel

Sociology for Social Workers and Probation Officers
Viviene E. Cree

Forthcoming titles

Integrating Social Work Theory and Practice
Pam Green Lister

Social Work
A reader
Viviene E. Cree

Building Relationships and Communicating with Young Children
A practical guide
Karen Winter

Sociology for Social Workers and Probation Officers

Second edition

Viviene E. Cree

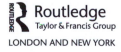
Routledge
Taylor & Francis Group

LONDON AND NEW YORK

First edition published 1999
by Routledge

This edition published 2010
by Routledge
2 Park Square, Milton Park, Abingdon, Oxon, OX14 4RN

Simultaneously published in the USA and Canada
by Routledge
270 Madison Avenue, New York, NY 10016

Routledge is an imprint of the Taylor & Francis Group, an informa business

© 2010 Viviene E. Cree

Designed and typeset in Rotis
by Keystroke, Tettenhall, Wolverhampton
Printed and bound in Great Britain
by TJ International Ltd, Padstow, Cornwall

British Library Cataloguing in Publication Data
A catalogue record for this book is available from the British Library

Library of Congress Cataloging in Publication Data
Cree, Viviene E., 1954–
    Sociology for social workers and probation officers / Viviene E. Cree. 2nd ed.
        p. cm.
    Includes bibliographical references.
    1. Social service–Sociological aspects. 2. Probation–Sociological aspects.
    3. Sociology. I. Title.
    HV41.C74 2010
    301–dc22   2010003587

ISBN10: 0–415–44621–X (hbk)
ISBN10: 0–415–44622–8 (pbk)
ISBN10: 0–203–84677–X (ebk)

ISBN13: 978–0–415–44621–1 (hbk)
ISBN13: 978–0–415–44622–8 (pbk)
ISBN13: 978–0–203–84677–3 (ebk)

For Kate

Contents

Contents

Preface

Setting the scene

It is ten years since the first edition of this book was published, and ten years since I first set myself the task of explaining sociology in layperson's terms to a social work audience. At that point, I acknowledged that there was a huge amount of sociological writing in the public domain, and suggested that this book might fill a gap in the sociological and social work literature, both by providing an introduction to sociological ideas and research and by considering the application of these concepts to practice with service users in social work and probation settings. The environment has changed in the intervening years – internationally, in the UK and, more parochially, in my own life. All of these changes have some relevance for this book. And of all these changes have relevance for a sociological understanding of social work.

Internationally, we have seen massive political, economic and social changes, all of which have had an impact on individual lives, societies and nations. These include (and not in any particular order):

- *Global climate changes*: increasing carbon emissions and greenhouse gases, accompanied by the melting of the Polar ice packs; increasing 'natural' disasters, such as floods and hurricanes.

- *Global economic changes*: major developments in the economies of Asia, alongside downturns in the US and UK economies.

- *Global political changes*: dramatic shifts leading on from the fall of the Soviet Union; the growth in membership and power of the European Union; major upheaval in Afghanistan and Iraq, accompanied by continuing unrest in the Middle East; the election of the first US African American president.

- *Global social changes*: the changes outlined above have led to a vast increase in the number of displaced people – asylum seekers and refugees, as well as economic migrants in search of work.

Nationally, the UK has inevitably both reacted to, and contributed towards, the global changes:

- The UK has experienced extremes of weather, including strong winds and torrential rain.

- The UK recession of 2008 and 2009, and the international financial crisis of which it was a part, have had serious consequences for the public sector, including health, education and social work services.

- A Labour government was elected in 1997, promising change. How far this has been achieved is a matter for debate, but some political changes are irrefutable, including the impact of devolution on all the countries of the UK. Scotland elected its first Scottish Parliament in 1999; the National Assembly for Wales' powers have increased in recent years in line with this; and the Northern Ireland Assembly assumed office in 2007. Discussions about some redistribution of power in England continue. (See Cree 2009.)

- Social changes have taken place across the board: people are living longer, including those with long-term illness and disability; children have been staying on at school and going to university in increasing numbers; girls have overtaken boys in examination results; more people are employed in part-time, insecure employment, often in the service sector, and many more people are self-employed; more people have come to the UK in search of work and a place of safety; more marriages are breaking down and more people are choosing to cohabit and have children without getting married; more people are home-owners, and more home-owners are getting into financial difficulty.

More personally, I have lived through changes in the last ten years which are indicative of some of these national and international transformations. I have been lucky enough to experience first hand the benefits of globalisation, through invitations to visit and teach at universities in different parts of the world; through opportunities to supervise international students who have travelled to the UK to study; and through the massive improvements which have been part and parcel of the revolution in information technology. I have also been fortunate enough (so far) to have been protected from the worst effects of the global economic downturn by having secure employment and the prospect of a pension in the future; this, in itself, is a huge privilege. And throughout this time, I have lived through upheavals including the deaths of my parents following prolonged illnesses; the breakdown of my marriage and the building of a new relationship; my children growing up and becoming independent adults; and the death of a dear friend, to whom this second edition, like the first, is dedicated. This is not intended to be self-indulgent whimsy. Rather, it is to locate myself, in the tradition of critical reflexivity, in the project of this book, and, at the same time, to encourage others to do the same: to make connections between the personal and the political, the individual and society, agency and structure. (For more on reflexivity, see David 2003, Hertz 1997, Ramazanoglu with Holland 2002.)

Just as my own life has changed, the profession of social work has changed and is changing. In Cree (2009), I argue that changes in social work reflect the wider changes taking place across three broad fronts: political, organisational and individual. Political changes in Europe, accompanied by devolution at home in the UK, have led to greater differentiation and, at the same time, paradoxically greater standardisation of services. The introduction of a new social work degree, alongside regulation of social service agencies and social service workers, demonstrate these changes. Meanwhile, the mechanism of the market has transformed the organisation and delivery of social work in the UK. At an individual level, those using services have increasingly come to be viewed as customers (with all the helpful and unhelpful consequences of this), just as social workers have increasingly found themselves in the roles of 'manager' and 'administrator', rather than those of counsellor or advocate which they would clearly prefer (see Cree and Davis 2007). Threading through all these changes are a particular set of discourses (ideas and practices), which attempt to determine what social work is and what it should be. In this new edition, I hope to show that sociology can help not simply to understand this, but also, perhaps, it can allow us to see how we might begin to do something about it.

Aims of the book

Sociology for Social Workers and Probation Officers examines a range of sociological concepts that are central to an understanding of the context in which practice takes place, and argues that socio-logical insight can inform and improve practice today. Howe distinguishes between theories *for* social work and theories *of* social work: theories *for* social work help to explain people and their situations and to inform practice; theories *of* social work say something about social work itself – What is it? What is it for? What should it be like? (1987: 166). This book offers a sociology *for* social workers and probation officers, looking at the ways in which sociological understanding might inform and improve professional practice.

The book explores the sociological ideas that influence practice across all service user groups (children and families, adult and community care, criminal justice and probation) and all practice settings (statutory, voluntary and private; health, education and criminal justice; multi-agency, day-care and residential). Social work as a profession has become increasingly fragmented in the UK in recent years, and it seems likely that further specialisation is yet to come. This does not, however, detract from the main purpose of this book. *Sociology for Social Workers and Probation Officers* remains relevant to all practitioners working in social work, social services, education, child care and probation, whatever their job title and organisational setting. I have chosen to use the generic term 'social work' throughout the book for the sake of clarity, but I am fully aware that this concept is likely to continue to shift in the years ahead.

Sociology for Social Workers and Probation Officers will examine key sociological themes within social work and probation practice, drawing attention to the often unexplored assumptions and ideas on which practice is based. Each chapter will focus on developing an understanding of the context within which practice operates (individual, family and community), while simultaneously analysing fundamental ideas about childhood and adolescence, crime and deviance, care and control. I will present different theoretical positions and encourage readers to reach their own views about the implications and usefulness of holding certain positions. I will also endeavour throughout the text to take an anti-discriminatory stance, pointing out the racism, sexism, heterosexism, disablism and ageism which permeate classical and present-day sociological and social work knowledge and practice.

The book is more than simply a review of sociological literature, or a re-statement of sociological theories. On the contrary, it is my intention to build and develop new knowledge about social work practice; knowledge which reflects sociological issues and concerns. I believe not only that this is the most helpful way to work with service users, but also that it may help to guard against cynicism, pessimism and 'burn-out' in our work, by encouraging us to look beyond immediate personal distress and the confusion of people's lives. C. Wright Mills, writing over fifty years ago, describes this as a 'sociological imagination'. He writes:

> The first fruit of this imagination . . . is the idea that the individual can understand his own experience and gauge his own fate only by locating himself within his period, that he can know his own chances in life only by becoming aware of those of all individuals in his circumstances. In many ways it is a terrible lesson; in many ways a magnificent one.

(1959: 5)

Mills's language may seem rather dated, but the issues that he raises are as relevant today as when they were written. He urges us to develop a self-consciousness about ourselves and our lives; to go about with our eyes wide open, willing to ask questions and make relevant connections between our experiences and those of others, between 'personal troubles of milieu' and 'public issues of social structure' (1959: 8). The study of sociology, then, is not simply an intellectual exercise. It is a way of thinking and being that encourages us to ask questions and strive to make changes to the society in which we live.

Structure and contents

Following the format of the first edition, the book begins with a chapter that sets out key sociological perspectives which will be developed throughout the book. Chapter 2 explores the family, giving attention to the ways in which ideas about the family (what it is and what people think it should be) influence professional practice with families today. Chapters 3 and 4 discuss childhood and youth; developmental stages that are central to social work practice, whether young service users are perceived as 'troubled' or 'troublesome'. Chapters 5 and 6 consider community, care and caring. Chapter 7, on health and illness, is a new chapter in this edition. Chapter 8 explores ideas of crime, deviance and social control. The book finishes, as before, with some pointers for a sociological social work practice.

The main chapters adopt a consistent structure throughout. Each begins with the exploration of a concept – its definition, and the ways it is discussed in everyday language – and examines implications arising from this. We then move into the main discussion, which is an analysis of the concept from different perspectives: historical, cross-cultural and sociological. At regular intervals along the way, implications for practice are considered. At the end of each chapter, suggestions are offered for further reading.

Definitions

As will be clear as the book unfolds, I am especially interested in how concepts are defined: by whom, and why, as well as the key question – why now? In *Discipline and Punish*, the French philosopher Michel Foucault (1977) argues that it is through discourses – that is, the ensembles of beliefs, concepts and organising ideas which make up and organise our relation to reality – that power and knowledge come together. Knowledge is not seen here as singular or uncomplicated; instead, Foucault argues that particular forms of knowledge are constructed and created through power. From this viewpoint, a concern with meaning is not a dry, academic discussion of semantics, but critical to understanding the everyday assumptions that underpin our thinking about the world. In an earlier work, *The Archaeology of Knowledge* (1972), Foucault raised a number of fundamental questions which I discussed in my analysis of the changing task of social work (Cree 1995). These offer a useful way into thinking about the very many concepts which we take for granted in our professional and personal lives. Foucault's broad questions (paraphrased in Cree 1995: 10–11) are as follows:

1. When did new ideas and practices emerge? Why should they have emerged at that moment?

2. Who is speaking, and what is said and not said?

3. Where does the discourse come from? From which institutional sites does it derive its legitimate source and point of application?

4. What positions can the subjects of the discourse adopt, and how does this relate to the changing positions of other groups?

5. How are the objects formed, and once formed, divided, classified and related to and from one another?

6. What are the concepts; that is, the perceived solutions/strategies which are presented to resolve perceived problems?

Each chapter in this book will, in its own way, attempt to address these questions, getting to grips with the contested nature of knowledge in social work, and demonstrating that some voices (notably, academic and professional perspectives) were traditionally the most influential in creating the theoretical concepts and practices which together made up 'social work'. More recently, 'voices from the inside' (that is, the perspectives of service users and their carers) are increasingly having an impact on building new understandings that challenge mainstream theory and practice (see Cree and Davis 2007, Doel and Best 2008).

Historical accounts

Historical accounts will be introduced in each chapter as a way of showing how society and social work have changed over time, as well as reminding the reader that things may not have operated in the same way in the past. In other words, a historical analysis allows us to see both continuities and discontinuities over time. It is important to acknowledge, however, that this is not as straightforward as it might seem. In an attempt to give the material a 'reader-friendly' structure, I have presented each chapter in a roughly chronological way, telling its 'story' coherently so that the reader can follow how one theoretical concept builds on, or reacts to, another. But ideas do not necessarily develop in a straight line. On the contrary, like all theorists, sociologists go back and forth and may even hold quite contradictory beliefs at the same time. Just as importantly, the history of ideas is not one of ever-greater enlightenment and understanding. Ideas that are currently cherished may, in practice, be less life enhancing and hold less explanatory power than ways of thinking that were valued in previous years. Foucault draws this conclusion in *The Archaeology of Knowledge*, where he rejects traditional, evolutionary, linear approaches to history, which present change in terms of continuity and transition. He writes:

> We must rid ourselves of a whole mass of notions, each of which, in its own way, diversifies from the theme of continuity . . . Once these immediate forms of continuity are suspended, an entire field is set free.
>
> (1972: 21, 26)

This gives a good indication about how I hope people will read this book. Readers are invited to follow the 'story' as it unfolds, but not to believe it as a story of progress or ever greater knowledge and insight. Instead, they must bring to the story their own knowledge and experience, all the while asking critical questions such as: Does this make sense? What are the implications of holding such a view, for individuals, for families, for communities and for society? Are they positive or negative, and for whom? (Adapted from Young 1981.)

Cross-cultural studies

In the same way that historical accounts remind us that there are alternative ways of thinking and acting, cross-cultural studies demonstrate the ethnocentricity of many of our ideas and practices. As we will see in the chapters that follow, it is often the case that our ways of thinking about the world and our models of practice are built on an assumption that 'our' culture and society is the 'norm'; all other cultures and societies are evaluated in relation to our own, and frequently found to be inferior for one reason or another. This is important because the often unacknowledged norm is most frequently that of the industrialised, developed world, and may, in social work textbooks, be simply the UK (or even England!). The developing world, by contrast, is presented as the exception to the rule; as somehow incomplete, in transition or at the very least 'other'. By opening the window onto different cultural contexts, I am endeavouring to show that there are other ways of thinking about key concepts such as family, community and caring which are just as valid as a developed-world perspective. Narrowing down the discussion further, it is my intention to highlight that different cultural contexts exist within the UK itself, so that we can begin to interrogate the majority community viewpoint, as well as learning about the experiences within different minority ethnic communities.

There is not space in this book, of course, to do justice to cross-cultural evidence in the round; this book is not, and cannot be, a social anthropological textbook. I can only give a flavour of what is available, in the hope that the general point will be understood. I believe that this approach is essential to the development of anti-oppressive knowledge in social work. Given what has already been said about the critical significance of the power to define the parameters of any discussion, it is vital that we always interrogate the context within which an idea or practice is located, and ask ourselves: what is being assumed, and whose interests are being prioritised? At the same time, we need to question whose ideas are being ignored or marginalised. The radical educationalist Paulo Freire (1970) used the term 'conscientization' to refer to the process of awareness and the development of the capacity to think critically about the relationship between social conditions, exclusion, wider society and the individual. This explains much better than I could why cross-cultural studies are important for social workers.

Implications for practice

Each chapter is punctuated by boxed sections, headed 'Implications for Practice'. This is the moment where I try to tease out the lessons for social work from the theoretical discussion. Inevitably, the implications that are addressed have broad relevance, rather than being related to specific settings or fields of practice. Given that the organisational context of social work changes at regular intervals, it is more helpful to draw attention to what can be seen as the bigger or more general issues. The final chapter in the book takes a further step back and offers a code of practice for a critical and reflexive sociological social work.

Use of evidence

As already stated, research evidence and statistics are presented throughout the chapters. But it is important to acknowledge that research is always tainted in some way by the predispositions, values and beliefs of those who fund it and carry it out (Gubrium and Silverman 1989). Because of this, it is unsurprising that it is impossible to step outside of ideology and uncover pure 'facts'. Similarly, statistics are notoriously unreliable and open to manipulation. A classic text by Huff (1973) points out that one set of figures can appear to give quite different information, depending on how the statistics are set out and how they are contextualised. I am therefore asking the reader to accept the evidence presented, but to do so critically, bringing a healthy scepticism to the material. The reader should be prepared to give the author the benefit of the doubt, but at the same time, never accept anything at face value, in this or any other piece of writing.

Terminology

One of the most visible changes in this revised edition is in the use of terminology. In an endnote to the first edition, I explained that I used the term 'black' to refer to 'the very many minority ethnic groups in the UK who experience discrimination and oppression on the basis of skin colour and assumed "racial difference". This includes people whose ethnic origins lie in South Asia, the Caribbean and Africa' (Cree 2000: 210). Although this was an acceptable position to hold in the late 1990s when the book was first written, it would seem insensitive today, if not downright offensive, to collapse 'the very many minority ethnic groups' into one grouping. Language and ideas have moved on apace since then, with much greater acknowledgement of the differences within and between ethnic groups, including the white majority.

In consequence, the term 'black' will be used in this edition in a more specific way, either historically (as in 'black movements', 'black consciousness' or 'black power') or politically, to refer to the shared experience of British people of colour as an oppressed minority group. Where 'black' is used in terms of ethnicity, it will refer only to people of African and African Caribbean or African American origin. The word 'Asian' as a 'catch-all' term for all people whose ethnic origins are in India, Pakistan, Bangladesh, China, Vietnam, etc. will be avoided where possible. This is in recognition of the reality that the term is, as Cullingford and Din aver in their study of ethnicity and Englishness, 'at once an opposite to something else, and a term of such variety that it is meaningless' (2008: vii). Consequently, whenever detailed ethnic background is known, it will be given. The growing number of people with mixed parentage in the UK will also, when possible, be defined as such, rather than as 'black', recognising their complex identities and cultural and ethnic backgrounds (Alibhai-Brown 2001, Tizard and Phoenix 2001).

There are times, of course, when it is impossible to get away from generic terms, because research does not always make the specificities clear, and the collection of ethnic information in official statistics has only recently become more detailed. The ethnic classification in the 2001 Census includes sixteen groups in comparison to the nine distinguished in the 1991 Census (Pilkington 2003: 26). Arguably, this is still too narrow to reflect the increasing complexities of the ethnic backgrounds of people in the UK today. In a touching prelim to her book on mixed parentage, Alibhai-Brown (2001) dedicates the book to her daughter 'who is Indian, African, Pakistani, English, British and a born Londoner' and to her son 'a young man of many places too, including his beloved Edinburgh'. This demonstrates well the point I am trying to make.

Another important term to consider is that of 'service user' or 'client'. The term 'client' was commonly used in social work and social policy texts until the 1980s to refer to the person who was in receipt of social work services. After this time, the term tended to be replaced by the arguably less patronising term, 'service user'. In the late 1990s, the terms 'customer' or 'consumer' became popular terms, particularly in the context of community care. By the early years of the twenty-first century, the title 'service user' became increasingly differentiated from 'carer', reflecting a greater awareness that the needs of primary service users and their carers might not be the same. More recently, a new term has emerged: 'experts by experience' (see Preston-Shoot 2005). This demonstrates the development of user perspectives in social work, and marks the realisation that service users are professionals in their own lives and experiences; their knowledge is just as valid as more mainstream, academic knowledge (see also Doel and Best 2008). For the sake of clarity, and because other terms may not be widely understood, I have used the phrase 'service user' in this book, except where I am quoting another person's writing. This follows the practice adopted in an earlier book (Cree and Davis 2007).

Context

I would like to end with a word or two about context. It has been suggested that a textbook is where things start, not where they finish (Bernardes 1997: xvii). Certainly, *Sociology for Social Workers and Probation Officers* should be regarded as a springboard for social work and probation students, practice teachers and practitioners. For this reason, each chapter is fully referenced so that readers may either draw on the material as set, or go to primary sources for further elaboration of specific themes or ideas. Each chapter also finishes with a short list of recommended texts that will give readers a good introduction to the subject under consideration. The book cannot, however, cover the whole field of sociology. In the interests of writing what I hope is a readable and manageable text, I have had to make decisions about what to include, and what to leave out. This has proved extra-ordinarily difficult, not least because my knowledge and understanding of sociology has increased exponentially since the first edition was published. What finally appears in the book, then, is a compromise between what I would like to write about and what I have time and space to write about. It is also a selection of some of the material that I have found interesting and relevant to my overall objective. I hope that readers will find the selection useful, but that they will also feel able to take forward the ideas and issues raised here through further reading and through making connections with their own experience.

The first edition was written with the aim of being a useful textbook for social work students and teachers based in the UK, and because of this, social work practice scenarios and government statistics, for example, reflected UK experience. This new edition continues to be largely set in the UK context, but I have tried, where possible, to draw on sociological insights from beyond the UK and US, and in this way to demonstrate a more comparative perspective that challenges traditional Western sociology's ethnocentrism.

Acknowledgements

I would like to express my thanks to all those who have made a contribution to the development of my sociological understanding over the years, including colleagues and friends at my own and other universities and practice agencies, members of the User and Carer Forum at The University of Edinburgh, and generations of social work students who have been the subjects and objects of my sociological journey, and have been so willing to share their thoughts and feelings with me.

Thanks also go to Grace McInnes at Routledge for her continuing support and for her encouragement in bringing together this second edition.

1 Sociological perspectives

Definitions

What is sociology?

This question has been asked by generations of sociologists, who all come up with slightly different answers. A simple definition is offered by Macionis and Plummer (2008), who suggest that sociology is 'the systematic study of human society'. It is, they continue, 'a form of consciousness, a critical way of seeing the social'. Moreover, it has 'the potential to change your life forever' (2008: 4). That is a big claim to make at the outset, but it is true nonetheless. Sociology starts with something we all know about: ourselves and society. It then sets out to examine this afresh: to encourage us to think about and 'unpack' our common-sense assumptions and attitudes about society and our place in it. It does so by, at times, taking a broad view, looking at structures and institutions within society now and across history. At other times, it takes a microscopic view, interrogating the minute processes and relationships that make up our daily lives. From this, we can see that we are both subjects and objects of the sociological enterprise, because we are members of a particular society, born at a given historical moment with a specific gender, class, ethnic, cultural and racial grouping. It is only by stepping outside our own lives and experiences that we can begin to see the patterns and the systems that govern our existence. The American author C. Wright Mills has called this process of stepping outside 'the sociological imagination'. He writes:

The task of sociology is that people should be enabled to grasp the relations between themselves and the way in which their society operates . . . The sociological imagination enables us to grasp history and biography and the relations between the two in society.

(Mills 1959: 8)

What is society?

If sociology is about analysing society, it raises the question: what is 'society'? Sociology emerged in the middle of the nineteenth century at a time of great social, economic and political upheaval in Europe and North America. Sociologists set out to make sense of the changes that were taking place around them, and to analyse the ways in which people were located in what was becoming a new urban, industrial and capitalist society. Sociologists began with the premise that this 'modern' society could and should be investigated, and in doing so they contrasted 'modern' society with the 'primitive' society that had gone before. 'Modern' for early sociologists thus signified progress, rationality, scientific reasoning and enlightened thinking; it also encapsulated the idea of a loss of traditional values and ways of life. 'Modern' was everything that 'primitive' was not.

Since the late twentieth century, the idea of society as a unitary phenomenon has been severely criticised. Pluralist approaches present society as a mosaic of competing worlds; power is understood to be spread across a wide range of social locations, and the task of sociology is to investigate the different interest groups and coalitions that come together at different moments. 'Post-modern' perspectives take this further, emphasising the contingent nature of our existence and the chaotic, unexpected characteristics of late capitalist (sometimes called 'late modern') society. Society is now perceived as complex and fragmented: just as we have more than one identity, so there are many

Table 1.1
'Primitive' versus 'modern' society

'Primitive' society	'Modern' society
Feudal	Capitalist
Agrarian	Industrial
Rural	Urban
Simple	Complex
Religious	Secular
Faith	Science
Superstition	Reasoning
Tradition	Progress

Table 1.2
'Modern' versus 'post-modern' society

'Modern' society	'Post-modern' society
Capitalist	Post-capitalist
Industrial	Post-industrial
Urban	Global
Complex	Fragmented
Secular	Pluralist
Knowledge	Relativity
Scientific facts	Beliefs
Truths	Contingencies

competing societies within which we live and move. 'Modern' society is again understood in opposition, this time to 'post-modern' society.

Although sociologists have increasingly seen society as multi-faceted, sociology's customary concern with issues of structure and power has not disappeared. On the contrary, many sociologists maintain that the identities and societies that we inhabit continue to be structured by wider experiences of class, gender, 'race', ethnicity, age, sexuality and disability, and by the power relations that flow from these (see, for example, Bauman 2006 and Bauman and May 2001).

Social work and sociology

The relationship between social work and sociology has been a changing one, reflecting broader debates about the nature of knowledge and the understanding of theory and practice within both subjects. Today, departments of social work and sociology in universities and colleges are likely to be separate units with distinct approaches and different personnel. This was not always the case.

When the Charity Organisation Society in Britain began the first academic institution devoted to the training of social workers in 1903, they named it the 'School of Sociology' (Smith 1965). This tells us a great deal about the ways in which sociology and social work were conceptualised in the early years of the twentieth century. Sociology and social work were seen as two sides of one coin: social reform in Britain and the United States was based on the assumption that sociology and social work went hand in hand, as the work of Charles Booth, Beatrice Webb and Seebohm Rowntree illustrates. They believed that in charting the living conditions of the urban poor their wider project for social reform and social welfare might be realised. This was the promise of the 'modern' age: that through scientific discovery and rational investigation the 'truth' might be uncovered, leading to an improvement in the workings of society and in the lives of individuals. Bilton *et al.* describe this succinctly: 'As a "modernist project", it [sociology] was committed to the idea that it was possible to produce reliable knowledge about society that human beings could use to shape their futures for the better' (2002: 24).

Social work in its early years was not, however, concerned only with large-scale social change. It was also much more routinely concerned with finding individual solutions to individual problems. The work of the Charity Organisation Society focused on individuals and their families, but still in the context of their social networks. Mary Richmond, writing what became a textbook for social work practice in Britain and the United States, suggested that sociology offered practical guidance to the carrying out of the social work task by helping social workers to make assessments of the situations that they faced. Richmond stressed the importance of *social* factors in the social worker's under-standing of the individual and she urged the collecting of 'social facts' or 'evidence' as a foundation of assessment (Richmond 1917). This is highly reminiscent of Durkheim's *The Rules of Sociological Method*, first published in 1895, in which he argued that the study of society is made possible by the collection of 'social facts'.

The relationship between social work and sociology has remained a live and contested issue for social work. Writing in 1931, MacIver argued that although sociology has no direct therapeutic implications for social work, it nevertheless provides 'the basis for the development of that social philosophy which must integrate the thinking of the social worker, which must control the direction and illuminate the goal of his activity' (quoted in Leonard 1966: 15). In practice, sociology has not provided social work with the underpinning social philosophy that MacIver envisaged. Instead, the knowledge base of social work has been dominated largely by ideas and practices that have their origins in psychological perspectives (Cree 1995, Yelloly 1980). Sociological voices have remained on the edge of mainstream social work theory and knowledge, struggling to be heard above the predominantly individual, psychological and correctional discourses in social work. Sociological ideas did, however, play an important part in social work thinking in the 1970s, when the radical social work movement looked to sociology to explain the workings of state capitalism and the role of social work within the welfare state (see Bailey and Brake 1975). The development of a feminist critique and black perspectives in social work in the 1980s also drew on a sociological framework of understanding (see Dominelli and McLeod 1989, Hanmer and Statham 1988). These ideas came under open attack in the 1980s and 1990s as part of a concerted attempt to discredit what were seen as 'left-wing' influences on social work practice. Educational institutions and social work agencies were pilloried for their 'political correctness' and there were indications that the teaching of sociology might be removed altogether from social work education (Jones 1997).

In reality, such pessimism was unfounded. The new social work degree programme, which was introduced in the UK in 2003 and 2004, has given renewed impetus to the teaching of knowledge based on sociological understandings. The National Occupational Standards for Social Work are built on an assumption that individuals must be considered in the context of their families, groups/networks and wider communities. Because of this, wider ecological, environmental and *sociological* explanations are considered relevant to assessing individuals' needs and strengths and providing and reviewing services. At a more detailed level, the standards spell out the need for students to have knowledge about the following sociological topics:

- demographic and social trends;

- social policy, criminal justice, housing, welfare rights, education, etc.;

- theories of poverty, unemployment, health, and other sources of discrimination and social exclusion;

- understanding why people use services;

- human growth and behaviour, and the factors that impact on this;

- mental health and well-being;

- social interactions and relationships;

- discrimination and oppression;

- difference and diversity;

- understanding of systems and organisations.

These topics are discussed further in Cree and Myers (2008) through vignettes which explore sociological perspectives alongside other kinds of underpinning knowledge, including psychological and service user knowledge.

Sociological ideas are also prominent in the re-emergence of a radical voice in social work in the UK. In *The Social Work Business*, Harris (2003) takes a fresh look at the role of social work, as it has been transformed over the last thirty years. Writing from a similar tradition, Ferguson and Woodward (2009) are highly critical of what they perceive to be a 'neoliberal approach' to social work and set out to demonstrate that a radical tradition can be developed in contemporary social work practice. The formation of a new collective in 2005, the Social Work Action Network (SWAN), gives further evidence of social work's continuing preoccupation with a radical agenda. This is discussed more fully in Chapter 5.

Chapter 5

My final assessment of the relationship between sociology and social work is, I hope, both positive and realistic. Sociology cannot be assumed to offer a single set of solutions to either society's or social work's problems, not least because there is a myriad of sociological perspectives, a host of possible ways of conceptualising the individual and society. The 'modern' dream of enlightened progress and increasing rationality has been exposed as a myth: theory, knowledge and ideas are all contextually and historically specific, conditional and open to challenge. Not only this; theory, knowledge and ideas can never be assumed to be neutral, value-free or apolitical. Foucault (1977) has shown that knowledge, ideas and practice are sites in which power is acted out; as a consequence, what we hold to be 'true', in terms of our understanding of the society in which we live, both reflects the state of contestation which is inevitably at the heart of the sociological discourse and at the same time sets the parameters and structures of that sociological enterprise. Sociology, then, in common with social work and all the social and human sciences, may be regarded as an integral part of the process through which society investigates, controls and manages (or using Foucault's terminology, 'disciplines') its citizens. In this way, both sociology and social work construct the 'individual' (and, in the same way, the family and the community) of whom the discipline then speaks (Gubrium and Silverman 1989).

This is why social work needs a sociological imagination. Social work's central purpose is to work on behalf of society to help individuals and groups who are vulnerable and marginalised. But the problems which these individuals and groups face may not be of their own making: the origins and maintenance of what are presented to us daily as individual problems may lie in structures of inequality in society. Explanations are therefore likely to be found not in individual psychology or in biology but in *social* practices and *social* structures. Social workers must be able to understand the connections between individual problems and society: between 'personal troubles and the public issues of social structure' (Mills 1959: 8). If social workers cannot make these connections, there is a very real risk that, by pathologising and blaming individuals and families, they will perpetuate the oppression and discrimination that characterise the lives of users of social work services.

Sociological insights may be useful at an institutional and organisation level, as well as at the level of knowledge creation. Questions raised by sociological thinking may provide planners and managers of services with a framework for reviewing structures and systems which operate so that services can be planned and managed in a thoughtful and critical way. A sociological imagination may allow planners to look at a situation from the vantage points of competing systems of interpretation (Berger 1967). Better still, a historical sociological analysis may allow decision makers to see the connections between personal activity and social organisation over time (Abrams 1982).

This is not to suggest, however, that social work is a kind of applied sociology, or that social workers can lead service users to a new kind of consciousness through sociological understanding. As Davies wryly comments, 'sociologists ask questions; social workers must act as though they have answers'. The social worker, he continues 'is a revolutionary irrelevance – a mere employee in the welfare indus-try, with a range of quite specific skills to learn, tasks to perform, services to deliver, a professional identity to maintain, and a career to pursue' (1991: 7). But even within this circumscribed existence, the social worker has choices to make and a degree of autonomy of action. It is crucial that the social work practitioner acts in a way that seeks to empower rather than to oppress those with whom they are working. At the same time, social workers must be encouraged to reflect on their own experiences and their own practice; not just in the narrow sense of developing skills, but in terms of understanding the role of social work within the state and the scope they may (or may not) have for negotiation and creativity within this. Social workers must learn to 'unpack' or deconstruct their attitudes and values, and to examine the theoretical frameworks that structure their thinking and practice. They must begin to see the connections and interplay between themselves and others, as well as between others and their social structures. This is central to a critical social work practice (Fook 2002).

To argue that social workers need a sociological understanding does not, of course, imply that other understandings are unimportant. Social workers should also understand the influence of psychological approaches on social work: psychodynamic, developmental, cognitive and behavioural. There are occasions when sociological and psychological explanations will be at variance with one another; for example, in some studies of crime and deviant behaviour (see the practice example at end of this chapter). There are also large areas of overlap between the interests and concerns of psychologists and those of sociologists, particularly around socialisation and the family. In recent years, post-modernist and post-structuralist sociologists have become increasingly interested in subject areas which in the past were considered the domain of psychology, including sexuality, identity and psychoanalytic approaches (see Turner 1996, Ussher 1997, Ramazanoglu and Holland 2002).

Social work has itself been a subject of sociological investigation, with studies of professionalisation and bureaucratisation, organisation, managerialism, social work practice, social work education, and social control in social work (for example, Davies 1991, Day 1987, Dominelli 1997, Heraud 1970, Sibeon 1991). Social work's abiding interest in sociology is similarly demonstrated in two more recent textbooks on the topic (see Cunningham and Cunningham 2008, Llewellyn, Agu and Mercer 2008).

The discipline of sociology

Sociological textbooks make different claims as to the origins of sociology. Some look as far back as to the philosophical writings of classical Greece, and the beginnings of debates about social differentiation, social inequality, conflict, and the links between human nature and society. Others argue that its origins lie in the social and political upheaval which characterised Western industrial societies at the end of the eighteenth and beginning of the nineteenth centuries.

The eminent sociologist Anthony Giddens (2006) agrees that human beings have always been curious about the sources of their behaviour. But he points out that for thousands of years this was most often understood and expressed in religious terms, passed down from generation to generation. Giddens asserts that the study of society is in fact a relatively recent phenomenon, dating from the late 1700s and early 1800s. This was the time of the so-called Enlightenment, when scholars, artists and thinkers from Scotland, France and Germany came together to spread 'the light of knowledge and rational understanding in order to break with the gloom of tradition and superstition' (Pryke 2002: 93). They believed that in doing so, 'humanity as a whole could raise itself up economically and morally from the poverty and ignorance that had hitherto characterised life' (ibid.). As part of this movement, philosophers and economists began to write for the first time about society as an entity in itself and about the 'social' basis of behaviour. These ideas were taken up and developed by the early sociologists some years later.

The foundation of sociology as an academic discipline is usually attributed to the French scholar Auguste Comte (1798–1857), who is credited with inventing the name 'sociology'. Comte believed that the search for order and progress in the social world would be achieved not by investigation of human nature, but by scientific experimentation and by the analysis of what he called 'social facts'. He argued that society could be studied scientifically through systematic research (he called this approach 'positivism'), in the same way that the physical world was explained by natural science. Although Comte's work was highly influential in its day, we must look to the end of the nineteenth century to find the broad expansion of sociology as a discipline in its own right. Sociology advanced at this time out of a need to understand the changes that had accompanied the process of 'modernisation'

in society (see earlier discussion of the usage of the term 'modern'). Urbanisation, industrialisation and the revolution in France had brought in their wake an increase in crime, deviance, suicide and disorder. There was a crisis in religious faith, as new ideas from science challenged established beliefs and practices. Liberalism was seen as failing to cope with the challenges of the 'modern' world. Sociologists set out to describe and explain the changes and, at the same time, to offer solutions. The three 'founders' of sociological theory, Emile Durkheim (1858–1917), Karl Marx (1818–1883) and Max Weber (1864–1920) were all engaged in this enterprise, but from different perspectives and reaching very different conclusions, as will be explained in more depth in the next section of this chapter.

Sociology has continued to develop from this time, sometimes building on early approaches and at other times seeking to find new ways of making sense of the set of problems and relations which are part and parcel of living in a 'modern', 'late modern' or even 'post-modern' society. This means that there is no single 'Sociology', with a capital 'S', any more than there is one 'Society', because sociologists are constantly in the process of redefining, contesting, changing and developing

sociological knowledge. Moreover, there can be no end-point in this, as old theories and ideas are re-worked and new ways of thinking which engage with, and challenge, existing knowledge are introduced. (The section New Directions in Sociology will explore this further.)

Traditional sociological frameworks

Traditional or 'classical' perspectives in sociology can be broadly divided into three main traditions: functionalism (drawing on the work of Emile Durkheim), Marxist perspectives (building on Karl Marx's ideas) and the interpretive paradigm (originating in Max Weber's work). Confusingly, these perspectives are often given different names, as we will find out.

Functionalism

Functionalism, the standard sociological approach between the 1920s and the 1950s and still popular today, set out to explain how society holds together and how it changes over time, particularly in the context of the shift from feudalism to industrial society. Functionalism offers an equilibrium model of society: society is understood as a complete system made up of interconnected and interdependent parts, all working together to achieve the maintenance and continuity of the whole. Just as all the parts of the body work together to maintain it, so it is the 'function' of the institutions in society (the family, education, religion, political systems, the economy) to contribute to the maintenance and survival of the wider social system. Social order and individual well-being are seen as one and the same thing: individuals need the control and regulation that keeps society in order, because without it, they would be unhappy and unfulfilled. Happiness and social order are therefore seen as being based on a core of shared values, which are taught from birth and maintained through social institutions.

Emile Durkheim (1858–1917) is widely regarded as the principal figure in the establishment of the functionalist tradition in sociology. He set out to create a new understanding of society, as a corrective to the biological and psychological approaches of his day which saw behaviour largely in terms of the actions of individuals. He argued that, in essence, society is bigger than the actions of the individuals within it; it exists 'beyond ourselves' and is also 'in ourselves'; what he called 'sui generis'. Macionis and Plummer explain this simply:

> Society is more than the individuals who compose it; society has a life of its own that stretches beyond our personal experiences. It was here long before we are born, it makes claims on us while we are alive, and it will remain long after we are gone. Patterns of human behaviour form established 'structures'; they are 'social facts' that have an objective reality beyond the lives and perceptions of particular individuals.
>
> (2008: 109)

Durkheim believed that human behaviour should be understood in terms of 'social structures' and 'social facts', not individual motives or choices. Social facts are collective ways of thinking, feeling and acting that are acquired through learning and training; they constrain and regulate our thoughts, emotions and behaviour. Some social facts are institutions (beliefs and modes of behaviour); others are collective representations (shared ways of thinking such as myths, legends and religious beliefs). Some are written down in laws and religious texts; others are less obvious but no less powerful (Fulcher and Scott 2007). Durkheim illustrated this in a story about his own life:

> When I fulfil my obligations as brother, husband or citizen, I perform duties, which are defined, externally to myself and my acts, in law and custom. Even if they conform to my own sentiments, and I feel their reality subjectively, such reality is still objective, for I did not create them; I merely inherited them through my education . . . The church member finds the belief and practices of his religious life ready made at birth; their existence prior to him implies this existence outside himself.
>
> ([1895] 1964: 1–2)

These 'duties' are also described in the same work as 'the ties that bind'; they 'make us a unitary aggregate of the mass of individuals' [1895]. The law and morality are important not only for the good functioning of society; they are also vital for human happiness. Durkheim thus insists that human happiness is realised, not through the satisfaction of individual wants and needs, but through the creation of social harmony. He believed that the 'science of sociology' could play a major part in helping to achieve social harmony, by 're-establishing social integration and moral consensus in the modern industrial world' (Bilton *et al.* 2002: 470).

Durkheim proposed that in order to be seen as a science, sociology had to collect evidence using the same methods as the physical sciences: through direct observation and investigation. (This is the essence of what is known as 'positivism'.) Durkheim's best-known book is his 1897 study of suicide, republished in 1952. In this, he set out to prove that a positivist, sociological approach was not only feasible, but provided a powerful tool for analysing something which, until then, had been seen as a highly personal act; that is, the decision to take one's own life. Durkheim studied suicide rates and observed that they differed from one group to another and from one social situation to another: Protestants were found to be more likely to commit suicide than Catholics; those who were single, divorced or widowed were more likely to commit suicide than married people; there was a decline in suicide rates in times of war; and suicide rates increased at times of economic crisis. From this, he demonstrated that suicide rates were higher amongst people who either experienced 'anomie' (lack of social regulation) or 'egoism' (lack of social integration). He concluded that even the most personal of our actions (suicide) was a 'social', not an individual, act, and so required a sociological explanation. Durkheim also studied crime as a social, not an individual, phenomenon. He pointed out that crime

Chapter 8

has positive as well as negative functions, because it sets the boundaries for what is acceptable (and unacceptable) behaviour. Furthermore, when someone does something illegal, others come together in outrage against this, which in turn helps to sustain conformity and stability, thus strengthening society (Durkheim 1964).

The functionalist sociologist to have had most impact on social policy and social work is the US scholar, Talcott Parsons (1902–1979). Developing Durkheim's ideas, Parsons argued that what held society together was a 'normative framework' of cultural values and social norms which people learned through a process of socialisation; it was this framework which shaped people's actions, and hence their realities (1949). Parsons was interested in a range of topics of concern to social work, including the family, gender relations and illness, all of which will be discussed more fully in later chapters.

Critical overview

There are, as we can see, a number of assumptions implicit in a functionalist approach, all of which have been challenged by subsequent sociological perspectives. First, it is assumed that all the parts of society (the social institutions) work together to the same end; that there is compatibility between institutions. But is this ever truly the case? Is it not conceivable that, for at least some of the time, there might be divergence between institutions, such as, for example, between the family and organised religion, or between the law and the police, or between education and politics? This leads to a second assumption: that there is agreement about means and goals in society – there is a value consensus, held by all – at least to some degree. Again, what if this is not the case? How do we reconcile issues such as disagreements between citizens and policy makers about nuclear power, about capital punishment, or about war? Can we be sure of a value consensus about any of these important issues, and if we cannot, what does this tell us about a functionalist perspective? Finally, there is an assumption that order and stability are essential for the survival of society and that social control must play a part in maintaining that order. But social control of whom? And whose order is being sustained? There is no recognition here of the choices and behaviours of individuals; of the ways in which different groups may have their own values and perspectives which are at odds with those of 'mainstream' society; or of the impact of differential power and opportunities for setting the core agenda in society.

Marxist perspectives

Marxist perspectives were increasingly influential in sociology during the 1970s. Like functionalism, they set out to explain how society works and how change had come about from feudal to industrial society. Again in common with functionalist perspectives, Marxist approaches begin with the starting point that society is best understood as an objective whole; individual actions are explored in terms of the social structure in which they are located. But this is where functionalist and Marxist approaches diverge. From a Marxist point of view, society is not seen as a consensus. Contradictions are held to be endemic within capitalism, just as conflict between diverse and opposing interest groups in society is held to be inevitable. Social control is seen as functional only in terms of propping up existing privileges and inequalities within society.

Marxist perspectives originated in the writing of the philosopher and economist, Karl Marx (1818–1883). Like Durkheim, Marx was inspired to build a science of society, but he did not describe himself as a sociologist. Sociology was still very new at this time, and his ideas were not picked up by sociologists until the next generation (Fulcher and Scott 2007: 28). Marx's goal was not simply to explain the development of industrial society, but to make sense of the development of *capitalist* society. Macionis and Plummer (2008: 102) put this in context. They point out that Marx spent most of his adult life in London, then capital of a vast British Empire. Here he was surrounded by the contradictions that were part and parcel of the new capitalist environment: the extreme affluence of some people, and the abject poverty of others. He struggled with fundamental questions: 'in a society so rich, how could so many be poor?' Just as importantly, 'how could this situation be changed?' Marx argued that the early stages of industrialisation had transformed a small number of people into a class of private property owners: the capitalists who owned the means of production. At the same time, most of the rest of the population had become industrial workers (the so-called proletariat, who sold their labour for the wages they needed to survive). Marx saw an inevitable conflict in this, as capitalists sought to maximise profits and keep costs down, and workers sought to increase their wages and standard of living.

In his analysis, Marx argued that there are two fundamental components of any society: the base and the superstructure. The base comprises the forces and social relationships of production; that is, the economy and class relations. It is the foundation on which a superstructure of social institutions is built, including the family, the education system, ideas and beliefs ('ideologies'), the law and the political system. In this way, the base is believed to determine all other relationships and institutions in society. Marx also gave attention to what this meant for individuals. He argued that through a process of socialisation, people are encouraged to hold ideas and values that support the *status quo*: they are indoctrinated into a 'false consciousness' which allows them to accept their subordination. Macionis and Plummer explain:

> Marx was saying, in effect, that industrial capitalism itself is responsible for many of the social problems he saw all around him. False consciousness, he maintained, victimises people by obscuring the real cause of their problems.

> (2008: 103)

But Marx was not pessimistic about the possibility of change. On the contrary, looking back over history, he noted that there had always been class conflict: between masters and slaves, nobles and serfs, and now between capitalists (or 'the bourgeoisie') and the proletariat. At the start of the *Manifesto of the Communist Party* (1848), Marx and Engels declared: 'The history of all hitherto existing society is the history of class struggles' (quoted in Macionis and Plummer 2008: 103). From this point of view, not only was class conflict inevitable, but industrial capitalism laid wide open the inequalities inherent in the capitalist system. Because of this, it held within it the seeds of its own destruction; as 'class consciousness' developed, so the proletariat would rise up and overthrow capitalism (Marx and Engels 1976).

Critical overview

Marxist approaches have been criticised for being too simplistic and too mechanistic; they are said to underestimate the importance of ideology as a force in its own right and to ignore the importance of other inequalities, such as those of 'race' or gender. Nevertheless, it is important to acknowledge that Marx himself was led to say 'I am not a Marxist' because he was unhappy about the claims being made in his name (Fulcher and Scott 2007: 30). Conflict theories and critical perspectives both developed as a challenge to what has been called 'crude' Marxism, taking on board some of the lessons of the interpretive paradigm, while at the same time drawing on a Marxist analysis of structure. Ralf Dahrendorf (1957), for example, explored conflict from the standpoint of the unequal distribution of 'authority': those in power have a vested interest in holding on to their privileges; those who are ruled have an interest in seeking to alter the distribution of power. Because of these differences, Dahrendorf argues, people tend to form 'social classes'; these interest groups 'come into conflict with one another and are the actual driving forces in social change' (Fulcher and Scott 2007: 57).

Critical theorists have developed Marx's ideas further still; Marx himself believed that a critical, self-conscious approach was essential for understanding society and for changing it. Fulcher and Scott

(2007) point out that authors like Antonio Gramsci, writing in the 1920s, had a huge impact on radical thinking in the 1960s and 1970s. Gramsci (1971) criticised Marxism's insistence that ideology is subordinate to, and subsumed by, the economic system. He argued instead that ideology has power in its own right and that individuals must be led to socialism through ideology. Another critical theorist, Jürgen Habermas (1981a and b), has been highly influential in arguing that both structural and interactionist approaches are necessary; that neither alone provides a satisfactory base for social theory. He argues that only an interest in 'emancipation' (what he calls 'critical-dialectical thought') can liberate people from ideology and error, and bring about the self-determination and autonomy that was Marx's ultimate goal of human history (Fulcher and Scott 2007: 59). Critical writing has developed greatly in recent years, moving beyond class-based explanations and taking on board lessons from feminism and the anti-apartheid and black movements (see Davis 1997, Hall 1991, Harding 1987, Hill Collins 1990, and Smith 1988). This writing continues to assert that knowledge is structured by existing sets of social relations and that these sets of social relations are oppressive in nature. But current analysis, instead of focusing on class as the main centre of oppression, explores the intersections of oppression based on class, gender and 'race' (for example, Harvey 1990).

The interpretive paradigm

The interpretive paradigm offers a very different way of conceptualising society from those proposed by the structural approaches of functionalism and Marxist perspectives. Interpretive, 'interaction' or 'action' perspectives no longer assume that the whole of society is a unitary social system. Instead, the focus is on the small-scale interactions between individuals and groups within society, and the ways in which meanings and definitions are constructed in particular ways at particular times. Interpretive approaches, therefore, are interested to interrogate individuals in order to find out why they behave in a certain way, and to investigate the areas of ambiguity and negotiation that are central to all our thoughts and actions.

Max Weber, a German economic historian, lawyer and sociologist (1864–1920), is the lead figure in the development of interpretive perspectives in sociology. Like Durkheim and Marx, Weber set out to understand and explain the changes that were taking place in the development of a new industrial society. And in common with Marx, he believed that the essence of capitalism is the pursuit of profit. But this is where any agreement ends. Weber was highly critical of what he saw as Marx's over-emphasis on economic interpretations of historical development. In reviewing the shift towards modern society, he argued that ideas and values were as important as economic factors in bringing about social change; more than this, he believed that beliefs could transform society. Weber explored these ideas in a series of empirical studies. His most influential work was a study of religion, *The Protestant Ethic and the Spirit of Capitalism* (1974), first published in 1902. Here Weber argued that modern society was the product of a new way of thinking, not just of changes in technology and economics. For Weber, it was religious values, especially those associated with Puritanism, which were fundamental in creating a 'capitalist outlook' (Giddens 2006: 18). From this, he went on to suggest that values influenced economic behaviour and not vice versa (Weber 1974). For Weber, it was rationality that was the driving force behind capitalism: modernity was to be understood as 'the triumph of rationality over all other forms of action'. The major problem for modern industrial society was not, then, economic inequality but 'the stifling regulation and dehumanisation that comes with expanding bureaucracy', leading to what Weber calls an increasing 'disenchantment with the world' (Macionis and Plummer 2008: 109).

Weber was not, however, interested only in analysis at the macro level. He also rejected Durkheim's and Marx's notion that structures in society have a life of their own, external to individuals. Weber's own assessment was that 'individuals have the ability to act freely and to shape the future', just as social structures are formed by 'a complex interplay of individuals' actions' (Giddens 2006: 18). This, he argued, was where sociology needs to start. Individuals are creative actors whose actions determine both present society and the course of history. This does not imply that there are no constraints on individuals: constraints do exist, but what is significant is how people perceive those constraints. Weber emphasised the importance of understanding the subjective meaning that every 'actor' brings to a social situation: each social situation is established and sustained by the meaning brought into it by participants. It is this unique ability of human beings, to interpret the world around them and choose to act, which Weber sees as the key concern of sociology. Sociology should seek to understand the theories of the actors themselves (*Verstehen*) instead of constructing expert theories about social systems. The principal concepts used by social scientists (capitalism, bureaucracy, the nation state) are, for Weber, no more than 'ideal types'; they are 'analytical devices that are constructed by social scientists in order to understand the more complex reality that actually exists' (Fulcher and Scott 2007: 40). This does not suggest that they have no meaning or worth. If constructed well, with large enough sample sizes, they can be useful tools. But, Weber warns, they will always be from one-sided, value-relevant standpoints; there are no universal truths valid for all time.

Critical overview

Fulcher and Scott observe that Weber's argument is difficult to follow at times, not least because he rejected the idea that we all experience the world in the same way (2007: 40). Nevertheless, his insights have been highly influential for the development of feminist and post-modern perspectives in sociology. For example, it is rarely acknowledged that it was Weber who brought the notion of patriarchy, or rather, patriarchal authority, into sociology, to be developed by Sylvia Walby in 1997 (Delamont 2003). Although there are a number of theoretical perspectives that can be described as interpretive sociology, the best known of these are symbolic interactionism, phenomenology and ethnomethodology.

Symbolic interactionism grew up in the 1920s and 1930s, in the work of American sociologists including William Thomas, Charles Cooley and George Herbert Mead. This approach emphasises the flexibility of individual responses to social situations; its central concept is meaning and the variability of meaning in everyday life. George Herbert Mead (1934), for example, argued that individuals give meaning to the world by defining and interpreting it in certain ways; in doing so, they are using definitions ('symbols') that are available to them in their culture (Fulcher and Scott 2007: 52). Mead also saw 'the self' as a social construct: the way individuals act and see themselves is, at least in part, a consequence of the way other people see and react towards them. In this way, individuals learn to behave differently in different situations. Erving Goffman (1922–1982) developed this idea further,

describing social interaction as a form of theatre in which we all play out roles in the drama of life, presenting different versions of ourselves to different people in different settings (Goffman 1969). These ideas have been extremely influential in understanding crime and deviance, as we will explore in Chapter 8.

Phenomenological approaches, originating in the ideas of Husserl and Shutz in the 1920s and 1930s, and later developed by Berger and Luckman (1966), investigate the ways in which the everyday world comes to be seen as normal, 'natural' and taken for granted. They argue that we are born into a pre-constructed social world, which has both objective and subjective meaning. We take it for granted and build our views and interpretations on the basis of this construct, this 'thing' that we do not question. What happens next is that the 'thing' starts to take on a life of its own, and seems to have a greater

unity than it actually does (an example of this might be the concept of 'the family' which we will consider more fully in Chapter 2). Fulcher and Scott explain: 'When we give a name to something, we make it appear as something that is separate from us, external to us, and that is solid and substantial' (2007: 54).

Ethnomethodology, while continuing to accept that individuals construct their social world, is particularly concerned with the underlying rules that govern everyday behaviour. For example, Garfinkel (1967) is interested in how people account for their actions and interactions: what they choose to leave in, and what they choose to omit. There is no such thing, he argues, as a complete story: we cannot understand action and interaction until we know the context, the background, the knowledge and assumptions that underpin it. Bilton explains this as follows: 'Whereas symbolic interactionism focuses on the importance of *Verstehen* . . . ethnomethodology attempts to show how *Verstehen* works' (Bilton *et al.* 2002: 506).

Interactionists of all perspectives have been criticised for failing to take account of the reality of power in society. Because groups and individuals have differential access to the process of creating meaning in a situation, explanations based on meaning may lose sight of the broader issues of power and inequality. Nevertheless, they have proved a powerful corrective to the determinism of large-scale structural theories.

New directions in sociology

Although classical perspectives have not disappeared from sociological writing, more recent sociological perspectives, often building on earlier traditions, are much more likely to emphasise that there are multiple ways of thinking about the social world. Not only this; it is argued that some of the familiar sociological methodologies have privileged certain groups and certain voices (that is, those of white, Western, heterosexual men) at the expense of others. In consequence, sociology has offered an incomplete analysis; it has also, at times, missed the point completely, as we will see.

Feminist perspectives

From the 1970s onwards, feminism has acted as a commentary on, and corrective to, mainstream or 'malestream' (male-oriented) sociology, contributing to the development of sociological knowledge while simultaneously challenging and confronting the ways in which that knowledge is created and recreated. Feminists have drawn attention to 'androcentric' (male-centred) language and practices in conventional sociology and have explored what a feminist sociology might look like. For some feminists, this has meant building a sociology set apart from conventional sociology, centred on women's experience and a feminist standpoint (Harding 1987, Smith 1988). For others, the task of feminist sociology has been to 'gender the social': to work within and beyond sociology to explain and to understand gender relations, at the same time as extending the parameters of sociology into previously untheorised areas, including housework (Oakley 1974 and 2005), sexuality and hetero-sexism (Lees 1986, Lind 2004), violence against women (Dobash and Dobash 1979 and 1992). This work has effectively transformed a sociology that was previously mainly concerned with 'public' issues into one that now recognises the existence of 'private' issues and 'personal' lives (David 2003, Maynard 1990).

Feminism is, of course, not one single ideology or one simple movement. There are as many feminisms as there are sociologies, so that we can find proponents of liberal, Marxist, socialist, radical, black, psychoanalytic, post-modern and post-structural feminism, and, more recently, eco-feminism. Within each broad grouping, there are significant differences in approach and orientation as well as areas of overlap and agreement. Some feminist approaches, for example, share with Marxist approaches their insistence on the impact of overriding structures in society, both economic and patriarchal (see Barrett and McIntosh 1982). Others (for example, Skeggs 1997) argue that concepts such as class have little meaning in many working-class women's lives. While Marxist feminists accept the dual importance of class and gender in society, radical feminists have argued that patriarchal structures have the central power to determine the nature of women's experience in society. Other feminist perspectives are more interested in developing the understanding of individual action and meaning (an interpretive approach) rather than taking on board large-scale 'grand' theory. What has united feminists, however, has been a shared experience of gender oppression and a will to change this. Writing in 1994, Kelly, Burton and Regan propose:

> Feminism for us is both a theory and practice, a framework which informs our lives. Its purpose is to understand women's oppression in order that we might end it.
>
> (1994: 28)

Contemporary feminist sociologists have had to face up to the reality that some of the building blocks of the feminist enterprise do not seem to be on such solid ground as they did in the early days of the women's movement. Black women, gay women and disabled women have all pointed out that 'woman' is not tenable as a single category, and some feminists have even suggested that the idea of 'man' may be similarly problematic (Cavanagh and Cree 1996). Some feminist sociologists have sought to find ways of understanding the contradictory nature of women's oppression (for example, Hill Collins 1990 and 2005, Maynard 2002). Others have confronted liberal feminism's complicity in racism, colonialism, and the oppression of black women. New feminist writing explores the absences and exclusions within feminist scholarship, highlighting that feminism 'must be constantly challenged and transformed by the conflicts and divisions between women who identify with it' (Ahmed *et al.* 2000: 4). One example to have emerged in the twenty-first century is 'aboriginal' or 'indigenous' feminism, which asserts that a feminist perspective is not, as previously argued, incompatible with a valuing of aboriginal culture and belief-systems (Green 2007). The developments within feminist sociology do not, however, mean that 'old-style' gender oppression has disappeared. On the contrary, feminists across all traditions highlight the reality that women's lives continue to be structured by oppression based on gender, as the following chapters will ably demonstrate.

Black perspectives

Just as women have highlighted the implicit sexism in sociology, black women and men have drawn attention to the racism that permeates conventional sociology. Racist assumptions are, it is argued, like the letters running through a stick of seaside rock; they are present in all the structures of society and in the values and beliefs that we hold to be true. Sociology, it is argued, is built on the experience of white, Western men; everything else becomes 'other', either treated as a variation from the 'norm' or ignored completely. Not only has sociology disregarded a large proportion of the world's population in the so-called developing world, it has, like feminism, tended to ignore the experience of indigenous black people living in Britain and in the United States (Maynard 1990).

Black perspectives, like feminist perspectives, are many and varied within sociology. Black and white sociologists have been concerned to explore both 'race' and racism, as well as prejudice, discrimination and the legacies of colonialism. Some (for example, Wilson 1980) have focused on the question of class and 'race', arguing that traditional Marxist approaches do not explain sufficiently the experience of African Americans who have been, to all intents and purposes, a separate class in the United States. Others (for example, Hill Collins 1990) have struggled to interrogate the experiences of black women and the notion of a black consciousness within feminism. In her more recent book, Hill Collins (2005) takes this argument further, arguing that the black community will not be able to meet its progressive political agenda, or tackle issues such as the HIV/AIDS crisis, if it does not also value the marginalised perspectives of women and those who are lesbian, gay, bisexual or transgender (LGBT). Post-colonial authors (such as Said 1993) have challenged the superiority of 'white' or dominant thinking and urge that we need to listen to 'the voices of people who have been hidden from sight through colonialisation' (Macionis and Plummer 2008: 336). Building on an interpretive paradigm, some sociologists have examined the nature and persistence of prejudice, drawing on the work of

W.I. Thomas (1863–1947), who argued as early as 1931 that 'if men define situations as real, they are real in their consequences' (republished 1966: 301).

Contemporary sociologists have inevitably turned their attention to the impact of 'race' and ethnicity, racism and nationalism in late modern or post-modern societies. Macionis and Plummer optimistically suggest that most Western societies are, to differing degrees, 'pluralistic in several respects'; living with difference is, after all, 'the goal of multiculturalism' (2008: 338). But in many other respects, Western societies are far from pluralistic. On the contrary, they remain environments of division and segregation; places of 'haves' and 'have-nots', where those who 'have' work hard to safeguard and secure their superior position. Looking at the UK, it is evident that black people and minority ethnic groups are more likely to be disadvantaged across a wide range of social indicators: poverty, unemployment or low wages, poor housing, ill health; the list goes on (see Goodman *et al.* 1997, Shaw *et al.* 2007). Large-scale migration to the UK in recent years has done little to improve this situation. Instead vast numbers of migrants, encouraged to enter the UK as part of a reserve army of labour, find themselves discriminated against in law and excluded from participation in civil society (Toynbee and Walker 2008). Subsequent chapters will explore all of these issues in more depth.

Post-modernism and post-structuralism

Post-modernist perspectives in sociology are prefaced by the assumption that the society in which we are living is qualitatively different from the society envisaged by the early sociological writers. Whereas early sociologists sought to describe and explain the conditions of 'modernism' (that is, industrial, urban, technical, scientific, bureaucratic, rational society), post-modern writers (for example, Bauman 1992, 2006 and 2008, Kumar 1995, Parton 1996 and 2004) conceptualise those in the West as living in a 'post-modern' society, or at the very least in an advanced form of 'modernism', in which the certainties of the old world have gone. Today's society is envisaged as a pluralistic, individualistic one; a 'multiplicity of voices'. There is a contingency about our being, because everything is fluid and changing. We inhabit a host of different identities of class, 'race', ethnicity, gender, age and sexual orientation, and we may choose which identity to forefront in different situations.

This is a politics of 'difference'; not of class or of gender (Butler 1992, Hekman 1990, Weedon 1987). And there is no single, 'true' theoretical perspective – no 'grand theory' – which can explain and interpret our experience. The consequence is that life may feel fragmented and disparate: we do not always know who we are and how to behave. Post-modern writers argue that there is no 'master identity' which determines everything else, just as there are no universal categories of experience and explanation and no 'grand narrative' of history as a story of ever-unfolding progress and advancement towards an ideal, rationally organised society. Mouzelis suggests with more than a hint of irony that 'given the fragile, chaotic, transient and discontinuous character of the social, any holistic theory that imposes an order and a systemness on the social world, in fact, exists only in the confused minds of social scientists' (1995: 42).

Post-structuralists, in common with post-modernist writers, reject the 'essentialism' of conventional sociological writing. While structuralists like Saussure (1974) believed that the meaning produced by language is fixed, post-structuralists view meanings as multiple, unstable and changing (Featherstone and Fawcett 1995). Michel Foucault (1926–1984) argued that there is no such thing as set or objective meaning; instead power, language and institutional practices come together in 'discourse' at specific moments in time to produce particular ways of thinking (Foucault 1977). For Foucault, discourse is more than simply verbal representation or even ways of thinking and producing meaning. Discourses are ways of regulating knowledge: 'practices that systematically form the objects of which they speak' (1972: 49).

Globalisation

One of the key features said to be characteristic of post-modernity is 'globalisation'. Fulcher and Scott (2007: 624) state that globalisation refers to 'a complex of interrelated processes' which are demonstrated in four key ways:

1. the destruction of distance;

2. the stretching of relationships beyond national boundaries;

3. a growing awareness of the world as a whole;

4. an increasing interdependence between different parts of the world.

Globalisation brings with it scope for a greater understanding of the needs and problems of different cultures and societies throughout the world. It also, however, poses potential threats. As transnational companies operate in an increasingly sophisticated global market, so poorer countries can be exploited for the benefit of richer countries and an economic crisis in one place can quickly have an adverse impact on another. Moreover, traditional customs and patterns of consumption and distribution may be undermined. Kumar is more hopeful: he argues that globalisation can lead to particularisation and diversity, not just standardisation and uniformity, as critics of globalisation claim. This is because, to continue to be successful in a world market, capitalism needs to diversify and individualise its products (1995: 189).

Risk

Another central preoccupation of post-modern writers is the notion of 'risk'. It is argued that society is not only inherently more risky today than in the past, but that our expectations that something can, and should, be done about it have increased accordingly. Beck (1992) argues that we live in a 'risk' society; that industrial society brought with it new and damaging risks that modernity sought to regulate and manage. In post-modern times, risks have become more difficult to calculate and control; they are global and at the same time local, or 'glocal' (1999: 142). 'Risk society' therefore equals 'world risk society', in which human experience is characterised by unintended consequences and greater knowledge does not ease this state of affairs; instead, more and better knowledge often leads to more uncertainty (1999: 6). 'Expert' and lay voices now compete with one another as the outcomes of modernity are challenged on all fronts, in a process which Beck calls 'reflexive modernisation'. On a similar theme, Bauman (1997) argues that post-modernity is governed by the 'will to happiness': the result, however, is a sacrificing of security and increased anxiety, as the world is experienced as overwhelmingly uncertain, uncontrollable and frightening.

'Post'-theories and social work

Post-modern and post-structural approaches have had a major impact on research and scholarship over the last twenty years. Sociologists like Bauman (1993) have interrogated social work and social workers, arguing that social work is essentially a moral endeavour that is currently being strangled by rules, regulations and organisational structures which inhibit rather than encourage its moral purpose. Social work authors such as Howe (1994) and Parton (1994 and 2004) have also used post-modern ideas to interrogate social work in general, while Parton, Thorpe and Wattam (1997) used this approach to explore child abuse and child protection. I drew directly on a Foucauldian framework myself for a historical analysis of the development of social work (Cree 1995). What these accounts share is an acceptance that social work is a creature of modernity: it grew up alongside the social sciences as a means to explain and improve the human condition. Social work theory and practice is presented as fragmented and unclear, demonstrating all the uncertainties and ambiguities of post-modern life.

Post-modern and post-structural ideas have not been universally accepted within social work. As we shall see in subsequent chapters of the book, post-modern perspectives have been criticised for lacking an adequate analysis of power and for featuring a relativism that encourages pessimism and despair. Smith and White (1997) argue that a post-modern analysis in social work is 'ethically flawed'. They continue:

> In minimising the continued role of the state, and in collapsing all ideology and subjectivity into discourse, the often grim, lived realities of oppressed groups may be reduced to 'difference' and, in the process, pressing (emancipatory) social imperatives may become obscured.
>
> (1997: 293–4)

In spite of this critique (which Bauman would undoubtedly have some sympathy with), Sue White has gone on to undertake research that draws heavily on post-modern ways of thinking about social work's current preoccupation with the quest for certainty, individualisation and regulation (see Taylor and White 2006, White, Fook and Gardner 2006, White and Stancombe 2003). Moreover, recent discussions of risk and protection in social work are also underpinned by post-modern thinking (for example, Cree and Wallace 2009).

Looking ahead

I would like to finish by re-stating the reasons why a sociological approach is both helpful and necessary in social work. I will also locate myself within the sociological tradition, setting out my own position in terms of the sociological perspectives discussed in the chapter and in the book as a whole. The chapter ends with a practice example that is designed to illuminate the distinctiveness of a sociological approach to an everyday social work task.

Research into service users' views of social work practice has consistently highlighted that effective practice depends on the combination of good interpersonal skills and clear, systematic, organised practice. Based on conversations with service users and practitioners around the UK, Cree and Davis (2007: 149–56) found that good social work:

- is responsive;

- is about building relationships;

- is person-centred;

- is about support which is both emotional and practical;

- is holistic;

- is about balancing rights, risk and protection;

- is knowledgeable and evidence based;

- is future orientated;

- is there for the long term.

If we are going to achieve any or all of these characteristics, as social workers we need to have a good grasp of what we know (and don't know), and a clear route map which justifies and explains to ourselves, as well as to others, why we are taking a particular course of action (and not another). This might be called a belief system; it might also be thought of as a theoretical perspective. In this context, 'theory' is not some abstracted phenomenon consigned to a top shelf in a library, with little connection with the 'real world'. Instead, theoretical ideas are the basis of all behaviour: everything we do in life, and hence in social work, reveals something about who we are and how we see the world. As social workers, we must be prepared to step back and examine afresh everything we hold dear, questioning not just the origins of our beliefs, but also what the consequences might be of holding such a view or position. Bauman and May assert that sociology 'defamiliarizes' things: it distances us from our comfortable, common-sense views and makes us more sensitive to the ways in which these opinions are formed and maintained. Although this 'defamiliarization' might be unsettling, it can, they argue, have clear benefits:

Most importantly, it may open up new and previously unsuspected possibilities of living one's life with others with more self-awareness, more comprehension of our surroundings in terms of greater self and social knowledge and perhaps also with more freedom and control.

(2001: 10)

In the first edition of this book, I described my own perspective within sociology as a critical post-modern one, drawing on insights from both critical and post-modern perspectives. There I stated that in keeping with a critical tradition, I accepted the importance of analysing individuals within wider social structures and systems of power relationships, particularly those of class, 'race', gender, age and disability. At the same time, however, I said that I valued the interpretive position because of its insistence on the centrality of human agency: the capacity which individuals have to bring choice and meaning to their lives. Moreover, I found post-modern approaches made sense of the contemporary world, and I felt encouraged by the possibilities that post-modern analysis offers; as I wrote, 'if all things are contingent, then resistance and change may indeed be possible' (2000: 23). Ten years on, I continue to hold to a critical post-modern position, whilst acknowledging that the structures of inequality are so ingrained and self-perpetuating that the idea of fluidity promised by post-modern approaches now seems less than convincing.

Box 1.1   Sociological perspectives: a practice example

You have been asked to carry out an initial investigation on a fourteen-year-old white boy, who has been truanting from school and has recently been apprehended trying to sell stolen goods.

A psychological approach might focus on the boy himself: his age and developmental stage, his family relationships, his early childhood experiences, his psychological needs, his relationships with siblings and peers.

In contrast, a sociological approach would explore the larger questions about the structural place of young white men in society, looking at masculinities, class and structural disadvantage, education and youth unemployment, the construction of 'whiteness', the organisation of white working-class families and communities, poverty, marginalisation and inequality. Sociologists may also question why young people are targeted for special scrutiny or condemned as 'dangerous' in society. Finally, they may wish to draw attention to the political context and values of consumerism and individualism within this.

Recommended reading

Bauman, Z. and May, T. (2001) *Thinking Sociologically*, 2nd edn, Oxford: Basil Blackwell. An easy-to-read, stimulating text.

Mills, C.W. (1959) *The Sociological Imagination*, Oxford: Oxford University Press. A classic text, well worth a read in spite of the passage of time.

A number of very large sociology textbooks geared mainly at undergraduate sociology students are published each year. I strongly advise potential buyers to look at these in a bookshop or library and choose the one they find most accessible in terms of its structure and language. Recently published books include:

Bilton, T., Bonnett, K., Jones, P., Lawson, T., Skinner, D., Stanworth, M. and Webster, A. (2002) *Introducing Sociology*, 4th edn, Basingstoke: Palgrave Macmillan.

Fulcher, J. and Scott, J. (2007) *Sociology*, 3rd edn, Oxford: Oxford University Press.

Giddens, A. (2006) *Sociology*, 5th edn, Cambridge: Polity Press.

Macionis, J.J. and Plummer, K. (2008) *Sociology: A Global Introduction*, 4th edn, Harlow, Essex: Pearson Education Ltd.

Marsh, I., Keating, M., Punch, S. and Harden, J. (eds) (2009) *Sociology: Making Sense of Society*, 4th edn, Harlow, Essex: Pearson Education Ltd.

2 Family

Introduction

The family occupies a central position in social work theory and practice across all sectors: not just education or children and families, but also in work with adults and in criminal justice. Much of what we think and do as social workers is underpinned by what may be unrecognised and unchallenged assumptions about the nature of the family and its relation to society. It is important, therefore, to look critically at the family and at our ideas and beliefs about it so that social work policy and practice can reflect a deeper understanding of the contradictions and complexities which characterise both family life and the relationship between the family and the state.

This chapter begins by considering what we mean by 'family', clarifying the differences between family, household and kinship structures, and identifying the persuasive nature of familial ideas and practices. The main body of the chapter examines historical, anthropological and sociological approaches to the study of the family.

Definitions

Why define the family? After all, we have all grown up in a family, of one kind or another. But that is the point: *of one kind or another*. Conventional wisdom (as well as much classic sociological writing) often seems to suggest that 'the family' is one entity or institution; that 'the family' can be equated with the 'nuclear family', consisting of a heterosexual couple living together with their children. This is the assumed norm which has dominated advertising, housing and social policy at least since the Second World War: it is the 'cereal packet norm family' of husband at work, happy smiling wife at home and two children, most often presented as a boy and a girl (Leach 1967). Yet huge numbers of families do not fit this 'ideal', most obviously lone parent families. The most recent census confirms that less than a quarter of the population lives in a nuclear family. As family households have declined, so there has been a matching rise in one-person households. The proportion of people living alone in Great Britain has doubled from 6 per cent in 1971 to 12 per cent in 2008; 30 per cent of all households in 2008 were single-person households; the largest increase was among those who are below state pension age (ONS 2009).

But I have allowed a common error of logic to slip in here, because I started talking about one thing (the family) and ended up talking about another (households). This lapse, whether deliberate or accidental, is something that we see frequently in the broadsheets, the popular press and in politicians' speeches, usually in the context of a tirade about the loss of traditional family values. Families and households are clearly not the same thing. Hill and Tisdall (1997) similarly observe that when we speak about 'lone parent families', we most probably mean 'lone parent households'. Unless one parent is dead, children are likely to have two parents in their family, although they do not all live together, and this, as we know, is a far more likely scenario.

Muncie and Sapsford (1999) agree that it is important to distinguish between the family and the household. The family, they suggest, is generally seen as a group of people bound together by blood and marriage ties, but not necessarily located in one geographical place; parents may separate and children may leave home or go to boarding school, but they still see themselves as a family. The household, in contrast, is usually considered to be a spatial category where a group of people (or one person) is bound to a particular place. But Muncie and Sapsford acknowledge that there are difficulties with this definition. What about situations where extended family members live together under one roof, but do not see themselves as one family? There are other problems too. While the distinction between family and household may work as a factual statement, it may not fit how people *feel* about who is in their family; for example, unmarried heterosexual couples or same-sex couples who have registered their civil partnership under the 2004 Act. Statistics demonstrate that the proportion of children living with cohabiting couples increased from 8 per cent to 13 per cent between 1997 and 2008 (ONS 2009), and 8,700 civil partnerships were formed in the UK in 2007. It is also possible that a person living alone, perhaps with a pet to care for, may see herself or himself as part of a family. And where do friends fit into this characterisation? Many people may see their friends as their 'chosen' family, as the discussion of cross-cultural studies later in this chapter will show.

Giddens defines the family as 'a group of people directly linked by kin connection, where the adult members take responsibility for caring for children' (2006: 206). 'Kinship ties', he continues, 'are connections between individuals, established either through marriage or through the lines of descent that connect blood relatives' (ibid.). But what about couples who live together and do not have children? Can they not also be 'a family'? And what is the special significance of 'kin connection' or the concept of kinship more generally? Studies of kinship demonstrate that historical and cultural differences lead to hugely differing expectations of kinship and parental responsibilities (Allan 1996). This means that, although it is not difficult to identify those who are related to us (our aunts and uncles, brothers and sisters, parents and grandparents, nephews and nieces, in-laws, cousins, second cousins, etc.), the list itself, whether large or small, tells us nothing about either the quality of kin relationships or the variability of kin obligations. Finch and Mason's (1993) study of kin relationships and responsibilities finds support for the supposition that kin relationships are a significant source of assistance for many people. But their study also makes it clear (as will be discussed more fully in

Chapter 6) that kinship commitments cannot be guaranteed automatically. Rather, they are built up over time in the context of relationships between people and are the subject of negotiation and compromise (1993: 169). This suggests that we should not make any assumptions based on preconceived ideas about 'family' or 'kinship'.

The notion of family and kinship becomes even more complicated when we consider the rebuilding of families after divorce; four in ten marriages in Great Britain are now remarriages for one or both parties (ONS 2009). What used to be called 'stepfamilies' are more likely to be described today as 'reformed', 'reconstituted' or 'blended' families, and in these situations a complex mix of inter-relationships can occur, with multiple parental and grandparent figures, as well as a range of biological and step-siblings, cousins and other extended family members. Recent studies of adoption also pose a challenge to conventional thinking about family and kinship. Most importantly, they highlight that the notion of families 'of choice' offers little insight into the complex family arrangements that follow on from adoption. Current adoption practice suggests that there should, as far as possible, be openness in adoption, so that adoptive children are able to maintain a relationship with their birth parents after adoption. This opens up a whole new set of possible family relationships, which Jones conceptualises as 'retained families' (where the link between adoptee and birth parents is maintained despite legal adoption and physical separation), 'estranged families' (where the link between adoptees and birth parents is lost through legal adoption) and 'gained families' (when the adoptee and adopters move from a relationship between strangers to a relationship of intimacy) (2009: 226–7). Jones argues that what makes a family is not either biological connectedness or a legal order. Instead, 'family' is created and sustained through daily living and through 'family practices'.

What this discussion reminds us is that 'the family' is, of course, more than simply a practical living arrangement or a grouping focused on the upbringing of children. It is a social institution, steeped in all the beliefs (religious, secular, intellectual and moral) that any one society at a given moment has about the family: what the family is and what it should be. Debates about the family, therefore, are never neutral: when social commentators bemoan the breakdown of the family, or when politicians declare their party to be 'the party of the family' (as both Labour and Conservative governments in the UK have done), they are referring to the 'traditional' nuclear family. All other types of family are, by default, defined with reference to this. The term 'the family' thus carries with it a collection of very specific meanings and assumptions about men and women, about children, about work, about sexual behaviour and about caring.

It was feminists writing in the late 1970s and 1980s who first drew attention to the fact that most writing on the family (sociological literature included) was imbued with a set of very specific ideas about how roles and responsibilities within families should be organised – they called this 'family ideology' or 'familial ideology' (sometimes 'familism'). Vernonica Beechey suggested that two assumptions underlie familial ideology:

> The co-resident nuclear family . . . is normatively desirable . . . the form of sexual division of labour in which the woman is the housewife and mother and primarily located within the private world of the family and the man is wage-earner and bread-winner and primarily located in the 'public' world of paid work is also normatively desirable.
>
> (1986: 99)

We might add a third, implicit assumption to the above; that is, that heterosexuality is 'normatively desirable'. In reviewing the continuing prevalence of familial ideology, Abbott, Wallace and Tyler (2006) point out that it is successful precisely because it is predicated on the assumption that the family is biologically determined and that the particular forms of family life are therefore 'natural'. Family ideology is demonstrated (and institutionalised) in a range of practices which uphold and promote that view of family life. Feminists and lesbian, gay, bisexual and transgender (LGBT) sociologists have pointed out that social policies, and the whole welfare state, have been built on the assumption that the heterosexual nuclear family is the best arena for raising children and is good for society as a whole (see Lind 2004). In addition, it has been argued that social work practice has been structured around an outmoded, patriarchal, white and middle-class concept of family life (see Barrett and McIntosh 1982, Brook and Davis 1985, Wilson 1977).

Implications for practice

- It is important that we are clear what is being talked about – family or household? Nuclear or diverse?

- Remember that whoever is talking, they are likely to have a particular angle or vested interest, drawing on deep-seated attitudes and personal experience, and that this may be stated or implicit, just as with 'facts' or research evidence on families.

- Familial ideology remains powerful in the public, personal and professional psyche, in spite of the diversity of relationships and family arrangements.

Historical accounts

Much of what we know (and think we know) about families in the past derives from the work of the historian Philippe Ariès (1914–1984). Ariès's 1962 account of the differences between the medieval family and the industrial family set the tone for historical and sociological analysis of the development of the 'modern' family. Ariès depicted the medieval family household as a stable economic unit, in which three or more generations of one family worked and lived together alongside various apprentices, lodgers, servants and other unrelated adults. There was, he maintained, little notion of private space as something to be valued or sought after, and scant evidence of love and affection between husbands and wives or between parents and children. Ariès contended that industrialisation and urbanisation destroyed the extended family household unit and put in its place the 'modern' family; that is, small-scale, intimate, child-centred family units in which home and work were separate from one another, and geographical mobility commonplace.

Whilst Ariès's account may indeed have 'set the tone', it has not gone uncontested. Laslett (1972) challenged Ariès's portrayal of medieval families, arguing that over the centuries households in Britain have generally been made up of nuclear, not extended, families. He studied the parish records of 100 English country villages from 1564 to 1821 and found that the large extended family households described by Ariès had never been common, because of late marriage and shorter lifespan. Moreover, he identified that the mean household size in England (including servants) remained more or less constant, at about 4.75, from the sixteenth century right through the industrialisation period until the end of the nineteenth century, when a steady decline set in, falling to a figure of about 3.00 in contemporary censuses. This suggests that although the English family did get smaller, industrialisation cannot be held to be the simple explanation for this. In addition, Laslett's research indicated that historically most people did not live in households made up of three or even four generations, as Ariès had suggested. Instead, they lived in one- or two-generation families.

Hareven (1996) confronts another myth about the medieval versus the modern family. She points out, perhaps surprisingly, that there was widespread geographical mobility in pre-industrial societies. Far from inhibiting the extended family arrangement, industrialisation actually led to an increase in co-residence, as incoming migrants to cities and towns lived with relatives, at least during the initial settling-in stages. Hareven argues that most of the migration to industrial centres was carried out under the auspices of kin; villagers 'spearheaded migration for other relatives' by locating housing and jobs for them. In this way, migration often strengthened family and kinship ties by developing new functions for kin in response to the changing economic and employment conditions (1996: 24). Similar patterns can be found in subsequent periods of migration to the UK; for example, immigration from the New Commonwealth in the 1960s and 1970s, and from former Eastern European countries in the 2000s.

Hareven is critical, too, of the implicit assumption that the family is a passive institution that is acted upon by urbanisation, industrialisation or whatever. She argues instead that the family is an active agent, involved in planning, initiating and even sometimes resisting change (1996: 26). Her research on Manchester demonstrates that before industrialisation whole family groups were involved in home-based 'cottage' industries founded on weaving or spinning; after industrialisation, workers took their skills with them into the factory setting, where again families worked together. Kin control over factory production weakened after the First World War, because of a shift towards a regime of labour surplus (1996: 30). She writes: 'Familial and industrial adaptation processes were not merely parallel but interrelated as a part of a personal and historical continuum' (ibid.). Hareven concludes with a call for an approach to family history which acknowledges that household structures change over time, so that one individual might live in many different family groupings over a lifetime.

Young and Willmott's (1957) classic study of post-war Bethnal Green in East London provides further evidence to dispute any simple characterisation of changes in family life as being explainable only (or even largely) in terms of industrialisation. Young and Willmott set out to investigate the impact of post-war housing and planning policies on family life. They did this by examining two very different communities: Bethnal Green, a poor, working-class neighbourhood in the East End, and 'Greenleigh', their pseudonym for Debden in Essex, a council housing estate 20 miles from Bethnal Green, and fairly typical of the estates to which former Bethnal Green residents had been re-housed. Young and Willmott described Bethnal Green as 'a village in the middle of London', and identified a community in which working-class people (albeit poor and living in sub-standard housing) still lived in close proximity to extended family members, and saw each other frequently. A complex network of relatives, held together by the powerful mother–daughter bond at the centre, provided mutual support and a sense of community. In contrast, the atmosphere at Greenleigh was said to be very different. They found people cut off from relatives, suspicious of their neighbours, and lonely. They concluded that it was not industrialisation that had transformed the family, but well-intentioned housing and planning policies. Moving people out of slums into new blocks of high-rise flats or out of London altogether had not given proper regard to the networks of relationships and had, in turn, left communities feeling uprooted and disorientated. Support systems had broken down, with disastrous effects on the quality of people's lives.

Young and Willmott have been criticised for presenting a romanticised and sentimental picture of working-class family life in Bethnal Green. Subsequent sociological studies have suggested that the reality of people's lives was much less cosy. For example, Cornwell (1984) argues that there is a difference between what people say in public about their family lives and what they feel in private; Young and Willmott's study demonstrates, she suggests, the public face of family life. Nevertheless, their study has continued to be hugely influential, impacting on whole generations of sociologists, planners and community workers (Day 2006). Young and Willmott maintained their interest in family life and communities in subsequent research (1960 and 1973), looking again at working-class communities and also at more middle-class suburbs. Here they reported that married couples were now more likely to be living independently of their parents, and often at a geographical distance from them. Because of this distance, couples had to rely on each other more, and built shared friendships in place of the segregated activities and friendships of the past. Women (including those with children) were more likely to be working outside the home, while at the same time men were experiencing periods of unemployment. Young and Willmott (1973) suggested optimistically that these changes might lead to the development of a 'symmetrical family', with more egalitarian and democratic relationships between husbands and wives, and both partners contributing to decision making and financial resources.

Michael Anderson (1983), in a seminal essay exploring 'what is new about the modern family', introduces another angle on the history of the family. He writes:

> . . . however hard we look, the stable community in which most of the population grew up and grew old together, living out their whole lives in one place, seems to have been very rare in most if not all of non-Highland Britain at least since medieval times.
>
> (1983: 68)

Contrary to the popular view, he asserts that the twentieth century produced more stable communities than had probably been found for hundreds of years, thanks to rent restrictions, the expansion of council housing and a fall in the population growth rate. Similarly, although migration in the past may have been over a relatively short distance, better communication and transport systems suggest that the possibility of keeping in touch today is 'at least as good as in the past' (1983: 69). In reviewing the historical evidence, Anderson concludes that many of the features that we think of as 'new' are a feature of the post-1945 period, rather than a product of industrialisation. Because of this, they do not necessarily tell us about families in the more distant past.

In reviewing the historical evidence as a whole, Gillis (1997) argues that the family is a historical construct; it is also a very powerful myth, integral to the culture of late capitalism. Gillis distinguishes between families we live 'with' and families we live 'by'. The former are the families as defined by the census and social survey research, namely co-resident members of households who define themselves as related to one another. The families we live 'by' are not found in statistical surveys, but are instead mental constructs that often overlap with the families we live with and include not only a far more extended array of kin, but both the dead and the unborn. Families we live 'by' occupy a much larger space than the household, and are extended over time, belonging to the past and the future as much as to the present. These 'imagined' families are no less real than the people we live with on a day-to-day basis and are made real through a set of cultural practices that includes family photography, reunions and vacations, as well as weddings, funerals and graduations. This takes us into the realms of anthropological evidence.

Cross-cultural studies

Just like historians, anthropologists have contributed much to the development of ideas about 'the family'. George P. Murdock, writing in 1949 (reprinted 1965), examined the evidence from 250 societies throughout the world and claimed that:

The nuclear family is a universal social grouping. Either as the sole prevailing form of the family or as the basic unit from which more complex familial forms are compounded, it exists as a distinct and strongly functional group in every known society.

(1949: 2–3)

Murdock's research was highly influential in providing the evidence upon which functionalist sociologists such as Parsons (1955) built their conceptual frameworks. However, Reiss (1965), a contemporary of Murdock, challenged his findings by presenting his own investigations into some of the societies explored by Murdock. In reviewing Murdock's work, he argues that although societies containing nuclear families may be surprisingly common, that is quite different from demonstrating that this is always the case or necessarily the case (1965: 447). He concludes that what is universal about the family is not the nuclear family as such, but the raising of children. He writes: 'The family institution is a small kinship structured group with the key function of nurturant socialization of the newborn' (1965: 449). Oakley's 1972 review of anthropological evidence on family and kinship systems confirms that there is widespread variation between societies in terms of family patterns and behaviour considered suitable for men and women. Most importantly, she asserts that men and women are not universally in all cultures divided into hunter-gatherers and carers of young children.

Contemporary studies of family and kinship have been concerned with exploring not just the differences between and within cultures, but also the meaning of these differences to individuals and groups. Such studies suggest that who counts as a relative (and who does not), and what obligations, rights, privileges and responsibilities (if any) flow from this are found to 'vary very widely and depend on numerous factors' (Allan 1996: 26). Carsten (2004) uses three vignettes (two concerned with fertility treatment and donor insemination and the third with adoption) to interrogate this further, and in doing so, seeks to find out what has happened to kinship at the close of the twentieth and beginning of the twenty-first centuries. She concludes that 'it is a fiction that kinship ever constituted some kind of intransigent rock on which more malleable and dynamic forms of sociality were superimposed' (2004: 186). Further, she writes, '. . . the boundaries of what is constituted by biology or kinship are not set in stone, but may shift or merge in relation to each other' (2004: 188). Her solution is not to abandon the nature–culture divide, but instead to interrogate it so that a new kind of comparative understanding of kinship might be achieved.

Implications for practice

- Historical and anthropological evidence demonstrates that 'the family' is a historical as well as a social construct; it changes over time and across different societies and cultures.

- Our views on families of the past and families of different cultural arrangements are often suspect (seen through the lens of nostalgia or racism) and need to be checked for their validity in practice.

- Gittins (1993: 8) concludes that there is no such thing as *the* family, only *families*. This is a helpful reminder for social work with families.

Traditional sociological approaches

The family has been one of sociology's primary concerns since the beginning of sociological theorising. As we will see, functionalist and Marxist perspectives both saw the family as a key institution, central both to the needs of individuals and to society. Interpretive approaches also accepted the primacy of the family, but were more interested in what this meant for individual family members.

Functionalist perspectives

Functionalist approaches to the family held sway in sociology between the 1940s and 1960s, and remain popular today, particularly in North American sociology. A functionalist perspective, as outlined in Chapter 1, presupposes that social institutions develop to meet the needs of society; that they play a positive part in maintaining the social equilibrium and harmony of that society. Functionalist writers therefore stress the positive benefits of families, arguing that families exist because of the functions the family provides for individuals and for society. Furthermore, it is suggested that families are 'still evolving today in order to help us cope with our changing economic and social environments' (Cheal 2002: 10).

Developing ideas that originated in the work of Durkheim, Talcott Parsons (1902–1979) pioneered the functionalist approach to the family in the post-war period in the United States. He writes:

> The basic and irreducible functions of the family are two: the primary socialisation of children so that they can truly become members of the society into which they have been born; second, the stabilisation of the adult personalities of the population of the society.
>
> (1955: 15)

The significant word here is 'irreducible': Parsons asserted that without the nuclear family, children would not be adequately socialised to become members of society and the personalities of adults would not be 'stabilised'. Parsons (1964) argued that the sexual division of labour is central to the success of the nuclear family: there must be one primary wage earner and one principal home-maker so that conflict and competition between men and women is reduced. Work and family commitments are presented as separate and gendered: 'expressive' women and 'instrumental' men inhabit different spheres of domestic (private) and work (public) life; the specialisation which is at the root of domestic relationships thus mirrors the differentiation inherent in industrialisation, and the home is seen as a place where the breadwinner can let off steam and relax away from the pressures of work. Just as importantly, Parsons (1964) argued that a 'good marriage' is one that includes children, because parental functions reinforce the functions that partners have in relation to one another as spouses.

The family is not only seen as important to individuals, however; functionalists claim that the nuclear family is 'uniquely well adapted to meet the needs of industrial society' (Bilton *et al.* 2002: 232). Parsons (1955) argues that modernisation brought institutional differentiation to family life, as specialised institutions emerged to meet particular needs, and the family lost some of its former functions. Parsons views this process of transformation positively, proposing that the new (nuclear) family form met the needs of the new, industrial economy for a mobile and adaptable workforce. At the same time, the new institutions (education, health and social welfare agencies) each played an important role in supporting 'ailing families' and preventing others from getting into difficulty (Bilton *et al.* 2002: 233).

Parsons's ideas were hugely influential in his day, reproduced in textbooks and taught widely beyond sociology (Delamont 2003), and functionalist approaches have had an enduring place in the public and sociological imagination. Political, religious and social commentators, as well as some sociological theorists writing today, continue to rail against the presumed breakdown of the nuclear family and the so-called 'evils' of lone-parent families, divorce, absent fathers, working mothers and teenage pregnancy. For example, in *Families without Fatherhood*, Dennis and Erdos (2000) claim that since the 1960s there has been a weakening of the norms of the 'traditional family' with, they suggest ominously, 'damaging consequences'. Others have expressed concern about the encroachment of 'the state' into the lives of individuals and families, suggesting that this has led to dependency amongst recipients of welfare services and an erosion of personal and parental responsibility. The solution for the politician and the functionalist sociologist is a return to the 'traditional' nuclear family. This view was evidenced in then prime minister Margaret Thatcher's famous assertion in 1987 that 'There is no such thing as society; there are only individuals and families' (cited by Muncie and Wetherell 1995: 62). It is also demonstrated by Davies, Berger and Carlson (1993), who call for a return to the 'stable nuclear family rooted in a coherent sexual ethic'. They write:

> The only institution which can provide the time, the attention, the love and the care . . . is not just 'the family', but a stable two-parent mutually complementary nuclear family. The fewer of such families that we have, the less we will have of either freedom or stability.
>
> (1993: 7)

Such views expressed both in Britain and in the United States have led to demands for the withdrawal of state benefits to lone mothers as the 'only way of re-establishing the traditional norms of married parenthood' (McIntosh 1996: 148). New agencies have been created to reinforce the importance of families taking care of their own, and at the same time to reduce the dependence of lone parents on the state. The UK Child Support Agency, first proposed in a 1990 White Paper, *Children Come First*, was set up in 1993 with the aim of enforcing absent parents (most commonly fathers) to pay main-tenance for their families. The 1980s and 1990s in the UK saw a number of changes in the organisation and delivery of health and welfare systems aimed at reinforcing the role of the community; hence shifting responsibility back onto families, and often (but not exclusively) onto women in families. (This theme is picked up in Chapter 6.)

Functionalist approaches to the family have not gone unchallenged in sociology. By the late 1960s, new approaches had emerged which drew attention to the importance of social class in understanding the family as an institution and a living arrangement.

Marxist perspectives

Although Marxist and functionalist perspectives both see the family as central to the operation of society, Marxist approaches present a very different set of understandings about the family. Where functionalists stress the benefits of the family for society, Marxist writers concentrate on the ways that the family perpetuates social inequality. The starting point of a Marxist approach is that the family is ultimately dependent upon the dominant mode of production (here the capitalist economy) for its existence and form. As a consequence, dominant class interests have a central impact on family structure and functioning.

One of the earliest accounts of the development of the modern family is presented by Engels in *The Origin of the Family, Private Property and the State* (Engels 1902 [1884]). Drawing heavily on Marx's notes relating to the work of a Victorian anthropologist, Lewis Morgan, Engels argued that mono-gamous marriage and the nuclear family emerged because of the development of private ownership of property (see Bernardes 1997). Marriage enabled men to protect their inheritance, since through it they could ensure that their heirs would succeed them. The role of women was, in turn, a form of prostitution, since wives 'sold' their sexual and reproductive services and their fidelity in return for their material care by their husbands (Muncie and Sapsford 1999). Engels believed that only a truly communist society, where property and tasks were shared, would guarantee the end of exploitation in the family (Marsh *et al.* 2009). Engels's analysis has been described as pioneering in its appreciation of the control of women's sexuality, but at the same time flawed in its conceptualisation of civilisation (Muncie and Sapsford 1999).

Marxist perspectives stress that the nuclear family services the interests of capital in three principal ways: by producing and reproducing labour power; by producing a site for the maintenance of a reserve army of labour; and by facilitating the consumption of vast quantities of consumer goods (Knuttila 2005).

1. *Production and reproduction of labour power*: capitalism needs healthy, mobile workers for its production systems; it also needs class divisions to be reproduced. Labour power is produced and

reproduced by the family, which provides workers with food and rest and at the same time socialises children into values which maintain the capitalist system and provide a refuge from, and counterbalance to, the oppressions of the workplace. The family is, then, a 'haven in a heartless world' (Lasch 1977). It both encourages and maintains the capitalist system.

2. *Reserve army of labour*: women in the family have a special part to play; firstly, as suppliers of unpaid domestic labour at home, and secondly, as a reserve pool to be drawn into the workforce at times of labour shortage.

3. *Unit of consumption*: the family is an ideal unit of consumption for goods produced outside the home. Institutions such as the media sell us an image of family life and encourage greater consumption in the family: consumer durables (from washing machines to lawnmowers to mobile phones) are sold to families as 'must-haves'.

This is not, to suggest, however, that Marxist accounts of the family have ignored the potential conflicts within the nuclear family system. As early as 1976, Zaretsky argued that the pressure to create a refuge from capitalism places a heavy burden on family members, and particularly on women. He sees the housewife as a 'classic expression' of the contradiction in the family: 'her family's income may rise, technology may lessen the burden of work, but she remains oppressed because she remains isolated (1976: 141). Sennett's (1992) account of the inevitable 'destructive *Gemeinschaft*' in familial relationships provides further support to this analysis. (See Chapter 5 for a fuller discussion of the use of the term *Gemeinschaft*.)

There are clear connections between functionalist and Marxist analyses of the family. Both see the nuclear family as the product of the 'modern' age, sustaining and supporting the industrialised, urbanised way of life. Both also identify in the nuclear family a place of personal freedom and retreat from the pressures of the workplace. But where functionalists see the family in positive terms as supporting economic structures, Marxist accounts view the family as an instrument of class oppression. It is one institution among many which promote dominant societal values and perpetuate both structural inequalities and the exploitation of subordinate groups, such as women and children. This theme is developed in later feminist analyses of the family.

Interpretive approaches

In contrast to the broad view taken by much functionalist and Marxist writing, interpretive approaches focus at the micro level on the interactions between family members, and on the meaning of the family for different members.

Phenomenologists such as Berger and Kellner investigated the role played by marriage in the social construction of reality. For them, marriage 'serves as a protection against anomie for the individual' (1971: 23); it is a place where the relationships of adults in society may receive validation. The family, likewise, is the place where children learn to internalise what will become their everyday common sense. The centre of analysis here is the process of socialisation: the ways in which children come to acquire the symbols or meanings of their given culture.

Another micro-level approach, social exchange theory, suggests that people are motivated by self-interest and act rationally, weighing up the rewards and costs of likely actions (see, for example, Blau 1964). A decision to get married, to start a family and even to get divorced is viewed as a utilitarian decision; the persistence and endurance of the family is explained in terms of the appeal to self-interest of the family. Some exchange theorists are also interested in the impact of negotiations and 'exchanges' at the level of social groups and organisations (see Klein and White 1996: 74–6). There is, however, a fundamental problem with this approach. An exchange framework, operating as it does on the assumption that human beings are autonomous, rational actors, takes no account of power differentials within families or of the impact of wider structural forces or ideologies on individuals. Radical psychiatrists such as Laing writing in *Politics of the Family* (1971) and Cooper in *Death of the Family* (1971) adopt a more critical perspective. They explore the destructive nature of family relationships, uncovering the reality that the intensity of family relationships can be damaging: love may be used as an emotional weapon to manipulate and smother children and partners.

Early interpretive approaches have been criticised by feminist researchers for 'obscuring asymmetry in relations between women and men, and for encouraging a benign view of family life that ignores the capacity of men to impose their definitions of reality upon women' (Cheal 1991: 138). Feminist researchers have therefore developed this approach to include an analysis of power within this.

New directions

Feminist approaches

It is widely accepted that feminism has been the single most important phenomenon to influence family theorising (Bernardes 1997: 42). Feminist analyses of the family take up the issue of exploitation, conceptualising the family as an institution that oppresses women; it is therefore a locus of struggle (see also Nava 1983, Wilson 1977). Writing from a range of different perspectives, feminists have brought to public attention a number of critical realities about family life, including domestic violence, rape within marriage, child sexual abuse, the sexual division of labour, housework and childcare issues. Underpinning the feminist critique of the family is the rejection of the functionalist notion that 'the family' is one unified interest group. Instead, feminists have pointed out that the family is a place where relationships are characterised by an unequal distribution of power, responsibilities and resources and 'where people with different activities and interests . . . often come into conflict with one another' (Hartmann 1981: 368).

Women, work and the family

Marxist and socialist feminists (for example, Barrett and McIntosh 1982, Beechey 1987, Smart and Smart 1978) have argued that the family is the central location of women's oppression. They point out that capitalism has had a profound impact on women in the family, demonstrated in the emergence of the notion of the 'family wage'. This, it is argued, benefited both capitalists and the organised (male) working class, by giving men social and economic power in the home. Women, in contrast, were not thought to be entitled to a 'family wage' for their work outside the family, so their low wages could be justified and their choices and economic power restricted (Abbott *et al.* 2005). In recent years, Marxist and socialist feminist analysis has explored the ways in which work outside the home has been restructured to take advantage of women's lower wages, again furthering women's oppression in the family.

Socialist feminists have also given significant attention to women and men's unpaid (domestic) work within the family and household. This began with Oakley's path-breaking study of housework in 1974, which identified for the first time the gender differentiation within household duties, and argued that these were a subject worthy of sociological concern. Some feminists put these ideas into practice and have experimented with alternative family arrangements and collective households. One of the discoveries made by women involved in new collective households was that their lives changed little: they still found themselves largely responsible for childcare and housework duties, as Segal (1983) reveals in an entertaining depiction of life in a 1960s commune in London. Again, more recent research has explored the reality that women's shift into the paid workforce over the last twenty years or so has not been accompanied by a male takeover of housework (Oakley 2005).

Women, the family and patriarchy

Radical feminists explain women's subordination in terms of the relation between women and men, and emphasise men's power over women, instead of capitalist domination. Radical feminists point out that patriarchy (the domination of women by men) existed long before capitalism, and so cannot be explained by the development of capitalism. The family, instead of being viewed as the glue which holds industrial capitalism together, is now seen as the principal institution which props up patriarchy (Delphy 1984, Delphy and Leonard 1992). It does so by securing personal domestic services for men, and by socialising girls and boys into gender-specific roles. Other feminist scholars, for example Walby (1990, 2009), challenge this, arguing that the idea of patriarchy as a total system cannot explain the differences and changes that have taken place in gender relationships over time. Walby suggests that we should think in terms of patriarchal structures, not patriarchy, suggesting that there are patriarchal structures other than the family which require attention, including trade unions and the state.

Violence in the family

A major theme to emerge in the sociological literature on families has been the realisation that families, far from being 'a haven in a heartless world' (Lasch 1977), can be dangerous places. A much-quoted assertion by the US sociologist, Richard J. Gelles, states that: 'The family is the most violent group in society with the exception of the police and the military. You are more likely to get killed, injured or physically attacked in your own home by someone you are related to than in any other social context' (quoted in Macionis and Plummer 2008: 589). Research into violence in families appeared in the late 1960s, beginning with the investigation of violence against children (then called 'battered baby syndrome'), and moving on to encompass violence against women in the home (sometimes called 'domestic violence'). Today, it is acknowledged that abuse in the family takes many forms – emotional, psychological, sexual and physical – and affects all family members, including children, partners and older people (now known as 'elder abuse').

Much of the research on family violence over the last forty years has drawn directly or indirectly on feminist analyses of gender relations and power within families. Feminism has been crucial in exposing hidden violence within marriage and rejecting the idea that it is simply a normal part of married life (Fulcher and Scott 2007: 480). It has also offered an explanation for family violence, based on ideas of patriarchy and patriarchal structures. The opening of women's refuges in the UK in the early 1970s demonstrates the beginnings of a shift in awareness and attitudes towards violence in the marital relationship. Early feminist perspectives sought not only to challenge the behaviour of individual men, but to put this in the context of an understanding of patriarchal structures (in this case, the family). For example, Audrey Mullender argues uncompromisingly that both masculinity and male sexuality are socially constructed to be oppressive, so that men's abuse of women is 'an extension of normal, condoned behaviour in a context of social inequality, not individual deviancy . . . Men wield power over women and all men benefit from this' (1996: 63). Liz Kelly takes a similar approach to the sexual abuse of children in families. In her study of sexual violence, Kelly (1988) explores the links between different forms of sexual violence (rape, child sexual abuse and domestic violence), and uncovers what she sees as similarities between the myths and stereotypes surrounding forms of sexual violence and the institutional responses to abused women and girls. She concludes that all these forms of sexual violence are rooted in one and the same thing; that is, male power in a patriarchal society. She puts this strongly: 'Men's power over women in patriarchal societies results in men assuming rights of sexual access to and intimacy with women' (1988: 41).

The radical feminist approach to domestic violence has not been without its critics, even within feminism. Some have challenged the focus on men's violence, pointing out that women can also be violent in marital relationships and towards children. It is also acknowledged that abuse can and does happen within gay and lesbian relationships, as well as between older and younger people (see Phillipson and Biggs 1995). The feminist historian Linda Gordon (1988) raises this issue when she considers the case of women who abuse children. She writes:

> The role of women as child abusers is important because child abuse is the only form of family violence in which women's assaults are common. Studying child abuse thus affords an unusual opportunity to examine women's anger and violence. Unfortunately, feminist influence in anti-family-violence work has not historically supported such an examination, because of an ideological emphasis on women's peaceableness and a rejection of victim-blaming that have pervaded much of feminist thought.
>
> (1988: 173)

Feminists working from an interpretive approach have stressed that the best way forward for understanding the family is to look in detail at the experiences of family members, interrogating the feelings and relationships within families. In a ground-breaking study, Jessie Bernard (1972) argued that within every marriage, there were two very different relationships: 'his' marriage and 'her' marriage. This idea was developed further by Kate Cavanagh and her colleagues in a study of 122 men who had used violence against their partners (Cavanagh *et al.* 2001). Drawing on Erving Goffman's (1971) idea of 'remedial work', the researchers suggested that the men in the study used various tactics ('accounts, apologies, and requests') to impose their own definitions on their women partners, in order to neutralise or eradicate the women's experience of abuse and control the ways in which the women interpreted and responded to it. They conclude that their findings highlight the need for further investigation of how men's and women's accounts, definitions and responses to violence are interactionally connected through men's attempts to define the violence in exculpatory and expiatory terms, and in women's resistance to such definitions and their implications.

Issues of power and gender remain very much to the fore in feminist writing about the family (see Fawcett, Featherstone, Hearn and Toft 1996), but now there is much greater acknowledgement of the complexities and contradictions within relationships between family members, as will be demonstrated by the post-modern and post-structural approaches described later in this chapter.

Black perspectives

Black and Asian writers have drawn attention to much of the implicit racism in theorising on the family. Typically, sociological approaches take as their norm the white, Eurocentric family (sometimes explicitly, but more frequently in an unspoken, unacknowledged way). White patterns of family organisation and white cultural and historical influences provide the setting for discussions. Black and Asian families, which may have very different forms of organisation, history and traditions, are treated as exceptions to that norm; incomplete and at odds with the white family, rather than of value in their own right. Elliot (1996) puts this in the context of the old 'host–immigrant' model of ethnic relations: the host society is viewed as culturally homogeneous, while minority ethnic groups are depicted as immigrants, strangers, bearers of dangerous, alien culture. Such inherent racism leads to inaccurate and incomplete theorising. On the one hand, it may encourage writers to stereotype families, seeming to suggest that there is only one white or one black family and ignoring the diversities of class and ethnicity. It may also lead writers to miss the complexities of experiences of family life. For example, Marxist and feminist sociologists who have portrayed the family as an institution of oppression have failed to see that it may also be a primary avenue of support for family members living in a hostile, racist society. Bhavnani and Coulson (1986) take up this point:

> Whatever inequalities exist in such (black) households, they are clearly sites of support for their members. In saying this, we are recognising that black women may have significant issues to face within black households.
>
> (1986: 88)

Black perspectives today take as their starting point the differences between black and Asian people as well as their shared experience of oppression: differences of age, gender, ethnicity, culture, religion and class. For example, recent evidence demonstrates that there is widespread variation in family composition amongst different ethnic groups, with Asian and Asian British families most likely to be married, whereas the highest percentage of lone parents (48 per cent) is to be found amongst black and black British families (ONS 2009). Moreover, class-based analyses of the family encourage us to examine the ways in which the white nuclear family has been (and is today) supported and maintained by the labour of black people. Black working-class women work long hours as domestic servants caring for white children and doing housework for white families. While South Africa under the system of apartheid may have been a particularly extreme example of the practice of exploiting black women in the family, many white families in the major cities of Europe and the United States have, in recent years, been maintained by the labour of black women and women from former Eastern European

Chapter 6

countries. These women, while supporting white families (through their work as nannies, carers and cleaners), may at the same time be forced to neglect their own children in the process. (Brittan and Maynard 1984, Graham 1991 and Gregson and Lowe 1994). This theme is explored further in Chapter 6.

Post-modern and post-structural perspectives

Post-modern and post-structural approaches emphasise the instability of theories about the family. It is argued that a grand theory of 'the family' is unworkable; instead, new ideas emerge, become popular for a time and disappear, and theoretical frameworks have a tendency to break down when applied in particular contexts (Cheal 1991: 155). Post-modernism focuses on different kinds of families and on individualisation: on the individual adaptations and individualism that characterise some families, accompanied by greater fluidity and different identities of sex and gender roles. Post-modern writers also examine the contradictions within families, and the continuities, as well as the changes that have taken place. From this perspective, it is acknowledged that there are very many families which do not fit the traditional pattern for a range of reasons. These families may include people who choose not to get married, or where women with children work full time, or men take the role of home-maker and stay-at-home father. There are also ever-greater numbers of people who are 'living apart together' (Levin 2004): people who have committed relationships (married or not), but who are unable to live together under one roof; perhaps because work takes them to different cities, or because of responsibilities for children following divorce. This reminds us that just because a person is living alone, they are not necessarily without a family or long-term or casual relationship. There are, in addition, 'families of choice' – strong, supportive networks of friends, lovers and even members of families of origin – which 'provide the framework for the development of mutual care, responsibility and commitment for many self-identified non-heterosexuals (lesbians and gays, bisexuals, homosexuals, 'queers': the self-descriptions vary)' (Weeks, Heaphy and Donovan 1999: 111). These 'chosen' families are actively created as a means to maintaining a non-heterosexual lifestyle that affirms this identity and, at the same time, provides a 'new way of belonging' in the social world (Weeks *et al.* 2001: 46).

Intimacy, relationships and family practices

Recent sociological analysis of families starts with the idea that intimate relationships have changed and are changing. Giddens (1993), for example, argues that the notion of romantic, 'till death do us part' love has been replaced by 'plastic sexuality', in which people choose when, where and who to have sex with, and 'confluent love', where people only stay with a partner if the relationship is working; this is an 'until further notice' relationship. Similar ideas are explored by Beck and Beck-Gernsheim, by Jamieson and by Bauman. Husband and wife sociologists Beck and Beck-Gernsheim argue that our age is filled with colliding interests between family, love, work and the freedom to pursue individual goals; love is, then, 'a search for oneself, a craving to really get in contact with me and you' (1995: 175). Jamieson (1987 and 1998) also explores emotional bonds, suggesting that there has been a shift in focus from 'the family' to 'the good relationship' as the centre of a meaningful life. Developing this theme, Bauman (2003) suggests that in a world of rampant individualisation, relationships are a mixed blessing, filled with conflicting desires which pull us between two polarities: of freedom on the one hand, and security on the other. Our response to this is to place value on the quantity of our relationships, not the quality of them, hence we are constantly texting and phoning each other; without the constant circulation of messages, we feel excluded.

Sociologists have also moved away from thinking about what a family 'is', to exploring what a family 'does'. The starting point is an acknowledgement that the family is not a fixed entity. Instead, for many people, old relationships break down and new family relationships need to be redefined and re-established; family members have to work hard to build and sustain these relationships. David Morgan (1996, 2002) invites us to consider how people 'do' family, asserting that 'family' can be found in the routine ways in which people's actions create some activities, spaces and times as 'family' (what he calls family 'practices'). So he suggests that what you ate for breakfast and how you ate it tells the observer far more about family living than the rituals of weddings and funerals. Similarly, he argues that it is possible to explore how people 'do' other kinds of intimate relationships, including 'practices of friendship' and more general 'practices of intimacy'. A whole new sociology of friendships (and more recently, of acquaintances) has arisen following this approach. There has also been some exploration of family practices in minority ethnic families, such as those of South Asian Muslim families in Britain (Becher 2008). Finch develops the idea of family practices in another direction, proposing that the sociology of contemporary family relationships needs to be developed to recognise the importance of 'displaying' as well as 'doing' family. She argues that it is often the 'display' of an activity or action which makes it a family practice:

> Relationships do not exist as *family* relationships unless they can be displayed successfully . . . They need to be understood and accepted as such by others, and the way in which I relate to relevant others needs to be recognised as 'family like'.
>
> (2007: 79)

This is of major relevance to social work, as we reflect on how we expect families with whom we are working to 'do' and 'display' family in very particular (often white, middle-class, heterosexual) ways.

The policing of families

Post-structural writers, in rejecting any monolithic ideas of 'the family', have been concerned to understand the ways in which different discourses (knowledge, ideas and practices) come together at particular times in history to create and support particular ideas about 'the family'. Foucault (1977) argues that our understandings of the 'family' (its concept, its purpose and our expectations of it) are constituted by the very discourses which describe and explain it (Howe 1991: 153). In exploring the changing nature of discipline and power, Foucault (1977) identifies a shift in European societies, beginning in the seventeenth century, in the ways in which power was exercised over life ('biopower'), including sexuality. From then on, the control of citizens was no longer achieved by coercion or by the threat of the scaffold, but by new systems of classification and surveillance of social, and specifically sexual, behaviour. Central to this was the process of 'normalisation' – that is, discipline through the family, the school and the community – watched over by new *social* professionals: social workers, health visitors, doctors, teachers, psychologists, armed with their new *social* science knowledge and practices. The new social experts held a dual function: their role was to treat and simultaneously to define and judge the family (Howe 1991). In a seminal book, the French sociologist Jacques Donzelot (1980) clearly abhors what he sees as this 'policing of families'. He looks back to a patriarchal past where men were truly the heads of households and the state rarely intervened in family life. He contrasts this with the contemporary situation in which 'the family appears as though colonised' and there is now 'a patriarchy of the state' (1980: 103). This view has, inevitably, been contested by feminist scholars, including Barrett and McIntosh (1982). It is also criticised by Rose (1999), who argues that the state no longer needs to police families, because the self-regulation of family life is complete; families now share with government the idea of what a 'good family' is, and police themselves accordingly.

Social policy and legislation in the UK evidences the complex and, at times, conflicting relationship between the state, social work and the family. Marsh *et al.* point out that British government policies have 'placed both the family and paid employment centre stage as moral driving forces behind strong communities' (2009: 450). In this way, parents are told that raising children is a vitally important job – they are the key socialisers of the next generation – but at the same time, they are urged to engage in paid work outside the home. These contradictory demands place considerable pressure on working-class parents. The Children Act (1989) and the Children (Scotland) Act (1995) similarly demonstrate a rather Janus-faced approach. Both pieces of legislation stress the importance of keeping families together, and set out their objective to strengthen parents' responsibility for their children. However, both Acts also state that the welfare of the child must come first. This may inevitably lead to decisions being taken that effectively break up family units by removing from home children thought to be at risk.

Social work is, without question, one of Foucault's 'disciplinary mechanisms' of society; the expansion of social work has gone hand in hand with the increasing involvement of the state in surveying and controlling the lives of citizens. The purpose of social work's intervention in the family is to ensure the protection and well-being of children, while at the same time maintaining the legitimacy of the liberal state. Social work operates at a midway point between the individual and the state, between the private and the public spheres, acting as a bridge between the two. For Parton (1991), this is social work's 'crucial mediating role': it is social work which sets the standards of what constitutes 'normal family relationships' and what is 'good enough' parenting (1991: 214). But again, this is neither uncontested nor set for all time. Historical accounts illustrate that there have been very different solutions to perceived problems in family life over the last 100 years or so. In the late nineteenth century in the UK, protecting children meant removing them from their poor families and transporting them to new lives overseas in Canada, Australia and New Zealand (see Colton, Drury, and Williams 1995, Mahood 1995, Wells 2009). In the 1950s and 1960s, it meant placing deprived or illegitimate children for adoption with predominantly white, middle-class married couples (see Triseliotis 1980). Meanwhile, agencies such as Family Service Units and local authority social work services have struggled to keep so-called 'problem' families together since the 1940s. (For a fuller account of the historical development of social work with families, see Cree 1995, Holman 1988, and Parker *et al.* 1991.) Waterhouse (2008), in a discussion about changing standards of 'good enough' parenting, argues that social work's view of what is acceptable behaviour in the family is affected as much by public opinion as by its own internal, professional judgement. High public and professional tolerance reduces the numbers of children requiring investigation, registration and follow-up; low tolerance the reverse. 'Whatever benchmark is employed', she writes, 'universal standards for bringing up children and accepted limits of "good enough" parenting are likely to change over time' (2008: 21).

There is one last issue to be considered here. It has been contended that Donzelot and other writers influenced by Foucault have understated the significance of resistance in relation to surveillance and control in the social regulation of families. Dingwall, Eekelaar and Murray (1995 [1983]) in their influential investigation of child abuse argue that 'resistances' lie in both the culture and the structure of the social worker–service user relationship. They note that social work encounters with service users are characterised by 'the rule of optimism': an acceptance of parents' accounts and an acknowledgement that a charge of mistreatment is 'a matter of almost inconceivable gravity' (1995: 218). In addition, the structural constraints on social work agencies mean that they do not have the power of a family police force as envisaged by Donzelot. Taken together, Dingwall *et al.* assert that 'these restrictions constitute a powerful acknowledgement of the continuing force of family autonomy' (1995: 219). Two additional studies demonstrate that the relationship between social work and families is not a straightforward one of total imposition and restraint, but is instead one marked by negotiation and, at times, resistance. See Gordon's (1988) research into women victims of family violence and care-giving agencies and my own research (Cree 1995) into accounts of women using moral welfare agencies.

Implications for practice

- The social work task with families demonstrates its functionalist (and modernist) underpinnings. Social work aims to support and, if necessary, to re-educate families into the norms and values of society. Its focus is not the social and moral education of *all* families (as is the pattern for the provision of universal health and educational services). Rather, it is in the business of retraining and controlling society's casualties: those specific families who fall through the net of universalistic welfare. They may be 'problem families' (likely to be poor and socially disadvantaged, often lone-parent families, often from minority ethnic groups) or they may be families whose members have already experienced family breakdown (such as families with foster children, adoptive families, etc).

- But the social work task with families has changed over the years and is changing still. Since the 1980s, social work theory and practice with families has been under sustained attack from a group of academics, practitioners, researchers and service users concerned to bring about new Marxist, feminist, anti-racist, and, more recently, post-modern understandings to social work. Social work with families has therefore changed as society has changed; there is no one 'family social work' to be found everywhere, any more than there is one 'family'. The family as a living arrangement, as a set of relationships and as a social institution is constantly developing, as individuals negotiate and re-negotiate their lives, and as society and other social institutions act upon and engage with the family in all its forms.

Conclusion

This chapter has argued that the family is a key social institution, and that sociologists propose very different definitions of the family, leading to equally different theoretical conclusions. As social workers, we must forefront the reality that there is no singular 'family perspective' or 'family needs'. Instead, the experience of family life is mediated by structures and institutions in society: by 'race', ethnicity, gender, age, sexual orientation and social class; by the law, the education system and social policies; and by dominant ideologies which are inherently conservative in orientation, as well as being sexist, racist and heterosexist. Social work is inevitably implicated in this: we are part of the problem, but we can also become part of the solution, by choosing to critically examine policies and interventions to consider where and when 'traditional' family arrangements are being privileged over other family forms. We must also be prepared to value other family patterns, and work with service users to support them.

Recommended reading

Allan, G. and Crow, G. (2001) *Families, Households and Society*, Basingstoke: Palgrave Macmillan. A useful overview of demographic and sociological material.

Bernardes, J. (1997) *Family Studies: An Introduction*, London: Routledge. A readable book with lively opinions on the nuclear family.

McKie, L. and Cunningham-Burley, S. (eds) (2005) *Families in Society: Boundaries and Relationships*, Bristol: Policy Press. A collection of interesting chapters.

3 Childhood

Introduction

It is widely acknowledged that until the mid-1980s there was surprisingly little sociological interest in childhood. Where children appeared in the main body of sociological writing, this was largely in the context of a wider investigation of something else; most frequently the family, the community or the educational system. Children were not actually invisible in sociology; rather they were marginal – adjuncts of their parents, their carers or their teachers – with little recognition that they might have a place of their own in sociological knowledge and enquiry (Corsaro 2004). Moreover, sociological surveys and official statistics frequently did not consider even the presence of children in their data collection and analysis, further increasing their invisibility in sociological discourse (Qvortrup 1994). The 'adultism' (Alanen 1994) in sociology has had important consequences for sociology and for social work. Most importantly, the absence of children in traditional sociological discourse presented a significant gap in the knowledge and understanding of society. This can be likened to the historical position of women within sociology. As explored in Chapter 1, feminist sociologists argued that sociology was not simply sexist, it was flawed sociology; its knowledge base and its research practices lacked validity because they ignored or sidelined the experiences of women (Harding 1991, Stanley 1990). Similarly in recent years, sociologists who are interested in children and childhood have struggled to make sociology reflect better the experiences and perspectives of children and young people.

Chapter 1

The historical lack of a sociological analysis of childhood has had serious, and, I believe, damaging consequences for social work. Without a well-developed social analysis of children and childhood, the discourse around childcare has been created on the basis of ideas and models that draw largely on psychological foundations. The individualising approach in psychology may make it difficult to see that the issues and problems which children and young people face may be structural in origin, rather than rooted in individual personality or developmental stage. More than this, psychological discourses which aim to classify, divide up and control children may oppress children in practice (Mayall 1994). The implications for social work are self-evident. Most of what social work knows about childhood is informed by psychology: ask any social work student what they can tell you about children and young people and they will probably come up with notions about 'ages and stages' or 'needs of children', demonstrating little awareness of the partial and normalising nature of the frameworks they are using. Similarly, dominant theoretical perspectives in social work with children tend to be individualistic in nature, seeking causes and explanations in individual personality or family pathology rather than in structural issues such as class, poverty or inequality, as Parton (1985, 2006) demonstrated in his analysis of the construction of child abuse as a problem of damaged individuals and dysfunctional families. It would be wrong, however, to leave the story there. There has been an explosion in the empirical investigation and theoretical discussion of children and childhood over the last thirty years or so, and in consequence, social work and child care has much new material on which to inform its knowledge base and practice.

This chapter will examine two phases of sociological enquiry into childhood: firstly, sociology's early (and continuing) interest in socialisation; and secondly, sociology's more recent concern with childhood as a social institution. Before going on to consider sociological approaches to childhood, it is necessary to set the parameters of the discussion: to ask – what is childhood?

Definitions

Defining childhood is not as easy as we might expect. We can be fairly certain that childhood begins at birth, or perhaps even at the end of infancy. But when does childhood end and adulthood commence? By looking at this more closely, we find that definitions and expectations of age groups are not fixed and that they change over time as well as between and within countries.

Legislation exemplifies the lack of clarity about childhood by failing to delineate the childhood/ adulthood boundary in any precise way. This means that in the UK there are different ages for a range of behaviours which might be seen as 'adult': getting married, voting in elections, having sexual intercourse, driving a car, buying alcohol, claiming welfare benefits. There are also key differences between the countries in the UK. It is possible, for example, to marry at sixteen years without parental consent in Scotland; the comparable age is eighteen in the rest of the UK. There are also, significantly, different ages of criminal responsibility; that is, the age below which a child is considered to lack the mental capacity to commit a crime, and hence cannot be held guilty of an offence. Under the present law in Scotland, the age of criminal responsibility is eight years, soon to be raised to twelve; it is ten years in England, Wales and Northern Ireland. Ireland has the lowest age of criminal responsibility in Europe (at seven years): the age of criminal responsibility is twelve in the Netherlands and Canada; thirteen in France; fourteen in Russia, Japan, Germany and Italy; fifteen in Finland, Denmark, Norway and Sweden; sixteen in Spain and Portugal; and eighteen in Belgium, Brazil and Peru. In the United States, it is ten for federal crimes but is as low as six years in some states. The widespread variation shows that there is no consensus about what it means to be a child across different countries. This is not, however, a politically neutral state of affairs. On the contrary, there has been, and will undoubtedly continue to be, contestation over particular issues within this, as demonstrated in the successful campaign waged in the UK throughout 1998 to standardise the age of sexual consent to sixteen years for both homosexual and heterosexual sexual intercourse, and by Scotland's decision in 2009 to raise the age of criminal responsibility.

Regulations concerning the minimum school-leaving age also serve as a marker for current societal expectations of the boundary between childhood and adulthood. The school-leaving age in the UK has been raised on numerous occasions since the introduction of compulsory education in 1870. It is set to rise again from sixteen to eighteen years in England and Wales by 2013, reflecting government concern about the high numbers of young people who leave school and do not manage to secure either employment, education or training opportunities (known as NEETs: 'Not in Employment, Education or Training'). This is, of course, an initiative which is targeted predominantly at working-class children; middle-class children in the UK already tend to stay on at school until eighteen years of age. They are also, as research shows, more likely to go to university. Although participation in higher education (HE) in the UK has increased rapidly – the number of students in HE has quadrupled over the past four decades, from 621,000 in 1970–1 to more than 2.5 million in 2006–7 (ONS 2009) – socio-economic groups III, IV and V (skilled manual, semi-skilled and unskilled) remain seriously under-represented. Less than 24 per cent of students in HE come from socio-economic groups III, IV and V, although 40 per cent of all young people in the population come from these family backgrounds (Gilchrist et al. 2003, HEFCE 2003, Cree et al. 2009).

Expectations of childhood vary greatly among cultures, especially between rich and poor societies and between industrialised and developing countries. The childhood of children living on the streets of Brazil or India will, unquestionably, be very different to the childhood of children living in the West, whether in middle-class leafy suburbs or in working-class housing estates, as the cross-cultural studies will show. But there are also important ethnic and cultural differences for children who are living in the UK. For example, although the proportion of the UK-born population under sixteen years old is in decline, minority ethnic groups have an increasingly younger age profile. The highest increases in children under sixteen between 2003 and 2008 were for those in the ethnic groups: 'Other Black' (28.2 per cent), 'Other White' (26 per cent) and 'Other Asian' (24.6 per cent). This compares with a 6 per cent fall in the level of the population of 'White British' children under sixteen years over the same period (ONS 2009), suggesting that these children will have very different experiences of family life.

It should be acknowledged here that the international agenda on children's rights, illustrated in the United Nations Convention on the Rights of the Child (UNCRC) adopted in 1989, is built on the idea that childhood is universal in nature; not only this, the 'universal childhood' promoted by the UNCRC is Western in conception (Boyden 1997). It is worth taking a few moments to consider this further. The UNCRC starts from the premise that everyone under the age of eighteen years is a child; from the outset, this therefore sets the threshold higher than is common practice in many countries across the world. The UNCRC then goes on to assert that everyone under the age of eighteen has rights under the convention. These include rights to life; rights to a name, nationality and family ties; rights to be consulted about decisions that affect them; rights to be cared for and protected from harm; rights to health care, clean water and a decent standard of living; rights to a primary education; rights to relax and play, and to join in a wide range of activities. While we might wish to sign up to these requirements in principle, it is difficult to see how these 'rights' might be achieved in the developing world where large numbers of the adult and child population are dying from hunger, starvation, disease and war. Critics such as Boyden (1997) and others argue, furthermore, that the UNCRC and similar rights-based approaches bring a new set of problems to children, families and societies in the developing world, by transposing an individualising model of childhood and families onto a cultural context which has traditionally valued customary law and practice in family and community affairs. Some countries have, in consequence, introduced their own charters for children's rights. For example, the African Charter on the Rights and Welfare of the Child, which came into force in 1990, stresses both the rights and the responsibilities of children: just as parents have duties towards their children, so it is understood that children have duties towards their parents. In contrast, the word 'duties' only appears in the UNCRC in relation to parents' duties (see Burr and Montgomery (2003) for more information on this topic).

Implications for practice

- Social work operates with a set of assumptions about children and childhood that are rarely challenged for what they are; as social workers, we assess children, parenting and families on the basis of these 'taken for granted' assumptions.

- We need to find ways of acknowledging this and building new knowledge about children and childhood, by being open to the diverse experiences of children.

- A critical sociological approach helps us to do this.

Historical accounts

It was the French historian Philippe Ariès who first drew attention to the idea that childhood, rather than being 'natural' or innate, was socially constructed and that attitudes to childhood changed over time (Gittins 1998: 26). Ariès contrasts what he sees as indifference to children (or 'ignorance of childhood') in the tenth century with the 'obsession' with childhood in modern societies. He writes:

> In mediaeval society the idea of childhood did not exist; this is not to suggest that children were neglected, forsaken or despised. The idea of childhood is not to be confused with affection for children: it corresponds to an awareness of the particular nature of childhood, that particular nature which distinguishes it from the adult, even the young adult. In medieval society, this awareness was lacking. That is why, as soon as the child could live without the constant solicitude of his mother . . . he belonged to adult society.
>
> (Ariès 1962: 125)

Ariès based his ideas on the portrayal of children in medieval paintings and poetry. These portray children from about five years of age in adult clothes and taking part in the full range of adult activities. They were, Ariès contends, small adults to all intents and purposes, and, given high rates of child mortality, parents had no special emotional attachment to their children. Ariès identifies a shift from the end of the thirteenth century, when children started to become increasingly differentiated from adults, with their own clothing, literature and activities. The advent of formal education outside the home in the sixteenth and seventeenth centuries then consolidated the concept of childhood as a distinct phenomenon. Ariès identifies two distinct dimensions to the new consciousness about childhood. Firstly, he describes a new awareness of, and enjoyment in, children by adults; and secondly, he outlines a new conceptualisation of childhood as a time for physical, intellectual and social development.

Ariès is clear that the new understandings about childhood did not impact on all children at the same time. On the contrary, he perceives marked class and gender differences in the experiences of children. It was the new middle classes, he maintains, who were at the forefront of the drive to introduce education for boys. Upper-class boys in the sixteenth and seventeenth centuries received little formal schooling and could be army officers by the age of fourteen, and even as young as eleven years on occasions. In contrast, Ariès reports that girls from all classes had no formal schooling and many were married and running households by fourteen years of age. By the eighteenth century, most aristocratic children (both boys and girls) received some schooling, though girls finished earlier than boys. Working-class children continued to work to supplement family incomes late into the nineteenth century, and to have life experiences which were very similar to those of their parents. What this suggests is that the construction of childhood as a special category was targeted first and foremost at middle-class boys; subsequently, other children have been accommodated into this characterisation at different times and to different degrees. Ariès locates the lengthening of childhood in changes in ideological beliefs. Calvinism had stressed the notion of original sin: children were doomed to depravity unless controlled and trained by parents and schools. The Reformation brought with it ideas about a disciplined life, however, and in the eighteenth century, Enlightenment ideas placed on members of society the responsibility that they should seek to contribute to the good of society through attaining rationality: education was to play a major part in this.

Frost and Stein assert that Ariès has been 'central in helping us to build a conception of the historical variability of Western childhood' (1989: 12). However, his work has been seriously criticised on a number of fronts. Pollock (1987) asserts that childhood is not a modern concept, although what we expect of children has changed over time. Looking at children in Europe from 1500 to 1900, she argues that Ariès was mistaken in assuming that children joined adult society at the age of five years, or that parents were less emotionally attached to their children in the past. Thane (1981) is likewise critical of Ariès's views. She claims that Ariès underplayed both the importance of the Renaissance, along with the new ideas of individualism it brought, and the significance of economic change, or more specifically, the rise of capitalism. She links the emergence of modern age groups firmly to the birth and development of European capitalism, arguing that the new middle classes were striving to maximise their control over wealth and property, and at the same time that adult life was becoming more demanding, and more skill was required for those directly involved in commerce or in professional occupations such as the law. The consequence was the emergence of schooling and the lengthening of childhood. These pressures were, according to Thane, felt less acutely initially by either landowners or the landless labouring poor. She suggests that it was only when landowners felt the pressure of competition for power and wealth from the rising middle classes, and later still, when changes in economic and work practices led to the need for a different kind of worker, both literate and numerate, that education became more widely available. By the end of the nineteenth century, the new fear of the 'dangerous classes' led to the introduction of both factory and education legislation which aimed at taking working-class children out of the *adult* world of work and into the *children's* world of school. Thane thus concludes that there was a clear correspondence between the birth of capitalism, modern classes and modern age groups (1981: 11).

Jamieson and Toynbee's (1992) investigation of children growing up in rural communities in Scotland between 1900 and 1930 sheds further light on the real-life complexities that are concealed by the catch-all concept 'childhood'. Jamieson and Toynbee contend that the major feature in the lives of children of crofters and farm servants in the early years of the twentieth century was not separateness from adults: instead, children's lives were characterised by continuities between themselves and adults; they rose at the same time, worked together, and went to bed at the same time. Children had few toys and were expected to perform a variety of tasks for their parents, both inside and outside the house. Income earned by children was not for their personal consumption; it was a contribution to the family economy. Household membership carried with it 'expectations of contributing one's labour, in the same way that membership of the community created ties of economic and social reciprocity' (1992: 31). Although there were similarities between the lives of children and adults, Jamieson and Toynbee acknowledge that their lives were not the same. On closer inspection, it is evident that there was a clear demarcation between what were regarded as *children's* and *adults'* tasks; and within this, differences too between boys' and girls' jobs, reflecting the division of labour between adult men and women. Boys therefore did not drive cattle, look after cows or fetch water, but were expected to tether rogue sheep; girls never did this. Fishing was an exclusively male activity and it was rare for men or boys to do housework. The pattern of work connected with the collection of peat serves as a useful case-example of age and gender divisions. It was the men's job to mark and cut the peat, the women's job to carry it home, and the children's job to stack it.

This illustrates well the claim that childhood is historically variable, that it differs across class and gender, and that there are important continuities in experience between adults and children across generations. In an earlier publication, Jamieson and Toynbee (1990) pinpoint the post-Second World War period as a key moment in the creation of a new idea of childhood and a new relationship between parents and children. Changes in the nature and distribution of goods for consumption in the period after the end of the Second World War meant that working-class 'children's jobs' (daily shopping, collecting fuel, cleaning cutlery, polishing brasses) largely disappeared. At the same time, many more women were working, so that work around the home became a 'main leisure time activity for a significant minority of men and women' (1990: 95). New ideas also emerged in the relationship between adults and children, with parents seeking a more democratic relationship with their children, in contrast to the more authoritarian attitudes of the past. Jamieson and Toynbee locate these changes in increased affluence, the cult of leisure and the development of mass consumption, mass media and mass culture: the shift to the 'affluent consumer society' was associated 'not only with the multiplication of goods provided for children by parents, but also a reduction in the contributions made by children and young people to their family household' (1990: 102).

It is evident from the historical evidence that any idea of childhood as a fixed, chronological period with a universal, agreed conceptualisation is untenable. It seems likely that childhood, as it is currently envisaged in Western society, is a comparatively recent phenomenon, created by shifts in the socio-economic and political world, as well as by psychological ideas about the 'needs' of children as distinct from adults. A historical analysis also demonstrates significant points of connection and overlap between the experiences of adults and children. Frost and Stein (1989) assert that there is no such thing as *a* history of childhood. Instead, there have always been diverse experiences of childhood across class, culture and geography, and diverse accounts of family life, illustrating the capacity for both affection *and* cruelty across generations (1989: 18). Cross-cultural studies extend the discussion further.

Cross-cultural studies

Cross-cultural studies demonstrate that there are widespread differences in the social organisation of childhood in different cultural and ethnic settings. Hill and Tisdall (1997), for example, in their review of the evidence, identify that in some cultures children spend considerable amounts of time apart from adults, while in others they are involved in work-related activities alongside adults from an early age. (This connects with our earlier observations about children in rural Scotland in the early years of the twentieth century.) Boyden (1997) argues that the transition from childhood to adulthood across the world is fluid and changing. In countries like Peru and India, a significant number of heads of household are very young (from six to fourteen years), and in most developing countries many children still make up an important part of the workforce, even though more children have access to schooling. In her study of child labour in Nigeria, Okoli (2009) argues that child labour remains a fact of life and a way of life for children living and working in and around the cities' street markets. From her conversations with the children, we learn that they see work as both positive and negative; either way, it was part of their childhoods, even though most of them did also attend school. Furthermore, Okoli found that these children were not, as she had anticipated, homeless. Instead, most lived with family members and went home in the evenings after the markets closed. This finding echoes an earlier analysis of children in Paraguay in which Glauser (1997) argues that the term 'street children' needs to be deconstructed, because it does not correspond with the rich variety of children's lived experiences.

Cross-cultural studies also highlight differences in child-rearing practices. Again, Hill and Tisdall identify that there are communities across the world in which the care of young children, rather than being restricted to a nuclear family model, is shared among a wide set of people, often female kinfolk. Ideas of family identity in these settings, they argue, may be more important than those of individual personality (1997: 16). They also point to societies in West Africa where it has been common practice over many years for children to be fostered with relatives from five years onwards. This was not understood as an act of rejection on behalf of parents (as a white European perspective might assume), but was valued instead as a positive service to the children, who would be able to gain wider social links as well as specific skills in their new families. Such local customs have been challenged in recent years as Western ideas about 'good' childcare have been increasingly incorporated into daily lives. Wells (2009: 1) goes so far as to assert that in an increasingly globalised world, childhood is being reshaped by 'the increasing influence of international laws and international non-governmental organisations' (NGOs). She concludes that, in order to understand childhood, we must look to both local and global factors.

In looking at experiences across different countries, it is important to remember that there may be as many differences *within* countries (built on inequalities of class or caste, 'race' and ethnicity, gender, disability, etc.) as there are differences *between* countries. The childhood of someone who grows up in a privileged family in the United States or the UK may, arguably, have more in common with the childhood of a middle-class or upper-class person in Africa or Asia than with that of poor or working-class children from within their own countries. Wells (2009) is critical of what she perceives as the lack of theoretical interest in this. The sociology of childhood is, she asserts, largely built on the experience of white, middle-class children. (Feminist standpoint theory was similarly criticised for ignoring the diversities of women's experiences and for forefronting middle-class white women's lives.) Official statistics suggest that 15 per cent of children in the UK live in families where there is no person of working age who is in employment (ONS 2009); these people's childhood will undoubtedly be different from that of those born to middle-class professional parents. Rogers (1989) notes that the expectations and norms about childhood held by children growing up in minority ethnic families in the UK may also be very different to the traditional white, Eurocentric model. Although we need to be careful not to fall into the trap of stereotyping minority ethnic families, it is nevertheless important to draw attention to the continuing reality that there are different ways of thinking about children and childhood across different cultural and ethnic groups (see also Boushel 2000).

Hill and Tisdall (1997) stress the impact on black and minority ethnic children in the UK of growing up in a racist society. These children grow up legally, and in some respects culturally, British, but have their own distinctive religious and cultural influences; influences that are routinely marginalised, discounted and discriminated against (1997: 17). This means that oppression and discrimination may be a large part of their experience of childhood. More recent studies (see, for example, Mason 2003) have focused on the experience of transition experienced by all minority ethnic families, as first, second and third generation children struggle to find their place within a majority culture that remains hostile to them. Chahal (2000) argues that minority ethnic groups do not form a homogeneous mass at which policy initiatives can be aimed in equal measure; nevertheless, all minority ethnic groups continue to experience racist victimisation, particularly where families are isolated and removed from familiar networks.

Implications for practice

- Historical and anthropological evidence demonstrates that 'childhood' (just like 'the family') changes over time and across and within different societies and cultures.

- Our views of childhood in the past and of different cultural arrangements are often suspect, seen through the lenses of nostalgia, colonialism or racism.

- As social workers, we need to be prepared to hold up our assumptions both to critical examination in theory, and to validity in practice.

Traditional sociological approaches

As has already been stated, traditional sociology had little interest in childhood. But this did not mean that sociologists had no interest in children. On the contrary, they were extremely interested in children: but children as 'becoming adults', rather than as people in their own right. The familiar 'nature versus nurture' debate springs to mind here: how far is human behaviour seen to be determined by biology and instincts, and how far is it the product of internal and external controls? Classical sociologists argued that most of what we do is learned. We come into the world as helpless infants, and develop through learning what is required of us, by those around us and by society; it is the conscious element within this which makes us human (Fulcher and Scott 2007: 116). The concept that has been developed to explain the process of learning to adapt to and internalise society is known as 'socialisation'. It has preoccupied successive generations of sociologists, who have viewed it from a range of different perspectives.

Perspectives on socialisation

Macionis and Plummer (2008: 193) suggest that socialisation theory asks five broad questions:

1. Who is being socialised?

2. By whom?

3. How?

4. Where?

5. When?

Functionalists such as Durkheim and Parsons saw socialisation as a necessary process, which begins at birth, lasts throughout our lives, and continues until death. A distinction is often made between 'primary socialisation', which happens in the family in infancy and childhood and provides the basis for all future learning, and 'secondary socialisation', which happens when children are older and start to be influenced more by external individuals (such as the peer group) and by outside agencies (such as school, clubs and, later, the workplace). Functionalists believe that socialisation is important not just for human beings, but for society as a whole. Its job is to ensure that commonly held, societal values and norms are properly internalised; without it, human beings would experience depression, loss and disorientation ('anomie'), and society would fall into anarchy.

Socialisation is viewed in much less benign terms by those subscribing to a radical or conflict perspective. A Marxist or radical feminist viewpoint suggests that socialisation is enforced on individuals by the regulatory mechanisms of society, such as the courts, police, education, etc., either by rewarding certain behaviours and punishing others, or through the workings of patriarchy and the sexual division of labour. Socialisation is envisaged as a mechanism for enforcing social conformity, rather than transmitting the social consensus. The question asked is then whose norms are being encouraged and supported? And how does the *status quo* operate to retain and consolidate power, while at the same time managing to make alternative views and behaviours not just deviant but, at times, criminal? Examples of this might include the 'othering' of LGBT people or the tolerance of some drugs (such as tobacco and alcohol) and the criminalisation of others (including cannabis and heroin).

This conceptualisation of the socialisation process has been criticised for being determinist and absolutist in emphasis. For example, in an early influential essay Wrong (1961) described this as an 'over-socialized conception of man'. Critics have pointed out that socialisation is never a one-way street; there are always counter-cultures at odds with the 'dominant' view. Willis's celebrated study of working-class boys (1977) takes issue with those who see school as an inculcator of middle-class values that are supposedly absorbed unconsciously by working-class children. He points instead to the vast numbers of children who do not conform, and who actively resist attempts to incorporate them into a dominant middle-class culture. He argues that for many children their counter-culture is what matters most; that is, a working-class culture with profound similarities to 'shop floor culture' (that is, to the familiar ways of behaving – including the attitudes and the jokes – which are part and parcel of working on the shop floor). This is not a defeated culture, but one which has rules and skills all of its own.

Functionalist and radical perspectives have also been criticised for minimising individual 'agency' and the capacity of the individual to interact with and influence his or her social environment. Interpretive sociologists present socialisation as an interactive process. It is still accepted that we enter a pre-given social world, but individuals are no longer seen as wholly constrained by societal structures. Instead, it is pointed out that individuals (children and adults) try out new behaviour and build on previous experiences of given situations, bringing meaning and purpose to their actions. American social psychologist George Herbert Mead (1967) has had a major influence on thinking about the interactive nature of the socialisation process. His central concept, argue Macionis and Plummer, is 'the self, the human capacity to be reflexive and take the role of others' (2008: 197). Mead argues that there is no 'self' or personality that exists at birth. Instead, the self emerges from social experience; it is constituted throughout life, confirmed and transformed by a sequence of negotiations with others who are themselves on life's journey. The 'self' is understood to have two components: 'the self is subject' ('I'), as we initiate social reaction; and 'the self is object' ('me'), because in taking the role of another, we form impressions of ourselves. From this perspective, all social experience is the interplay of the 'I' and the 'me': our actions are spontaneous, yet guided by how others respond to us (Macionis and Plummer 2008: 199). Leading on from Mead, symbolic interactionists stress the importance of the 'roles' that we play: the primary task for a child in order to make sense of, and influence, the world is to learn to take the role of the 'other' (for example, mother, father, sibling). By adapting and submitting to the demands of the social world, the child learns to become a role player in different settings at different times. It is argued that each of us learns a slightly different combination of roles that will always be defined in slightly different ways (see Berger and Luckman 1966).

Some sociologists have criticised what is seen as over-determinism in the presentation of roles and how they work. Connell (1983), for example, argues that because we all hold countless roles, all bearing different expectations, no generalisations can be made here. He also disputes the claim that role (and the idea of the internalisation of role prescriptions) can explain social learning and personality formation. He writes that role cannot explain 'the opposition with which social pressure is met – the girls who become tomboys, the women who become lesbians, the shoppers who become shoplifters, the citizens who become revolutionaries' (1983: 202). In other words, role cannot explain resistance. Goffman is also interested in the ways that people actively resist, refuse or manipulate their given roles. In his (1968) study of asylums, he argues that even in institutions with the most rigid rules, there is still a process of negotiation; a twisting of the rules, an unwritten contract between warder and patient. This is possible because, as Goffman sees it, in any setting, each person is both an actor and an audience; we play parts in the drama of life, and work constantly to create specific impressions of ourselves in the minds of others, as they do in ours.

Grbich (1990) picks up this theme, arguing that socialisation is a map, not a blueprint: it can never be a single, total process, and expectations others have of us will always be conflicting, loose and obscure, differing from situation to situation. There are also many areas of life where there are no established rules and expectations, where we have to make independent assessments. In the 'post-modern' world, socialisation can never be a complete, all-encompassing process. Bauman writes:

> Being free and unfree at the same time is perhaps the most common of our experiences. It is also, arguably, the most confusing . . . much in the history of sociology may be explained as an on-going effort to solve this puzzle.
>
> (1990: 20)

Bauman goes on to explore more fully the idea of freedom and independence. We are free to make choices and decisions, but the choices and decisions we can make are constrained in various ways: by those who set the rules about the choices we can make; by qualifications and personal resources, financial and otherwise; by class, gender, ethnicity. The groups of which we are members enable us to be free and, at the same time, constrain us by drawing borders on that freedom. It is therefore important to ask whose interests are being met in the sustaining of particular inequalities, such as those based on class, gender and 'race'. There needs to be an adequate analysis of how power works in society; of how the *status quo* is maintained and why. The fundamental question for sociologists now changes. Instead of asking 'how does society socialise individuals?' it is necessary to ask 'who socialises society?' In an interesting illustration of these issues, Khan (2009) investigated young female domestic workers in post-apartheid South African society, throwing into sharp relief the complex interplay of gender, 'race', class and different cultural expectations in the socialisation of girls to become domestic workers. In an earlier textbook, Brittan and Maynard (1984) also focus on the origins of socialisation; in this case, the ways in which children acquire racist and sexist beliefs and attitudes. Brittan and Maynard argue that racism and sexism exist not because of socialisation; on the contrary, 'socialisation reproduces what is already there' (1984: 111). This does not lead them, however, to be despairing about change. Instead, they point to the capacity of the Black Power and Black Consciousness movements in the United States and South Africa to reclaim negative images of what it is to be black in a racist society and recreate them in a powerful and positive way. (See also Ogbar 2005 for a more contemporary analysis.)

Post-modern writers are not only interested in formal agencies of socialisation; they are also interested in the new carriers of culture and society, in this case, the television, the computer and, of course, the worldwide Web. Writing in 1987, Denzin described the contemporary post-modern child as 'a media child': 'he or she is cared for by the television set, in conjunction with the day-care center. Cultural myths are learned from television, including how to be violent and how to be a man in violent society' (1987: 33). This reality has been magnified greatly over the last ten years, and the situation is likely to continue. Ballantyne and Roberts (2009), describing the US experience, claim that by the time a child reaches eighteen years of age, he or she will have spent more time watching television than doing any other single activity apart from sleeping. There is persistent concern in the popular press and in more serious academic writing about the flood of messages children are receiving about themselves and about society from computer games, mobile phones and the Internet. Who is regulating the content of these media? Are traditional agents of socialisation (like the family) being undermined by this? Are the new technologies a force for good or ill? Who decides? These questions will continue to be asked in the years ahead.

Implications for practice

- Social work and criminal justice groups have a role to play as agencies of socialisation – our purpose is to encourage some behaviours (for example, 'good parenting'), while preventing others (such as child or adult abuse).

- In this, we should be clear about the potential we have either for perpetuating inequalities or for encouraging more progressive attitudes and behaviours, and we should also be aware that our room for manoeuvre is itself controlled and circumscribed; not just by society, but by all the complex interactions and relationships which exist between ourselves and others.

New directions

Since the mid-1980s there has been an explosion of interest in the sociology of childhood, as sociologists have sought to redefine children as the subjects of research in their own right and to understand the experience of 'modern', and more recently 'post-modern', childhood. This scholarship is best understood as going through two overlapping phases of investigation and analysis. In the first, sociologists sought to understand how and why it is that children and childhood have come to be constituted ('socially constructed') in the way that they have. In the second phase of enquiry, the notions of 'child' and 'childhood' (with a capital 'C') break down, to be replaced by ideas of fluidity, change and relativity. In reviewing these developments, Mayall (2002) acknowledges the contribution that feminism and feminist theory has made to the sociology of childhood; she suggests that the new interest in children and childhood mirrors feminism's earlier struggle to put women at the heart of sociological endeavour. As we will see, there are connections too between the collapse of the idea of 'woman' as a single category in feminism and the breakdown of the notion of 'child' and 'childhood' in the sociology of childhood.

The social construction of 'modern' childhood

The new sociology of childhood starts with the premise that children and childhood are not 'facts' in themselves, but are social constructions; as James and Prout assert, it is 'biological immaturity rather than childhood which is a universal and natural feature of human groups' (1997: 3). A social constructionist perspective suggests that everything we think about and expect of children and childhood is socially constructed. Qvortrup expresses this as follows, 'Childhood is the life-space which our culture limits it to be i.e. its definitions through the courts, the school, the family and also through psychology and philosophy' (1994:3), and, I would argue, through the debates and discourses which form the sociology of childhood itself.

In one of the earliest contributions to the new sociology of childhood, Judith Ennew (1986) argues that the most important feature of modern childhood is the idea of 'separateness'. She sees this in two parts: first, the idea that children should be 'quarantined' away from various 'nasty infections' of adulthood, such as sex, violence and commerce; and second, the notion that childhood should be a happy, innocent, free stage of life; a time of play and socialisation, rather than work and economic responsibility (1986: 33). Wyness summarises this simply: 'Childhood = Play; Adulthood = Work' (2006: 9). The idea of the 'playing-child' has not emerged accidentally. Instead, it is constructed by the very laws which both forbid children from working and prevent children from receiving welfare benefits if they are not working, and by the association of play with the idea of innocence.

While childhood has been constituted as a separate phase, so children's dependent state has been stretched out to be far longer than it was in the past: although children may reach puberty at ten or eleven years, they may not be seen to enter adulthood until finishing full-time education aged twenty-one and upwards. Sociological studies have sought to explore this 'lengthening' of childhood: to examine children's activities in school, employment and leisure, their relationships with older generations, their dependency and independence, their legal status, and the impact of gender, 'race' and class on their lived experiences (see, for example, Chisholm *et al.* 1990, Coleman 1992, Mayall 1994, Qvortrup *et al.* 1994). This research demonstrates that children's lives have become increasingly age-segregated, thus increasing both their isolation and their dependency. Moreover, children are spending more and more time in institutional and organised settings, from pre-school to school and after-school care. As a consequence, they can be understood as inhabiting a separate and exclusive sphere in which they are protected from, and at the same time controlled by, the adult world. Kitzinger (1990) highlights the increased risks for children in this, as they find themselves increasingly at the mercy of the very people who may also be their abusers. The separateness of childhood thus increases children's vulnerability, even as it seeks to minimise harm to children.

Ennew (1994) sees parallels between the 'curricularization' of children's lives and the compartmentalised lives inhabited by adults. Just as adults move from different spheres of home, work, shopping and leisure, so the school timetable has been extended outside the walls of the classroom and into the whole of children's existence. She argues that within their tight schedules, children make superficial and fragmented social relationships with other children and adults, and the idea of 'free time' disappears as they are confronted with the imperative to organise and structure their time 'constructively'. Ennew identifies this as a feature of modern lives: 'Leisure and play, far from being separate and different from work, are now timetabled according to the same criteria and the same units of time' (1994:132). The curricularisation of children's lives increases both the protection of children and their dependence on adults, as adults ferry children to and from the various cultural and sporting activities that fill their out-of-school hours. From this perspective, it is argued that childhood, far from lengthening, is becoming a shorter and shorter phase of a person's life (Qvortrup 1995: 195).

Frønes (1994) takes a different approach. He is interested in the extent to which children have increasingly become consumers in their own right, with their own special clothes, books, games and television programmes. He locates this development in the context of the emergence of the individual in modern society. This process, he suggests, involves two dimensions: individuation (that is, the tendency of the modern state and organisational system to treat the individual as the basic unit) and individualisation (that is, an emphasis on the individual as a psychological personality) (1994: 147). Qvortrup puts this graphically:

> ... children are being individualised in a way themselves – exactly as parents and other adults have been individualised. Children spend more and more time as representatives for themselves rather than for their family; they have their own ID-card, their own key, their own money, and some experiments have already been made with plastic cards to be used each day for children in kindergartens to control children's time use for economic reasons.
>
> (1995: 196)

The individualisation process can be clearly demonstrated in the movement for children's rights. From the 1970s onwards, campaigners for child liberation have argued that the separation of children's and adults' worlds is 'an unwarranted and oppressive discrimination' (Archard 2004: 71), and they have fought for children to be treated the same as other people (that is, adults), with the same rights and privileges, including the right to vote, work, own property, and rights to make sexual and guardianship choices. In contrast, those operating from a 'caretaker thesis' (Archard 2004: 77) have argued that children cannot be seen as self-determining agents; they cannot make rational choices and adults must therefore make decisions in their best interests; Pilcher (1995: 50) claims that the 'liberationist' perspective is gaining ground. She evidences this in the emergence of organisations which seek to listen to children's grievances, such as Childline; in the redefinition of corporal punishment as physical violence; and in legislation which promotes the rights of the child.

Oldman (1994) argues that children's experience is best understood as that of a subordinate class, exploited by an adult class. Their activities are structured so as to serve the economic interests of adults; their work at home and school is no less 'work' than that of adults. He suggests that the two basic mechanisms of the exploitation of children by adults are the unsupervised activity of children (which frees parents from childcare) and formal supervision outside the family (which provides adults with paid 'child work'). Mayall supports the notion that children see themselves as a minority social group. As she writes, 'All their accounts point to inequalities between their status and that of adults, and to commonalities between them in their childhood status' (2002: 122). She argues that children's lives are shaped by the 'generationing processes specific to various societies, as well as by gender, class and ethnicity'; but they inhabit a 'common domain' of childhood, under the 'supervision, control and protection of adults' (2002: 122–3). The commonalities, Mayall continues, override details of gender, ethnicity and age, and point to the need to develop a specific 'child standpoint'. Lavalette and Cunningham reject the characterisation of children as a subordinate class. They argue that it is misleading to suggest that all children have a common set of interests, and that they all find themselves excluded and disadvantaged. They assert that they cannot see any oppression affecting the lives of the Royal children of Britain, nor that they have anything in common with children who live in inner-city slums (2002: 27).

Deconstructing 'modern' childhood

Where does this take us? We have seen from anthropological research that the separation of children from work is far from the experience of most children growing up in the developing world, where their contribution to the family's livelihood is an absolute necessity. It is also questionable how much opportunity many children have for play; the idea of the 'play-child' is clearly a 'modern' Western construction that may have little relevance in poor and developing countries. Boyden (1997) is highly critical of the ways in which the 'official' view of childhood is being disseminated internationally to countries and cultures which may traditionally have very different ideas about the capabilities and competencies of children. Children on the streets, out of school and away from home are being targeted for intervention by welfare and aid agencies. Yet the activities of these children, from a different point of view, may be understood as mechanisms of survival, performing the important function of preparing them for adult life.

Picking up Lavalette and Cunningham's point, it is also important to think about how far the familiar accounts of children's childhoods fit with the experiences of working-class children in the developed world. Families on low incomes and without transport will be much less able to make use of the many and varied social and cultural activities that are routinely available to more mobile, middle-class families with greater disposable income. Research indicates that working-class children continue to take part in unsupervised play around their streets and neighbourhoods. Furthermore, it is middle-class families who make most use of external childcare resources such as nurseries and paid childminders. In a study published in 1987, Hill found that working-class families relied more heavily for childcare on the extended family network, including parents, siblings and close neighbours, suggesting that family members, rather than paid adult carers, continued to play a prominent role in their lives. More recently, research conducted by the National Centre for Social Research in 2004, 2007, 2008 and 2009 has shown that although more families are using childcare and early years provision than in the past, wealthier parents are twice as likely as those from lower-income homes to use formal childcare, and minority ethnic families use formal childcare less than any other group (Speight *et al.* 2009).

Sociologists have also questioned the extent to which adult control and curricularisation of children's lives is ever complete. Studies of children's unsupervised play activities demonstrate the continuing vibrancy of the parts of children's lives that have not yet been colonised by adults. Opie's (1993) research into children at play suggested that games, rhymes, jokes and songs in streets and play-grounds were still an important part of childhood. Ennew (1994) also identifies studies that suggest that children will resist and take charge of their own time, in whatever ways they can. The main force of their resistance, she argues, is to hide from adults what they do in their own time: that is, what children do when they tell us they are doing 'nothing'. Parents today are bombarded by a confusing array of messages which suggest that children are not safe on the streets or in the play park, and yet by keeping them 'safe' at home they run the risk of them being 'harmed' by computer games and obesity (see, for example, Palmer 2006). Moreover, children's unstructured play continues to be treated by politicians and the media as a threat to themselves and to others. The use of Anti-Social Behaviour Orders (ASBOs) and curfews on children bear witness both to a continuing street life for working-class children and young people, and to public anxiety about the potential 'dangerousness' of children's unrestricted time, particularly unscheduled time in the evenings.

What the discussion so far demonstrates is that any idea of a universal or essential childhood is not sustainable. Furthermore, we have already noted that 'childhood' is itself a relatively new, 'modern' phenomenon. During the nineteenth century, children were physically removed from adult life (from factories and streets) and taken into new controlled settings: schools, reformatories, children's homes and youth organisations. Pearson (1983) argues that it is not simply the behaviour of children that has changed over time; it is the public's reaction to that behaviour. In a vivid account of the nineteenth-century moral panics about working-class children, he demonstrates that what had previously been regarded as 'normal' childhood activity (that is, street-vending) became criminalised. He concludes that an examination of 'bad' children tells us more about current perceptions of safety, 'dangerousness' and law and order than it does about the children and young people themselves.

Although Foucault was not primarily interested in studying childhood as such, his analysis of what he sees as a shift in 'disciplinary mechanisms' in society (1977) provides further information about the development of childhood as a distinct, regulated phase. Foucault identifies a shift in techniques of punishment from the surveillance of bodies to the surveillance of minds; from the control of the problem to the control of the problem-doer (that is, the individual or the family); from a traditional form of law based on juridical rights to a colonisation by the 'psy' complex (psychological and psychiatric ideas and practices) and the criteria of 'normalisation'. The 'psy' discourse, according to Foucault, created the categories which it then used to classify and divide up individuals, and regulate and control behaviour. Developing these ideas further, Donzelot (1980) examines the development in the late eighteenth and early nineteenth centuries of a sector he defines as 'the social'; neither public nor private, independent from but connected with other sectors (juridical, educational, economic and political). A new series of professions assembled under the common banner of 'social work', and took over the mission of 'civilising the social body' (1980: 96). From Donzelot's perspective, then, children and the family are 'policed' today to a degree that would have been unimaginable in the past.

Teachers, health visitors, social workers, youth leaders, counsellors, psychiatrists, ministers of religion and childcare 'experts' all have a say in regulating childhood and in maintaining children as innocent, asexual, dependent and in need of protection, as do education and welfare systems. Theories of child development and socialisation thus constitute the childhood that we take for granted while simultaneously setting the parameters for 'normal' and 'abnormal' children's behaviour: in Foucault's conceptualisation, they create childhood.

It is not only ideas about childcare that have set the boundaries of childhood. In a ground-breaking book, Parton (1985, 2006) argues that child abuse tragedies have played a major part in educating society about what childhood is and what it should be. Each of the public inquiries into the death of a child rehearses again the familiar notion that good parenting and the love of children is the norm; any deviations from this are presented as individual aberrations that should be treated as such. The focus for social workers working with families and children has therefore been to identify the small numbers of children who are seen as 'at risk' in families, and allocate resources accordingly. (In their study of scandals in social work, Drakeford and Butler (2006) take this idea further, arguing that the role of the public inquiry is to tell 'the story' of a particular scandal, and that through this its meaning is fixed.) Considering child abuse further, Parton, Thorpe and Wattam (1997) suggest that a shift has taken place, from child abuse being constituted as an essentially medico-social reality with the expertise of doctors as central, to a position where it is now seen as a socio-legal problem, with legal expertise as pre-eminent (1997: 19). At the same time, there has been a move away from a discourse centred on child *abuse* to one that is built around the much broader idea of child *protection*: not only the protection of the child, but also 'the protection of parents and family privacy from unwarranted state interventions' (1997: 41). This illustrates the tension that has been around for at least the last 150 years between those who promote greater state involvement in the lives of families and children and those who believe that regulation is a matter for the individual, not the state (Cree 1995).

Reconstructing childhood

In their preface to the second edition of their classic textbook on the sociology of childhood, James and Prout identify an important tension in the sociology of childhood literature. As sociologists have moved away from the notion of an 'ideal' childhood towards an acceptance of the idea of 'childhoods', they are, they suggest, at risk of 'relativism . . . in the face of the political, social and economic maltreatment ventured against children on an international scale' (1997: xi). This is clearly an issue of fundamental importance to social work and social workers. Are children's needs always context-specific? If we accept this, how are we then to view cultural practices such as female circumcision in childhood or the use of child soldiers? This, James and Prout assert, is a crucial question given that 'there is now widespread acceptance of children's rights where the "best interests of the child" are taken as a baseline for social and political action' (ibid.). One way forward is to acknowledge that cultural practices, like childhood itself, are not fixed; they are open to change and negotiation over time, and we, as those who seek to protect and empower children, have an obligation to work with them to ensure that their own wishes and views are forefronted.

One further confounding factor must finally be considered. Lee points out that the late twentieth and early twenty-first centuries must be viewed as an 'age of uncertainty', when it is not only childhood which is open to negotiation and challenge; adulthood itself 'can no longer be regarded as the state of stable completion and self-possession on which being-hood once rested' (2001: 2). In this post-modern, globalised world, there are potentially unlimited ways of being and becoming human. Lee argues that the implication of this is that 'we must give a positive alternative to age-based discrimination by maximising our acknowledgement of human variation and by showing that there are many ways to "become human", some more or less available to children' (2001: 3). He calls, in the end, for an 'immature sociology', one which recognises that the world is 'unfinished', and that our task is therefore to show creativity and imagination in the face of this.

Implications for practice

- The way we construct childhood has real consequences, not only for children, but also for the agencies and institutions that work with children. Children are constructed as separate from adults: innocent, vulnerable and unequal. They are also increasingly constructed as individual consumers, with individual preferences and rights that must be addressed. These developments may be seen to have positive aspects for children who are the subjects of social work intervention. But we must not be complacent about any progress which may have been made. Children's rights continue to be exercised in a very limited, controlled setting; any decision making on the part of children takes place in a firmly adult-led, paternalist environment.

- Children's lives in Western societies today (and increasingly in the developing world too), as we have seen, are more tightly regulated and monitored by a whole range of educational and health professionals than ever before. As social workers we play a part in that regulation, whether through voluntary measures of support or through compulsory measures such as supervision or even the removal of children from home. This is one of the main paradoxes within the social work discourse. Social work is not about care *or* control: it is instead about care *and* control.

- With its traditional emphasis on individual (and family) pathology, social work with children has paid insufficient attention to issues of culture, class and gender, to discrimination and oppression on the grounds of 'race', sexuality and gender, and to growing inequalities in income and wealth. Children who use social work services are predominantly poor, working-class children, often from lone-parent families and from minority ethnic communities. They are also, as we have seen, structurally disadvantaged on the basis of their age. We must acknowledge and seek to counterbalance this.

- Following Lee's challenge, we must recognise that social work and child care is 'unfinished', and we too must try to work creatively and imaginatively and with integrity.

Conclusion

This chapter has covered a wide range of material in relation to childhood and children. I have argued that childhood is a social and historical construction; that it changes over time, and that it is specific in terms of class, 'race', gender and culture. Traditional sociological theories, based on ideas of socialisation and children as 'becoming-adults', have been criticised as functionalist and inherently conservative, working from the basis of a white, Western notion of an idealised childhood. I have suggested that more recent sociological perspectives offer new understandings of childhood as a separate, familialised and individualised institution. Because definitions of children and childhood vary historically, socially and culturally, it can be difficult to quantify the nature and extent of the issues faced by children and young people across countries and over time. However, there is an even greater sense that our historical perspectives on childhood reflect the changes in the organisation of our social structure (Jenks 2005). In other words, we build the frameworks that create the very concept of childhood itself.

I have asserted that social work practice with children has in the past betrayed its psychologically based, paternalist and adultist origins. Pringle (1996, 1998) argues even more forcibly that welfare systems may actually reinforce and maintain social oppression rather than challenging it. This is because welfare systems are structured by the same oppressive power dynamics as societies themselves. In his analysis of child welfare systems across Europe, Pringle concludes that both the European model of family support and the English model of child protection fail to address adequately the issues of structural social oppression that characterise the lives of children. I believe that the ways forward for social work with children lie in a genuine attempt on our part to confront both the diversities of children's experiences and the fact of their shared experience as members of an oppressed group in society. We must then attempt to redress some of the inequalities experienced by children: to seek to empower children to make realistic and positive choices, and at the same time to trust that children, given the freedom and space to be themselves, will spend their time in no less creative ways than we might expect of other human beings. We must also, I believe, seek to challenge poverty and discrimination in the lives of the children with whom we are working. By operating from a critically aware, anti-oppressive framework, I believe that there are possibilities for the development of a more empowering practice with children. Thomas concludes his study of decision making and children with the following plea:

... the question of what is a child's place, in the world and in the family, is one that deserves our attention. If we are to understand these things better, we need theories and research that are based on respect for what children themselves might have to say.

(2000: 201)

Recommended reading

Hill, M. and Tisdall, K. (1997) *Children and Society*, Harlow, Essex: Addison Wesley Longman. This remains a useful overview of the subject.

Lee, N. (2001) *Childhood and Society: Growing up in an Age of Uncertainty*, Buckingham: Open University Press. An inspiring, thought-provoking account.

Mayall, B. (2002) *Towards a Sociology for Childhood: Thinking from Children's Lives*, Buckingham: Open University Press. An insight into a range of current sociological concerns.

4 Youth

Introduction

Chapter 3 stated that the study of childhood and children has been neglected in sociological research and literature until recent years. Nothing could be further from the truth when considering sociological interest in youth and young people. There has been a huge investment of time and energy devoted to sociology's scrutiny of youth, much of this based on the assumption that youth and young people are problems requiring analysis. This chapter aims to 'unpack' ideas of youth as a social problem and young people as 'troubled' and 'troublesome', developing further the thesis that age is best understood not simply as a biological fact, but as a social, historical and cultural construction, mediated by relations of power in society.

The chapter will outline dominant approaches to youth and young people, drawing on influential psychological and sociological approaches that have set the parameters for past and current conceptualisations of youth. It will be argued that our common-sense ideas about youth are created by the coming together of psychological and sociological discourses which name and set boundaries on expectations and behaviours. The chapter goes on to discuss current themes in the sociology of youth. The chapter begins, as ever, with a question: what is youth?

Definitions

If it is difficult to make absolute claims about childhood as a fixed period in the lifespan, then this is even more evident with the notion of youth. We might expect youth to begin with the start of puberty. But when does puberty start? We know that the onset of puberty for Western children has fallen by several years because of improvements in diet and living conditions (Rosenfield *et al.* 2000). We also know that puberty is not a single moment and may, in reality, take place over many years, as physical and emotional changes interact with one another. There are, moreover, social and cultural differences in the way we view puberty, and how it is interpreted will depend on the society in which it takes place. As Ennew (1986) has identified, the onset of menstruation may be a cause for celebration, or it may be ignored completely, or it may be mourned, depending on historical, social and cultural perspectives. Marking the end of the stage of youth is equally problematic. In previous years, leaving home to get married might have marked the beginning of adulthood. However, official figures show that young people now marry later in life or not at all. For men, the average (mean) age at first marriage rose from twenty-four in 1970 to thirty-two in 2006; for women, the equivalent figure rose from twenty-two in 1970 to thirty in 2006 (ONS 2009).

It is worth reflecting, finally, on the choice of the word 'youth' as opposed to 'adolescence' as the title and theme of this chapter. The word 'youth' is a sociological rather than a biological category (Frith 2005). It is also a more neutral term, in comparison with the word 'adolescence', which, as we will discuss, carries with it a very particular set of ideas (predominantly psychological and Western) about the nature of adolescence itself.

Implications for practice

- Although it may be difficult to pin down youth as a chronological stage, it is without doubt a time in which real changes take place in young people: changes in physical capacities, intellectual abilities and emotional and sexual development. Yet no less significant is the context in which these changes are taking place; that is, the political and economic, social and cultural environment, which impacts on young people who are undergoing the transition from childhood dependency to adult independence.

- The words 'adolescence' and 'adolescent' carry so many implicit assumptions, it might be helpful to avoid these as terms to describe young people.

Historical accounts

Chapter 3

The period between childhood and adulthood varies considerably across cultures and historical times, as detailed historical work demonstrates. Ariès's (1962) inquiry into childhood, as discussed in Chapter 3, suggested that the medieval child in Europe passed from infanthood to adulthood without any intervening phase. In other words, they effectively became adults at the age of five years.

Another influential historian, Gillis, looks at this very differently. He does not dispute that it was common practice in pre-industrial Europe for children to leave home at a young age to live in other households as servants or apprentices. But Gillis argues that this does not imply that they had achieved adulthood. On the contrary, he sees it as evidence of a very long transition period, beginning when the child first became somewhat independent of its family at about eight years of age, to the point of complete independence at marriage or inheritance, ordinarily in the mid- to late twenties (1981: 2). Gillis argues therefore that pre-industrial society *did* recognise a stage in life that was different both from young childhood and from adulthood, and he sees this stage as characterised by a long phase of gradually increasing independence from parental control. Gillis goes on to assert that there were few distinctions between younger and older youth in this extended period of semi-independence, because there was no universal schooling to postpone entry into the world of work, and no clear break at the onset of physical and sexual maturity. Puberty and the menarche came comparatively late in pre-industrial societies (just over seventeen years of age in Norway in 1850) and physical growth was, Gillis maintains, slow, with young people not attaining full physical powers until their mid-twenties. Importantly, Gillis claims that there is no evidence to suggest that there was any difficult or emotionally disruptive time in the teenage years, such that we have come to associate with 'normal adolescence'.

Davis (1990), in his historical exploration of the condition of youth in Britain, argues that the age-grade of adolescence as a theoretical entity was established for the first time in the late eighteenth-century writings of the French philosopher and writer Jean-Jacques Rousseau. In his conceptualisation of the ideal boy ('Emile'), Rousseau is said to have laid the foundation for the idea of a life cycle divided into stages, each stage with its own physiology and set of tasks to be accomplished. He envisaged boyhood as a time of outdoor play, in which the boy should be free to roam outside in loose clothing in his 'natural' state. Formal education should not begin until the boy reaches twelve years of age. Puberty was presented as marking a major shift from the carefree time of boyhood, bringing with it the 'tumultuous change' of adolescence and new birth into manhood. Rousseau expressed this forcefully: 'We are born, so to speak, twice over, born into existence and born into life; born a human being, and born a man' (quoted in Davis 1990: 41). Adolescence was viewed as innately and inevitably troublesome and stormy, requiring correct handling 'in order to ensure the smooth development of the individual and the continuity of society as a whole' (ibid.). Rousseau recommended that each adolescent boy should have his own personal tutor to give him careful instruction and guidance, unlikely to be an attainable goal for any but the wealthiest of families. Rousseau was not only responsible for laying down the parameters of male adolescence. As well as writing about the ideal boy, 'Emile', he wrote about the ideal girl, 'Sophie'. Unlike Emile, Sophie was to be trained in the home from an early age into domesticity and motherhood. This was, according to Rousseau, her 'natural' state. Gittins observes that in this depiction, Rousseau was 'naturalising' difference between the male world of the outdoor/public space and the female world of the indoor/private one (1998: 152).

If Rousseau was responsible for making adolescence a theoretical possibility, it was the social and economic changes taking place in the eighteenth and nineteenth centuries that made adolescence a practical reality for an increasingly broad cross-section of society. Gillis (1981) indicates that the eighteenth century had witnessed a steady growth in education for children of the upper and middle classes. A drop in child mortality amongst the aristocracy and middle classes meant that children growing up in smaller families found themselves spending more and more of their lives in controlled environments, at home and at school. Boys were kept at home for longer before being sent away to boarding school at the age of thirteen or fourteen years, and they stayed on longer at school. Girls were kept at home until marriage. While wage-earning young people of the working class experienced a greater degree of freedom from parental control than before, others found themselves dependent for longer on their parents, as apprenticeships declined and secondary schooling increased.

Gillis argues that the reform of the elite public school consolidated the special character of adolescence. As head teacher of Rugby public school, Thomas Arnold introduced a new style of educational management in the 1820s and 1830s; a style that was to be duplicated at public schools throughout the UK. Arnold instigated a military-style regime that envisaged the public school as a total institution in which the masters had a firm grip over all aspects of the boys' lives, educational and social. Gone were the days when the boys were free to spend their time as they chose, attending classes and instruction for only two or three hours a day. Now the boys' lives were structured into different phases of organised activity; games and sport were seen as a central part of the institutional framework. In this, Gillis identifies the formation of a new cult of heterosexual masculinity in which physical strength, playing games and sports were applauded as virtues, while femininity (and homosexuality) were associated with weakness and emotion.

There was, however, a quite different set of influences that contributed to the formation of the discourse around adolescence. Davis (1990) argues that there have been 'cycles of anxiety' in the parent culture around the issue of what might be termed 'juvenile delinquency' from at least the sixteenth century onwards. (See also Pearson 1983.) The late nineteenth and early twentieth centuries witnessed one such explosion of public concern about the behaviour of young people in the United States and across Europe. Davis (1990) points out that while the 'official model' of adolescence was being developed amongst upper- and middle-class children in public and grammar schools, working-class, urban young people had been developing their own distinctive subcultures. They had a higher degree of social and economic independence than ever before, their own entertainment (public house, football ground and music hall) and their own style of dress. There was universal fear and antagonism towards these so-called 'hooligans' or 'juvenile delinquents', illustrated in press and government statements of the day. Concern for the behaviour of young people came to a head in 1904 in the publication by American psychologist, G. Stanley Hall, of a massive two-volume work entitled *Adolescence, its Psychology and its Relation to Physiology, Anthropology, Sociology, Sex, Crime, Religion and Education*, widely read in both the US and the UK. Hall took Rousseau's ideas about human development and about the special importance of a 'second birth' at puberty and re-worked these in the light of post-Darwinian biology and evolutionist philosophy (Davis 1990: 60). He also used the phrase 'storm and stress' to refer to 'adolescence' for the first time, drawing on ideas from the late eighteenth-century *Sturm und Drang* movement in German literature and music, which had emphasised the importance of giving free expression to powerful emotions through the arts. Hall suggested that the three key aspects of 'storm and stress' in adolescence were conflict with parents, mood disruptions and risk-taking behaviour. All three, as we will see, were themes that were developed in psychological writing on adolescence.

Cross-cultural studies

Studies of different cultures over the last 100 years or so have engaged in the familiar 'nature versus nurture' debate, and in doing so have highlighted the specificity of 'modern' Western ideas about youth and adolescence. In one classic example, anthropologist Margaret Mead spent nine months living with young women in Samoa, observing their behaviour and their interactions with others: boys, elders and younger children. Her objective was to answer the pressing questions of the day:

> Are the disturbances which vex our adolescents due to the nature of adolescence itself or to the civilization? Under different conditions, does adolescence present a different picture?
>
> (1928: 17)

Mead's subsequent portrayal of Samoan life has been criticised for being rather idealised and idyllic; she is said to have made uncritical assumptions about both Samoan and American adolescence (see, for example, Freeman 1983). Nevertheless, her findings, scandalous at the time, remain of interest. She reported no differences between girls before and after puberty, except in relation to bodily changes; they experimented sexually, only later settling down to marriage and the raising of children. From her observations, Mead concluded that the passage from childhood to adulthood in Samoa was a smooth transition and not marked by any of the emotional and psychological distress, role confusion and rebellion seen in the United States. She attributed this difference to cultural factors, arguing that because Samoan adolescent girls lived in a homogenous culture, they did not face numerous conflicting personal choices and demands. Mead argued that explanations for youth rebellion and conflict must therefore be sought in Western society and its organisation and age structure (specifically, conflicting standards and a surfeit of choices), instead of in young people or adolescence *per se*.

Banton's 1965 exploration of rites of passage in tribal societies also provides information about different patterns for understanding and organising the stage between childhood and adulthood.

Banton points out that the period between childhood and adulthood can be a very short one in tribal societies, marked out by highly structured ceremonies and initiation customs which act as rites of passage into adulthood. For example, he describes the initiation process that took place amongst the tribespeople in Sierra Leone in which young boys were taken out into the bush and given a series of tasks to accomplish over weeks or months. When they were brought back to the village, they were reborn as adults, and in some societies they were even given new names as confirmation of their new status as adults. Girls went through an equivalent, though less prolonged initiation. Banton argues that ceremonies and initiation customs like these help individuals to adapt to new roles, thus reducing the risks of role confusion or uncertainty.

More recent cross-cultural studies draw attention to the very different understandings of 'youth/ adolescence' in countries throughout the world. Brown *et al.*'s 2002 volume, *The World's Youth*, demonstrates widespread differences in transitions to adulthood, and different patterns of relationships between girls and boys and between adults and children. Whilst there are some common features which relate to biological, cognitive and psychological factors, these are, Brown and Larson argue, 'transformed and given meaning within distinctive cultural systems' (2002: 2). Other studies highlight the changes that have been taking place in developing countries, just as the socio-economic and political situations of these societies have changed. Morrow (2003) associates changes in the practice of initiation and in children's behaviour in Tanzania (as in other parts of Africa) with the pressure of schooling and the breakdown of traditional family practices. So, for example, initiation ceremonies happen earlier in order that they do not interfere with schooling, and, consequently, girls become pregnant at an earlier age than in the past. Other factors such as the devastating impact of HIV/AIDS are also, she argues, greatly affecting the work roles and responsibilities of older children, as they take on the care of younger siblings in child-headed households (2003: 273).

Implications for practice

- Historical and cultural analyses demonstrate that common-sense notions about youth and young people are inextricably linked to the social, economic and cultural conditions of the day. We are therefore likely to find very different presentations of youth and adolescence within different social, cultural and ethnic groupings today.

Psychological perspectives

Although our focus is, of course, on sociological understandings, it is important to first examine psychological discourses, because it is these that have provided the ideological backdrop through which the creation of adolescence was given meaning and purpose at the end of the nineteenth and beginning of the twentieth centuries. Psychological ideas have also traditionally had the greatest influence on social work theory and practice in relation to work with young people.

Freudian explanations

I have suggested that in the work of G. Stanley Hall we can see the beginnings of a psychological conceptualisation of youth as adolescence, and particularly as a time of 'storm and stress'. Freud's notion of a 'genital stage' offered a way of explaining why adolescence was, in his view, inevitably 'stormy'. Austrian psychiatrist Sigmund Freud (1856–1939) believed that human beings pass through five distinct stages of development from birth to adulthood, and at each stage there are driving forces or tensions to be overcome, often unconsciously. Coleman (1992) offers a useful summary of Freud's stages:

- *The oral stage*: from birth to about two years of age, during which time infants' mouths are the focal point of their satisfaction and comfort, and the breast and feeding form the centre of the child's world.

- *The anal stage*: at two years, when infants discover the pleasure of some control over their bowel movements and the 'elimination of waste'; toilet training becomes a major task and potential area of conflict.

- *The phallic stage*: from three to about five years of age, as children discover their sexuality. This is the so-called 'Oedipal stage', when boys and girls are said to learn what will be 'normal' sex roles and behaviour by repressing the Oedipal (sexual) urges that they have in relation to their parents.

- *The latency stage*: from the fifth or sixth year until puberty, there occurs a latency period during which the young person's energies are taken up with social and learning activities and psychic conflicts are temporarily laid to rest.

- *The genital stage*: beginning at puberty, around twelve years of age, until adulthood at around eighteen. There is thought to be a rapid recapitulation of the three earlier stages of emotional development (oral, anal and phallic) and the unresolved Oedipal situation re-emerges. This is a particularly risky time for young people, fraught with risks and challenges. The end result of this stage of struggle and conflict is the achievement of 'normal' sexual identity and adult personality; whether this is successful or not will depend on the outcome of the three earlier phases.

From this perspective, crises in adolescence are both normal and necessary (Coleman 1992). Anna Freud's writing (1937 and 1958) illustrates this viewpoint. She goes as far as to propose that it should be considered 'abnormal' if a child 'kept a steady equilibrium during the adolescent period . . . The adolescent manifestations come close to symptom formation of the neurotic, psychotic or dissocial order and emerge almost imperceptibly into . . . almost all mental illnesses' (Freud 1958).

Research carried out over the last twenty years by social psychologists presents a more circumspect picture of adolescence, suggesting that although it may be a time of psychological difficulty and 'storm and stress' for some young people, this is by no means the norm. A study conducted by Michael Rutter and his colleagues (1976) on the Isle of Wight was highly influential in challenging Freudian assumptions. Contrary to expectations, the study discovered that children aged ten years, fourteen-year-olds and adults suffered from psychiatric disorders in roughly similar numbers. Moreover, a substantial number of those who experienced psychiatric problems in adolescence had had problems since childhood; when psychiatric difficulties did emerge in adolescence, this was often in the context of other stressful factors in the environment such as parents' marital difficulties. Finally, the study found that only 20 per cent of teenagers agreed with the statement, 'I often feel miserable or depressed'. Rutter *et al.* (1976) concluded that the psychiatric importance of adolescence had probably been overestimated in the past.

Feminist sociologists have also sought to challenge the Freudian representation of adolescence, pointing out that it is, in reality, a masculine construct. Hudson argues that all our images of the adolescent – 'the restless, searching youth, the Hamlet figure, the sower of wild oats, the tester of growing powers' – are masculine images (1984: 35). This means that girls who behave in what is seen as an adolescent fashion will be thought of not only as displaying a lack of maturity (since adolescence is dichotomous with maturity) but, significantly, as not feminine. Thus girls who act out what are commonly regarded as adolescent roles, using challenging, non-conforming behaviour, risk far stronger retribution and measures of control than boys who exhibit similar behaviour. Hudson asserts that this has serious consequences for young women, who are caught between stereotyped images of adolescence and femininity, and are judged by two, incongruent sets of expectations. They are left feeling that whatever they do is always wrong: 'a correct impression', she concludes, 'since so often if they are fulfilling the expectations of femininity they will be disappointing those of adolescence, and vice versa' (1984: 53).

Social psychologists today acknowledge that there is widespread variability in young people's experience of adolescence; that there may be as many 'adolescences' as there are adolescents. Coleman and Hendry (1999) assert that empirical evidence demonstrates that there is too much individual variation for young people of the same chronological age to be classified together. Adolescence, they argue, should be viewed as a transitional process, rather than a stage or even a number of stages. The transition is influenced by both external and internal pressures; that is, by outside pressures from peers, parents, teachers and wider society, as much as from inside physiological and emotional pressures. Sociologists, as we will discuss, agree.

Developmental explanations

Alongside psychoanalytic interpretations, other psychological perspectives have explored human development in terms of stages of cognitive development (for example, Piaget), moral development (for example, Kohlberg), and identity development (for example, Erikson).

Erik Erikson (1902–1994) trained as a psychoanalyst, and, like Freud, has been highly influential in representing adolescence as a time of psychological difficulty. He proposed that human beings develop their identities through a series of psycho-social stages from birth to death: the so-called 'eight ages of man' (1968). At each of these life stages, the individual has to resolve a series of psycho-social crises and to establish appropriate social relations (see Black and Cottrell 1993). Identity development, for Erikson, is therefore a process of differentiation, as the separate self learns to accommodate increasing numbers of significant others. The stages are outlined as follows:

1. *First year*: trust versus mistrust.

2. *Second year*: autonomy versus shame and doubt.

3. *Third to fifth year*: initiative versus guilt.

4. *Sixth year to puberty*: industry versus inferiority.

5. *Adolescence*: identity versus confusion.

6. *Early adulthood*: intimacy versus isolation.

7. *Middle adulthood*: generativity versus self-absorption.

8. *Ageing years*: integrity versus despair.

From this brief outline we can see that Erikson affirms the idea that inner turbulence and identity problems are central features of the adolescent stage; young people are uncertain about who they are and what they will do with their lives. He describes adolescence as a period of 'psychosocial moratorium': a time of enforced role play and experimentation during which conflicts and contradictions of identity must be resolved. The primary developmental crisis in adolescence is a quest for identity: adolescence is about preparing for adult identity.

Critics such as Springhall point out that there is little real social scientific evidence that any but a small minority of those in their teenage years experience a serious identity crisis, though there is clearly some change in the concept of self-identity at this time (1986: 227). Feminist psychologists have also challenged the whole basis on which Erikson's analysis is built. In an influential rebuttal of Erikson's ideas, Carol Gilligan (1982) points out that Erikson's original research subjects were all men and boys, so that male behaviour and attitudes became the standard on which his developmental theory was based. When Erikson did conduct research on women, he discovered that their life cycle was different to men's; women did not seek independence and differentiation as their ultimate goal in the way that men did, and instead expressed a desire to remain associated with others. Erikson analysed this gender difference by stating that male identity is forged in relation to the world, while female identity is awakened in a relationship of intimacy with another person, so that during adolescence, men and women have different tasks to accomplish. Whether or not this is the case, the underlying message was clear. Full maturity was conceptualised as independence and differentiation (that is, stereotypically male qualities). Gilligan argues that this has led to an ill-placed esteem for ideas of growth and independence, and a denigration of the values of integration and dependency.

Erikson's work has also been criticised for assuming that there is such a thing as 'normal' development. Sociologists and anthropologists today are highly critical of what they see as the ethnocentrism in psychological writing about adolescence. Nsamenang is unequivocal:

> Adolescent psychology is a Eurocentric enterprise. Western social scientists . . . have demon-strated remarkable ethnocentrism and have, with few exceptions, presented their findings as relevant to the human race . . . The ethnocentrism has been so overwhelming that the majority of both scholars and lay persons are unaware that the field would have been different had adolescence been 'discovered' within the cultural conditions and life circumstances different from those of Europe and North America, say, in Africa.

> (2002: 61)

The social work academic, Lena Robinson, makes a similar point. She argues:

> The conventionally accepted paradigms and discoveries of Western psychology do not provide an understanding of black adolescents . . . Despite the diversity of the various schools of Western psychology, they seem to merge unequivocally in their assumption of the Eurocentric point of view and the superiority of people of European descent. It is not surprising, therefore, that the conclusions reached . . . are invariably of the inferiority of non-European peoples.

> (1997: 152)

Robinson proposes that 'negrescence' (literally, 'the process of becoming black' or, more concisely, the development of a black racial identity) offers a more meaningful way of understanding black young people's experience than conventional psychological theories on child development (2004: 155). Negrescence models are useful, she suggests, because they allow us to examine what happens to a person during identity change. She introduces 'the best known and most widely researched' model of black identity development: Cross's 1971 model of the conversion from 'Negro' to 'black', a model which has been adapted by subsequent writers to make sense of the experience of a wide range of minority groups. Cross suggests that a black person is likely to move through five stages in developing a racial identity:

1. *Pre-encounter*: the person views the world from a white frame of reference (Eurocentric), under-standing himself or herself and others from a white viewpoint and denying the existence of racism.

2. *Encounter*: some shocking event, personal or social, awakens the person to new views of being black and the world. This leads to an intense search for black identity, involving two steps: experiencing and personalising the event, followed by testing out new perceptions.

3. *Immersion–emersion*: a period of transition, where the person struggles to destroy their former view of the world, immersing himself or herself in 'blackness'. (Cross (1991) later writes that this stage can result in fixation and stagnation rather than identity development.)

4. *Internalisation*: the person can focus, again, on things other than being black, and achieves inner security and self-confidence about being black; the person feels more at ease with himself or herself.

5. *Internalisation/commitment*: the person finds activities and commitments to express their new identity (recounted in Robinson 2004: 155–6).

Studies of young people of mixed parentage provide further insight into adolescent identity development. Tizard and Phoenix (1993) review the evidence for identity confusion amongst black and 'mixed-race' children, and present findings from their own research study of fifty-eight young people whose parents were both black and white. They report that early studies carried out in the late 1940s showed a disturbingly high level of identity confusion amongst black children, who repeatedly misidentified themselves as white, and attributed 'bad' characteristics to black dolls in experiments. Subsequent studies showed changes, however, with black children more likely to present positive self-images. Tizard and Phoenix point out that 60 per cent of the young people of mixed parentage interviewed for their study had a positive racial identity; 20 per cent had a problematic identity; and another 20 per cent were in an intermediate category, not definitely positive about their racial identity. They conclude that it is difficult to make generalisations about young people and identity. Class differences, gender differences, different schooling and different family backgrounds make for very different experiences for the young people concerned. The experience of girls in a predominantly white, middle-class school, protected from racism, were therefore at complete odds with the experiences of working-class boys growing up in mixed communities, where both racism and a strong black culture were part of their day-to-day environment. Updating their findings in a second edition, Tizard and Phoenix (2001) note that for a time, those of mixed parentage were, for political reasons, unwilling to define themselves as anything but 'black'. Today they are much more likely to wish to affirm both their black and white origins. Tizard and Phoenix explain this in terms of the very different ways that children and young people of mixed parentage have been 'racialised' in comparison to their parents. This again points to the influence of wider social, economic and cultural influences.

Implications for practice

- A critical review of the psychological literature suggests that, although Freudian and developmental explanations undoubtedly contribute to social work's understanding of young people, social and societal explanations must also be taken into consideration.

- Social work theory and practice portray ambivalent views about youth, often promoting conventional (conservative and Eurocentric) notions about youth and adolescence while also stressing young people's right to self-determination. We need to find ways of opening up the discourse around young people.

- At the same time, all those who work with children and young people must question their own 'common-sense' ideas about youth and adolescence before offering any meaningful help to young people of whatever class, gender or ethnicity (and, of course, sexuality and religion).

Traditional sociological approaches

Sociological approaches stress the primacy of social understandings of young people's experience of youth. The focus shifts to the social world in which the young person is growing up: the family, school, peer group and community, and at a broader level, society and its structured inequalities. Early sociological approaches (between the 1950s and 1970s) in the US and UK sought to understand youth as a social category, exploring such topics as role, peer group, generational conflict, culture clash and youth culture. Underpinning all of this was an interest not in adolescent development, but in youth transitions.

Role-learning theory

As Chapter 3 has already indicated, a central concern of sociologists has been to understand the process by which maturing members of society incorporate specific societal expectations and come to take their place as adult members of that society (that is, 'socialisation'). Functionalist sociologists argue that social behaviour has to be learned; 'socialisation is, above all, the process through which individuals learn how to perform social roles' (Fulcher and Scott 2007: 125). Social roles are 'blueprints or templates for action' (ibid.); we learn how to behave through a complex system of rewards and punishments by others and by societal institutions and structures. Along the way, we internalise what is expected of us (Parsons 1951). It

is when we do not know how to behave, when roles are unclear or ill-defined, that individuals become unhappy and society begins to lose its cohesiveness, as Durkheim (1952) has suggested in his analysis of 'anomie' (to be explored further in Chapter 8), and as Parsons (1949) argued in his discussion of the sexual division of labour in the family, already discussed in Chapter 2.

Banton's (1965) analysis of the impact of changing roles on youth in industrial and pre-industrial societies illustrates another functionalist approach to role-learning theory. Banton argues that moving from one role to another is not easy in complex industrial societies. Changing roles requires knowing the rights and obligations of the role and changes in behaviour; it also requires other people to recognise that a change in role has taken place and to modify their behaviour in a corresponding fashion. Yet in industrial societies, there are no clear dividing lines between the roles of infant, juvenile and adult, demonstrated in the reality that children may well attend their parents' graduation ceremonies. This leads to strains on young people, who may look and feel physically mature, but are treated like children by their parents. Lengthening education, Banton argues, has exacerbated this discrepancy. Also, since knowledge is changing so fast, children may no longer see their parents as helpful role models, or even as having a good enough understanding of the present world to be able to advise them, so that children have different, competing and unclear norms of behaviour to follow.

Banton's work made a significant contribution to shifting the focus of attention in the study of youth from individual, psychological concerns to events and structures in wider society. However, he has been criticised for his rather idealised picture of industrial and pre-industrial societies, and for a rather static presentation of the ways that roles operate in society. Interactionist sociologists present a more dynamic approach to understanding roles, arguing that at any one time we play a number of different roles, and we make choices about how we will play or act out these roles (see Goffman 1969). This would suggest that there is no 'essential' problem with role for young people. This discussion is brought up to date by the provocative analysis by contemporary sociologist Frank Furedi (2009). He argues that we are currently experiencing a 'socialisation-in-reverse'. Children are held up as being much more knowledgeable than their parents about the social world (likely to be true, he admits, in terms of their understanding of music, fashion and digital technology). They are also increasingly being invited by officials, advocacy groups and educational experts to 'educate' or 'pester' their parents about everything from eating five fruits and vegetables a day to illegal parking outside schools. The effect of all this, Furedi argues, is a weakening of parents' authority, and hence, the weakening of the authority of all adults, including teachers.

Peer group

Returning to traditional approaches to youth, another preoccupation of sociologists (and social psychologists) has been with the peer group, and specifically with the idea that the peer group has had increasing importance for young people. Musgrave (1972) defines the peer group as 'a homogeneous age group', and argues that in such a grouping, young people gain experiences that would not be possible within the confines of the nuclear family. They are free to experiment, to have fun and to make mistakes, and most importantly, to practise relationships with members of the opposite sex. Smith describes this as 'the traditional, essentially structural-functionalist view of the influence of peers' (1987: 42). Peers are said to have an influence on socialisation in the spaces left by other institutions (principally the family and the school). The peer group is valued as a positive force, a place that provides support, security, understanding and a sense of belonging. This in turn is encouraged through the commercial exploitation of teenage purchasing power.

Smith makes an important distinction between sociological literature, which explores predominantly middle-class adolescents' peer groups, and criminological literature on juvenile delinquency, in which working-class peer groups are represented as 'gangs' – anti-school, anti-parent, or both (1987: 47). Smith argues from his own research that not all peer groups, and not all members of peer groups even amongst the working class, are anti-school. Smith is critical too of the omissions in sociological investigation of peer groups – specifically the absence of girls and young black people. He draws attention to studies which suggest that working-class girls' peer groups may be qualitatively different to those of boys. He pinpoints criminological studies that illustrate the ways in which girls' peer groups 'may reinforce passivity, dependence and compliance among their members', whilst boys' groups are said to do quite the opposite (1987: 56).

In an early feminist study, McRobbie explored girls' subcultures where she found strong supportive networks of friends amongst girls, and a real sense of solidarity between girls and their friends (with Garber 1976: 143). Her findings have been echoed in 1990s' ethnographical research, which suggests that girls' friendships are characterised by trust and loyalty. Griffiths argues that friendships between women are a major way in which girls 'maintain some degree of power and control over their lives in a society in which women still occupy a subordinate position' (1995: 171). Furthermore, Griffiths identifies conspicuous variations in the pattern of young women's friendships, so that they may be members of different groupings at school and at home. The school-based groups are likely to be single-sex, close-knit groups of pairs or more, whilst neighbourhood groups tend to be larger, and less clearly differentiated in terms of age, 'race' or gender. This research suggests that we should not make simple inferences based on the idea of 'a peer group', since young people are members of different peer groups, each serving different functions in their lives.

Generational conflict

A third and related theme in the early sociological writing is the notion that there is a 'generation gap' between adults and young people. It is argued that the peer group takes on greater importance for young people who are thrown together for ever longer periods with their own age group and are largely segregated from adults. They share experiences, circumstances and problems that separate them from the outside world (Eisenstadt 1956), and as a result generational conflict develops.

The 1976 study by the social psychologist Michael Rutter (discussed earlier) challenges the notion that young people's alienation from parents during the teenage years is the norm. His team found that parents continued to have substantial influence over the opinions and behaviour of most young people. Hudson (1984) supports this analysis. She highlights studies that demonstrate that teenagers generally choose friends whose values are similar to, rather than in opposition with, their parents. In her own study of fifteen-year-old girls, she found that most of those interviewed said that they generally agreed with their parents, and that disagreements were usually about trivial matters. She warns, however, that a discourse of adolescence framed by ideas of trouble and conflict leads parents, teachers and social workers to constantly expect trouble. Evidence from the Young People's Social Attitudes Survey first conducted in 1994 and repeated again in 1998 and 2003 confirms that young people's beliefs are not as radical as might be anticipated. On the contrary, their views are broadly similar to those of their families. Newman (1996) claims that children and young people are not yet storming the bastions of adult power:

They want parents to have a bigger say than themselves in the educational curriculum, they feel that drug use at school should be punished severely, they don't believe people should get married at a young age, leave school too early, or have sex below the current age of consent, and almost a third support current film censorship laws.

(1996: 17)

Culture clash?

While the relationship between white children and their parents has often been described in terms of a generation gap, the relationship between minority ethnic children and their parents has frequently been analysed as a 'culture clash': children challenging what are presented as the outdated customs and values of their parents. Brittan and Maynard (1984) see this perspective as implicitly racist; that is, a denigration of black culture. They assert that the focus should properly be on inter-generational conflict; on a rebellious period which any young person may go through, whether black or white.

Apter's (1990) research into relationships between black daughters and their parents makes a different point. She demonstrates that neither generation gaps nor culture clashes are necessarily essential features of so-called 'second generation' black families. She demonstrates that authoritarian parents with a strong sense of their own culture do not, as has been suggested, raise less self-confident or dependent girls. Instead they raise self-assertive, competent girls. Herbert (1997) similarly reviews the evidence for a generation gap and finds it unconvincing. He maintains that, if anything, the generations are drawing together rather than apart. Young people tend to agree with their parents on the important issues (specifically moral and political issues) more than do parents and their parents (grandparents); the family continues to be of critical importance to young people, though of course there may be differences of opinion over minor issues such as dress and hairstyle (1997: 90). Current research on culture suggests that ideas of a generation gap or culture clash may have even less meaning now than previously, as the commercial leisure and fashion industries target parents and young people alike as buyers of their products, whether music, clothing, food or films (see Jenks 2005).

Youth, youth culture and youth subcultures

Underpinning the functionalist sociological writing on youth in the years following the Second World War was the belief that youth and youth culture were both somehow qualitatively new and different from before. Youth was treated as if it was a 'new class' (Musgrove 1968). At the same time, ideas of 'post-war consensus', 'the affluent society', 'teenage consumers' and a new 'classless', meritocratic society contributed to the presentation of youth culture as a single, homogeneous culture, transcending all other cultural attachments of home, neighbourhood and class.

The Second World War is viewed as a crucial turning point in the development of British youth culture (Osgerby 1998: 17). In the decades that followed, a range of factors combined to highlight the visibility of the young as a distinct cultural entity:

- the post-war 'baby boom', which saw an increase in the youth population in the 1950s and 1960s;

- the Education Act of 1944, which raised the school leaving age to fifteen and led to an increase in young people attending age-specific institutions and awaiting entry to the adult world of full-time employment;

- the expansion of the youth service and the rise of 'myriad attempts to marshal the leisure time of the young' (Osgerby 1998: 19);

- the introduction of national service in 1948, which created a generation of young people caught in an 'interregnum' between leaving school and being 'called up' for two years at eighteen years of age (1998: 21); this ended in 1960, with the last period of service ending in 1962;

- the increased demand for the labour of young people and, with it, the increased spending power of youth;

- the rise of mass communications, notably television, which promoted youth culture.

Davis (1990) argues that the period's preoccupation with youth was essentially an ambivalent phenomenon. Youth culture was sometimes portrayed in positive terms: young people were held up as the future of the nation, bright, bold and independent. Youth was 'the great national resource which if correctly and sufficiently utilized could still provide the way out of the nation's troubles' (1990: 208). But youth was also presented as a negative, hostile presence; 'a portent of worse things to come' (ibid.) and a symbol of all that was problematic about post-war society.

The 1950s and 1960s saw the publication of a number of rather colourful sociological studies of youth culture. Research into the behaviour and rituals of teddy boys (in the 1950s) and mods and rockers (in the 1960s) began to demonstrate that the idea of a single 'youth culture' was not sustainable; instead, young people were seen to align themselves to different cultural groupings. By the 1970s, new perspectives drawing on a Marxist analysis dismissed the concept of youth as an entity in itself, and instead forefronted class as the dominant feature in the lives of young people. Marxist scholars argued that youth culture could only be understood as reflecting wider (parental) class structures in society. Willis's study of working-class boys' attitudes to school provides a classic example of this perspective. Willis (1977) asserted that the boys' counter-school culture, although markedly at odds with the middle-class values of school, had a great deal in common with the working-class 'shop floor' culture they would soon join as adult labourers. Their counter-culture in effect mirrored and anticipated working-class culture. Other studies have found that there are many similarities between working-class youth and parent cultures and that the differences between them have been exaggerated (see, for example, Humphries's 1995 oral history).

The Centre for Contemporary Cultural Studies (CCCS) at the University of Birmingham played a key role in the 1970s and 1980s in exploring youth and youth culture within a class analysis, examining the experiences of a number of youth groups including skinheads, punks and football hooligans. For example, in *Resistance through Rituals*, Clarke *et al.* (1976) argue that the idea of a homogeneous youth culture is an illusion – a 'social myth'. They write:

> ... what it disguises and represses – differences between different strata of youth, the class-basis of youth cultures, the relation of 'Youth Culture' to the parent culture and the dominant culture, etc. – is more significant than what it reveals.
>
> (1976: 15)

Clarke *et al.* propose that 'youth culture' must be deconstructed and replaced with the term 'subculture', reflecting the connections between subcultures and class relations, the division of labour, and productive relations of the society (1976: 16). Further, they warn against making assumptions about subcultures. Subcultures, they argue, may come and go. Some are regular and persistent features of the 'parent' class culture; others appear only at particular historical moments – 'they become visible, are identified and labelled (either by themselves or by others): they command the stage of public attention for a time: then they fade, disappear or are so widely diffused that they lose their distinctiveness' (1976: 14). Individual young people, similarly, move in and out of one or perhaps several subcultures; and the great majority of young people will not enter a coherent subculture at all. 'For the majority, school and work are more structurally significant – even at the level of consciousness – than style and music' (1976: 16). For those who do take part in subcultures, however, the subculture had particular functions as a symbolic form of resistance, allowing young people to 'work up' their own cultures 'as a way of handling a string of problems' (Macionis and Plummer 2008: 145).

CCCS researchers have been criticised for concentrating on the exotic and seemingly glamorous aspects of male working-class youth subcultures, and for failing to examine their negative aspects, or the personal responsibility that young people have for their actions (Hill and Tisdall 1997). Feminist sociologists have also highlighted the absence of girls in the youth studies, arguing that analyses of youth culture and subcultures serve to obscure the differences between young people, and more so, the power differentials between particular groups of young people, in this case boys and girls. McRobbie and Garber (1976) claim that the absence of girls from the whole literature is striking: where young women do make an appearance, they are usually seen in ways that are marginal, or that reinforce a stereotyped image of women. They conclude that girls negotiate a different space to boys, and offer 'a different type of resistance to what can at least in part be viewed as their sexual subordination' (1976: 221). Lees (1986) and Nava (1984) also provide a strong denunciation of the neglect of girls in the study of youth. Lees points out that young women in (male) youth studies are presented in terms of their sexuality rather than as human beings: as 'slag' or 'drag', 'virgin' or 'whore', 'girls flit in and out of the pages as sex objects in the boys' eyes' (1986: 16). This, she argues, is 'a crucial mechanism in ensuring their subordination to boys and men' (1986: 14–15). Lees argues that young people negotiate their sexuality and behaviour within powerful constraints; masculine and feminine behaviour is subject to different social rules and operates within different norms. Nava's study of youth clubs supports this proposition. She notes that the screening of power differentials leads boys to 'lay claim to the territory of the [youth] club, and inhibits attempts by girls to assert their independence from them . . .' (1984: 13).

Youth and delinquency

As already outlined, the sociological study of youth (whether focused on peer groups, cultures or subcultures) has been consistently framed in terms of an idea of young people as 'troublesome'. Young people are seen as posing a threat both to society and to the *status quo*. In his historical analysis of street crime and hooliganism, Pearson (1983) points out that it is commonplace to look back nostalgically to a 'golden age' of order and security, often described as 'twenty years ago' or 'before the war' (both the First and Second World Wars). This 'golden age' is held up as a period of peace and stability, with low levels of crime and high levels of popular respect for law and order. Pearson demonstrates that the notion of a tranquil past has no historical validity. On the contrary, documentary evidence suggests that there was widespread fear amongst the middle classes in the nineteenth century about working-class street crime, violence, vandalism, drunkenness and lack of respect for the police. In the 1850s and 1860s, this crystallised around the discovery of a 'new' street crime, called 'garrotting', in which the victim was choked and robbed. Pearson argues that the public reaction to 'garrotting' and an increase in policing led to the creation of a 'crime wave', much as the street crime of 'mugging' came to public attention in the 1970s (1983: 144).

Pearson goes on to ask why young people feature so heavily in criminal statistics. He concludes that biological explanations are not enough: they do not provide sufficient explanation for either crimes of violence themselves, nor for our preoccupation with them. He argues that the answer must instead be sought in ideology. The focus on young people, their leisure habits and pastimes at the end of the nineteenth century must, for Pearson, be understood as a concerted attack on working-class culture; as an attempt to control and contain the so-called 'dangerous classes'. The children of the urban poor epitomised the threat of proletarian revolution; they therefore needed to be educated and institutionalised into middle-class values. Working-class young people have continued to be seen as a threat and a danger, as subsequent moral panics about their behaviour reveal. Cohen's classic study of mods and rockers (1972) describes a specific moment when social reaction to the behaviour of particular groups of young people encouraged them away from intermittent deviancy towards a firm commitment to a deviant career: they effectively took on the personae of their stereotyped labels. Cohen points out that working-class youngsters had traditionally visited seaside resorts at holiday times, but at Easter 1964 in Clacton, the weather was cold and wet and tempers frayed. There were scuffles between local youths and visiting Londoners, and some beach huts and windows were damaged. The press reaction was furious, and for the rest of that year and subsequent years

in the 1960s, sensational press coverage accompanied disturbances at a number of British seaside resorts. Cohen demonstrates that media reaction played an active role in shaping events, leading to a 'deviancy amplification spiral' which consolidated and magnified the original behaviour. (This theme will be developed in Chapter 8.)

Chapter 8

Sociologists in the 1980s and 1990s argued that delinquency and social reactions to delinquent behaviour are rooted in gender and 'race' expectations as well as norms and assumptions based on class. Hudson (1989) asserts that people expect trouble from male youths: it is part of growing up and learning to be a man. Women in trouble, however, are consistently sexualised, and their behaviour interpreted on the basis of sexuality. Hudson expresses this as follows:

> What society expects of its white young men and views as normal behaviour is different more in degree than in kind from behaviour condemned as delinquent: these expectations contrast significantly with the agenda for young women who are expected to learn for a life of passivity, servitude and domesticity. Delinquency . . . provides one means for developing an identity as a man.
>
> (1989:37)

There are also significant differences in the experiences of young black people living in the UK, so that behaviour tolerated from white youth may not be tolerated from black youth. Hudson states that there is considerable evidence that state agencies are likely to perceive black youth's behaviour as

 problematic and in need of some form of controlling intervention more quickly, and more intensively. She suggests that this may be related to the readiness of professionals to mis-recognise and pathologise the culture of minority ethnic families. (Again this theme will be developed in Chapter 8.)

Chapter 8

New directions

Current sociological approaches to youth are concerned to understand youth transitions and the complex interconnections between age, class, gender, sexuality, 'race' and ethnicity for young people living in a complex and changing 'post-modern' society. They are also interested in the interplay between local and global cultures and contexts.

Youth transitions

A key idea running through all the sociological literature discussed so far is that the teenage years are characterised by transitions, as young people move from childhood into adulthood; from family of origin to adult sexual partnership(s); from school to work; from parental income to own income; from family household to own household (Hill and Tisdall 1997: 115). In the 1950s and 1960s, functionalist sociologists in the US and UK believed that a 'normative transition' existed, one made by all young people: they leave school, get a job, become engaged, get married and move into a new home. The transitions of specific individuals and groups were then compared alongside this 'normal' transition.

Later Marxist and feminist sociologists pointed out that there is no such thing as a 'normal' transition. They identified systematic variations in transitions: paths into adulthood could be longer or shorter, straightforward or more complex, depending on factors such as class, gender and ethnicity (see Abbott *et al.* 2005, Wallace 1987). Research drawing on an interpretive approach demonstrates that transitions are variable, reflecting other, more personal issues. For example, Banks *et al.*'s research (1992) on sixteen- to nineteen-year-olds in four British cities (Swindon, Liverpool and Sheffield in England, and Kirkcaldy in Scotland) uncovered widespread variation amongst the transitions of young people. While most young people did, as expected, undergo transitions that could be described as 'protracted', there were many different reasons for, and feelings about this experience. Some protracted transitions were said to be voluntary, others were enforced; some were thought to be positive, others negative. Experiences of boys and girls, although similar while remaining in education, were markedly different afterwards, with boys and girls heading for very different segments of the labour market. Young women also made more extensive contributions to household labour whatever their class, although this was accentuated in working-class families. This study brings back human agency to transitions research, suggesting that a structural analysis is not sufficient explanation in itself.

Debates about the nature of agency and structure in youth transitions continue to attend transitions research: how much freedom do young people have to make their own decisions regarding the transitions they make? Jones and Wallace (1992) assert that the actions of some young people should be understood as 'informed choice strategies' arising from opportunity; others are 'survival strategies' arising from constraint. Studies of the experiences of young minority ethnic people confirm this viewpoint. For example, Mirza's research on young African Caribbean women in Britain found that while still at school the girls had high aspirations for their future careers, regardless of their social class background. However, they were also aware that the labour market operated in racist ways. When Mirza followed up these young women four years later, she found them in a very narrow range of occupations, predominantly in low-grade office work, in spite of their earlier aspirations. Mirza identifies that the racially and sexually segregated workforce operated as a major constraint to these young women, limiting their opportunities. Reviewing the experiences of young black and Asian people more broadly, Morrow asserts that the expectations of parents, religious identity and cultural practices combine to structure their transitions as they 'juggle these sets of expectations with those of the wider society in which they are located' (2003: 286). She also draws attention to the important implications of findings from research on the transitions of young people who are disabled. Riddell shows that the transitions of young people with physical disabilities, learning difficulties and mental illnesses are affected adversely not just by the nature of their impairment, but by 'wider social and political factors which impinge upon their lives and have a profound impact on the way in which impairment is understood by themselves and others' (1998: 193–4). They are, she asserts, excluded from financial independence, paid employment, independent living and adult social relationships, and are treated in a patronising and infantilising manner.

Taken together, this research demonstrates that whilst young people retain some choice in the transitions they make to adulthood, these choices are at the same time affected greatly by wider structural factors such as social class, gender, ethnicity and (dis)ability. Barry (2005) argues that there needs to be much greater emphasis in policy terms on reducing the constraints of structural inequalities on young people; such an approach is witnessed in government initiatives that seek to increase the participation of young working-class people in higher education (see Department of Education and Skills 2006). Current sociological writing on transitions takes the discussion in a new direction, emphasising that what has affected youth transitions most in recent years has, in fact, been change, and the speed of change. Furlong and Cartmel argue that change has affected relationships with family and friends, experiences in education and the labour market, leisure and lifestyles, and the ability of young people to become established as independent young adults (2007: 1). As a result of the changes which have taken place, 'young people today have to negotiate a set of risks which were largely unknown to their parents'; Furlong and Cartmel argue that these are 'irrespective of social background or gender' (ibid.). Young people today lack the 'clear route maps' which previously smoothed the transition from childhood to adulthood. Increased uncertainty, they continue, is 'a source of stress and vulnerability' (ibid). Furlong and Cartmel locate these changes in the context of late modernity/post-modernity, where structural explanations are under attack, patterns of behaviour less predictable, and we are faced with a new and more diverse set of lifestyles.

Reflecting on this literature, Furlong and Cartmel offer a circumspect view. They suggest that post-modern writers have tended to exaggerate change; that there has always been choice and plurality in modernism, as well as a sense of uncertainty about the future. Moreover, they argue that while structures may appear to have fragmented, life-chances and experiences can still largely be predicted using knowledge of individuals' locations within social structures: 'despite arguments to the contrary', they conclude, 'class and gender divisions remain central to an understanding of life experiences' (2007: 2). In addition, inequalities associated with 'race' persist, in spite of the reality that the experiences of different ethnic groups can be 'quite distinct' (2007: 8). They sum this up as follows:

> ... the risk society is not a classless society, but a society in which the old social cleavages associated with class and gender remain intact: on an objective level, changes in the distribution of risk have been minimal although they can be more difficult to identify as the social exclusivity of pathways begins to disintegrate ... Whereas subjective understandings of the social world were once shaped by class, gender and neighbourhood relations, today everything is presented as a possibility. The maintenance of traditional opportunity structures combined with subjective 'disembedding' (Giddens, 1991) is a constant source of frustration and stress for today's youth.
>
> (2007: 9)

From classless to underclass

While young people were optimistically viewed as part of a 'classless' society in the post-war years, the focus more recently has been much less upbeat. Youth has been portrayed in the media as a part of the 'underclass'; separate from, and at the same time undermining, society as a whole. Within the underclass discourse, key figures have been given particular prominence: the young single mother, the absent father, the unemployed black youth, the working-class housing estate. Sociologists are deeply divided about the concept (and the existence) of an underclass, as illustrated in the commentaries on Murray (1994) and in MacDonald (1997).

Ken Roberts supports underclass theory, defining the underclass as follows:

1. The stratum should be disadvantaged relative to, and in this sense beneath, the lowest class in the gainfully employed population.

2. For the individuals and households involved this situation should be persistent, in many cases for the duration of their entire lives and, indeed, across the generations.

3. The underclass should be separate from other groups in social and cultural respects as well as in its lack of regular employment. For example, its members might live in separate areas, belong to separate social networks, and have distinctive lifestyles and values.

4. The culture of the underclass . . . should have become another impediment, and sufficient in itself even if other obstacles were removed, to significantly reduce its members' likelihood of joining the regularly employed workforce.

(1997: 42–3)

In an earlier book (1995), Roberts identifies what he sees as 'clear strands of evidence of underclass formation in Britain':

*   Long-term unemployment is common amongst certain groups.

*   Some young people do lose contact with mainstream social institutions and become invisible to official data collection, for example, homeless young people.

*   Some young people are unlikely to be recruited by any employer, because of their limited physical or mental abilities or persistent drug use.

*   Some young people do opt out into subcultural groupings: stealing and hustling become a way of life to them.

*   Finally, cycles do tend to repeat themselves: people with disadvantaged family origins tend to have children who repeat the cycle with their own children.

(1995: 101–4)

The contributors to MacDonald's (1997) edited collection present a robust critique of underclass theory. They point to the ways in which young people have been excluded from society, marginalised from economic structures and shut out from any feeling of social citizenship; far from choosing to opt out to live on benefits, the opportunities for them to join society have been progressively diminished. Writing in MacDonald's volume, Baldwin, Coles and Mitchell (1997) argue that underclass theories over-simplify the complex processes of social exclusion which lead heterogeneous groups of vulnerable young people along unsuccessful transitions (they include care leavers and those with special needs and disabilities in this). Jones (1997) meanwhile proposes that we need to replace right-wing representations of an underclass with a more sociological analysis of the interplay of structure and agency in shaping the risky housing transitions of youth.

Local subcultures or global youth culture?

Contemporary sociological writing on youth culture/subculture mirrors the key debates between sociologists interested in youth transitions. On the one hand, some sociologists have explored what they see as a new flowering of youth cultural studies, focusing on the 'rave' phenomenon, deadhead culture and 'post-political pop' (Epstein 1998, Redhead 1990). Here it is argued that as the dominance of 'common culture' breaks up, so 'style' and subculture are ways in which young people cope with their worlds. But now their worlds are fragmented, pluralist and individualistic, they are thoroughly 'post-modern'. Willis goes as far as to assert: '. . . "elite" or "official" culture has lost its dominance – the very sense, or pretence, of a national, whole culture and of hierarchies of values, activities and places within it is breaking down' (1990: 128). Garratt (2004) suggests that these subcultures are probably 'nothing more than a means to create and establish an identity in a society where they (young people) can find it difficult to locate a *sense of self*' (2004: 145). Subcultures may seem to be a challenge to adult society, but this challenge is symbolic rather than real, since it is based on aesthetics and fashion. Subcultures, he argues, have a positive value to the individual and society: 'They give young people the chance to express their difference from society, yet co-exist within it' (2004: 149).

But there is another trend pulling in the opposite direction; that is, the globalisation of culture. This means that at the same time that young people's lives are becoming more varied, so they are also becoming more homogeneous. Writing in an edited collection in 1992, Stewart argues that one of the most powerful influences cementing the 'shared' experience of young consumers has been the pervasiveness of American cultural norms and commercial brands:

> American brands such as Coke and Levis, or cultural icons such as Michael Jackson or Madonna, have established an almost universal appeal among young people the world over, to such an extent that they have become synonymous with youth and fully integrated into the mainstream culture.
>
> (1992: 224)

Of course, this is, arguably, an ethnocentric viewpoint. While it is undoubtedly the case that American (and, to a lesser extent, British) youth culture has been packaged and sold throughout the world, given the impact of global poverty and inequalities it is hard to see how far this has been a reality in the lives of many young people. As Saraswathi and Larson remind us, more than three-quarters of the population of the world live in developing countries, but they enjoy only 14 per cent of the world's income and 18 per cent of goods and resources (2002: 348). Where young people across the world are struggling to feed themselves and their families, it is difficult to see how we can talk about a 'global youth culture'.

Implications for practice

- Sociological studies have demonstrated that although young people inhabit the same structural position in terms of age, factors such as class, gender, sexuality, disability, 'race' and ethnicity have a profound impact on the life chances and situations of young people.

- We have also seen that there is no homogeneous 'youth' and no single 'youth culture'. Instead, young people in the developed world move in and out of groups and cultures, while young people in the developing world struggle to stay alive.

- Young people are not necessarily the delinquent, dangerous, troublesome underclass portrayed in the press. Yet numbers of young people are systematically excluded from society: from education, employment, housing and mainstream society. They have become the scapegoats of society, just as young people have been society's scapegoats in the past.

Conclusion

This chapter began by suggesting that young people have typically been regarded as a social problem: the 'troubled' and 'troublesome' of psychological and sociological literature. The reality is much more complex and contradictory. The social category of 'youth' is created, and at the same time contested, by the very discourses (ideas and practices) which set its boundaries. Beyond this, the experience of young people is immensely variable. Differences between young people are structured into society (through gender, class, sexuality, disability and 'race') as well as being specific to individuals' biographies, histories and personalities. Continuities and connections between adult and youth cultures must be understood alongside the changes and disruptions which both adults and youth experience.

The need for sociological insight into youth is unequivocal. Social workers work most frequently with those who have been disadvantaged in society: the poor, the working class, the young, the old, those with disabilities. It is crucial that in working with young people, social workers have an understanding of the structural basis of disadvantage and inequality, taking into account the continuing impact of changes in employment, social security and educational systems as well as the influence of structural factors such as class, age, 'race' and ethnicity, gender and sexuality. Social work services in the UK have increasingly been targeted at attempting to monitor and control young people deemed to be 'at risk' rather than meeting any broader imperative to counteract social inequality. This is a situation that those working with young people must seek to change, in partnership with young people themselves.

Recommended reading

Furlong, A. and Cartmel, F. (2007) *Young People and Social Change: New Perspectives*, 2nd edn, Maidenhead, Berkshire: Open University Press. Locates the study of young people in a well-argued structural analysis.

Pearson, G. (1983) *Hooligan: A History of Respectable Fears*, Basingstoke: Macmillan. A good antidote to the notion that 'youth' is a new problem.

Roche, J., Tucker, S., Thomson, R. and Flynn, R. (eds) (2004) *Youth in Society: Contemporary Theory, Policy and Practice*, 2nd edn, London: Sage. Offers a good overview of a range of issues facing young people.

5 Community

Introduction

Chapter 2

The theme of community has had a continuing presence in sociological writing since the early days of sociology. It is often portrayed with a nostalgic, 'soft-focus' lens, just as we have already discussed in terms of sociological writing about the family. It is also, like the family, held up as a potential remedy for a range of society's ills, and because of this, is a buzzword favoured by politicians of all affiliations. Perhaps surprisingly, statutory social work in the UK has, for a number of years, paid little attention to community, except in the very specific sense of 'community care'; that is, the management and care of individuals within the community. Social services have focused their efforts on individuals and families, leaving community development and community action firmly to the voluntary sector. There has, however, been a recognisable shift in recent years. Community has re-emerged on the policy agenda in the context of community programmes and community safety. Community is also appearing again on the curriculum of social work education courses, at the same time as a new radical social work coalition, made up of academics, practitioners, service users and students, is currently fighting to influence policy and practice agendas.

This chapter will begin, as in previous chapters, by exploring the meanings of community, before going on to consider the historical, anthropological and sociological bases of 'community', as the term exists in everyday usage, and as it permeates social work policy and practice.

Definitions

In common with the notion of 'the family', the word 'community' carries with it a host of ideas and assumptions that are largely taken for granted. Most of the time, when we think of 'community' we do so in positive terms: it is something (again, like the family) which acts as a barrier to, or defence against, the stresses and ills of modern living. It is 'a good thing', something that we value and something that is frequently perceived as having declined in the shift to a modern, industrial, urban society. But what is community?

'The concept of community', Hamilton writes, 'has been one of the most compelling and attractive themes in modern social science, and at the same time one of the most elusive to define' (1985: 7). Sociologists over the years have come up with very many different ways of describing community. In 1955, Hillery attempted to define community by examining its usage in sociological literature. He identified no fewer than ninety-four definitions, with little consensus between writers about what the concept meant. He claimed that 'beyond the recognition that "people are involved in community" there is little agreement on the use of the term' (1955: 117). More recent investigations have confirmed this conceptual confusion, with more than 200 definitions identified by McMillan and Chavis (1986). Some scholars have gone so far as to suggest that the term should be abandoned completely, because it is 'neither theoretically nor empirically useful' (Mooney and Neal 2009: 9). In spite of this, community as a concept and a reality has survived, and it remains a mainstay of sociological investigation today.

Although definitions vary in emphasis, many share common features. Three ways of characterising community emerge in the traditional literature. These are as follows:

1. *Community as locality*: community is defined as a physical-spatial entity; it is based on geographical location such as neighbourhood, village, town or place.

2. *Community as social network*: a community is said to exist when a network of interrelationships is established between people who live in the same locality.

3. *Community as relationship (or 'communion')*: community is defined as a shared sense of identity between individuals, irrespective of any local focus or physical proximity.

Some sociologists collapse the three definitions into one, assuming that locality, social networks and shared identity are necessarily contingent on one another. Others focus on one aspect, such as social networks, rejecting the usefulness of notions of locality or identity. Looking more closely, we find that communities may be very different to either or all of these representations; communities are highly variable and complex, as this chapter will demonstrate. Physical localities may be characterised by racism and exclusion of individuals and groups rather than networks of caring relationships or shared identities. Social networks may thrive across large geographical distances and may even be worldwide, facilitated by modern communication systems such as telephone, email and the Internet; meanwhile shared identity may have little to do with location or even with local social networks. The sense of belonging that people feel may derive from their connectedness to a totally different country or culture to that of their local neighbourhood, which might be a place in which their presence is tolerated but not welcomed (as is the customary experience of asylum seekers and refugees in the UK). As patterns of occupational mobility and migration increase, the fracture of community from locality seems all the more likely.

More recent sociological scholarship on community offers alternative ways of characterising communities. Fraser (2005), drawing on the work of Ife (2002), makes four key distinctions between different types of community. He identifies:

1. *Geographical communities*: where members are based in one region (this roughly approximates to the 'community as locality' above).

2. *Virtual communities*: where members' main form of contact is through electronic media.

3. *Communities of circumstance*: where people come together for a time around a common cause, such as bush-fires or floods.

4. *Communities of interest*: where identity groups come together to campaign for change in legislation or policy; for example, gay and lesbian groups or business lobby groups (this mirrors the notion of 'community as relationship' above).

Mooney and Neal (2009) contribute another two, more critical, definitions of community:

1. *Community as boundary*: community is understood as a form of exclusion; it is about keeping others out, as much as keeping people in; community is, from this perspective, a site of conflict.

2. *Community as a site of governance and policy intervention*: community is seen by government as a good way to deliver social welfare, to increase civic participation (citizenship), and so, to promote social inclusion.

It is clear from the discussion so far that when we think about community we enter the realms of discourses and ideologies – that is, the ideas, beliefs, values and practices that characterise community – rather than dealing with objective 'facts' about community. Symonds (1998) distinguishes between two parallel realities here. The first is the 'social lived reality' in which people work and live; a reality that recognises conflicts and difference, and is aware that community can be hostile and that social networks are not always supportive and friendly. The second is the 'dream' world of community:

> This community 'in the mind' is always warm, supportive, safe and secure. This picture has been transmitted culturally through literature, certain historical 'readings', sociology, and in television soap operas . . . the place of this dream community tends to be a small area inhabited by people who share the same culture, characteristics, history, language and understanding of their world.
>
> (1998: 12)

It is the 'dream' world of community which is invoked by US and UK politicians and intellectuals alike in the form of communitarianism (see Etzioni 1995, Murray 1990). Communitarians believe that community is in decline. They blame a long line of societal changes for this state of affairs: changing family structures, work patterns (including women's employment), suburbanisation, television and the mass media, and generational approaches have all 'played a part in breaking down social bonds, trust, volunteerism and engagement in social institutions' (Mooney and Neal 2009: 22). They would therefore like to see a return to 'old fashioned values and . . . sense of obligation' (Etzioni 1995: 117). Communitarians reject liberal/neo-liberal beliefs which place a high value on personal freedom and individual responsibility and oppose any notion that the state should take responsibility for the welfare of its members. They argue instead that we must rebuild the moral responsibility of citizens to their communities by strengthening community structures (that is, family, school and community organisations) and by giving control of communities back to local people.

This version of community has been at the heart of New Labour public policy in the UK ever since the Labour Party assumed government in 1997. It has been translated into a wide range of policies to tackle multiple problems, from health and social exclusion on the one hand to urban decline and crime on the other. As Karn outlines:

> In effect, communities represent a social institution that it is hoped will be able to cushion the worst effects of market economics . . . and act as a mediating institution between state and individual, offering a focus for a 'Third Way' of minimal regulation . . . It is this focus on empowering vulnerable communities and addressing social exclusion that gives this discourse a particular New Labour flavour . . .
>
> (2007: 19)

Karn suggests that the problem with this is that community is presented as both the object of intervention and the strategy to achieve its goals. This inevitably leads to confusion between means and ends. More cynically, it can be argued that the need for community has itself been created by successive governments' policies which have been designed to 'roll back the frontiers of the state'. There is another equally pressing problem, however. Although community may seem to be a positive solution, giving value to ideas of locality, neighbourliness and sharing, seen in a different light it may lead to unrealistic expectations of community support that do not take sufficient account of structural inequalities in society. It may also have more detrimental consequences. The sociologist Richard Sennett asserts (1973) that communities based on a belief in 'sameness' lead to conformism, an intolerance of difference, and the risk of confrontations with other communities. This demonstrates that how we define a situation or problem matters: ideology has real consequences, not only on our own work as practitioners, but on the lived experiences of those who use social work services.

> **Implications for practice**
>
> • Social workers must be able to distinguish between community as 'normative prescription' (what the writer believes it should be) and as 'empirical description' (what it actually is) (Allan 1991: 108). It is always political, used by those on the Left to emphasise collective identity control/government at a localised level, and by those on the Right to symbolise freedom from dependence on the state, individual choice and family responsibility.
>
> • We need to be aware that, because of its largely positive connotations, the word 'community' is added to a host of diverse activities and projects: community service, community homes, community workers, community development, community action, community programmes, community teams and community care all mean different things. The contradictions inherent in this must be acknowledged, because they have the potential to pull social work in very different directions.

Historical accounts

Conventional sociological perspectives are frequently premised on the assumption that communities in the past were more vibrant, more secure and more caring than they are today. But what evidence is there for this? There have, of course, been huge social, economic and demographic changes over the past 200 years or so. Mills (1996) outlines the scale of changes that have taken place in Britain. The Industrial Revolution, conventionally defined as the period between 1760 and 1830, led to the concentration of industrial activity on the coalfields and at the ports. Rural domestic industries declined rapidly, as did local self-sufficiency and agricultural employment. The population of England and Wales doubled between 1700 and 1800, and again between 1801 and 1851, and yet again between 1851 and 1911. Because much of the increased population was migrating to the towns in the nineteenth century, the population of most rural areas declined.

The massive growth in towns and cities provides the other side of the coin. The concentration of large populations in small areas led to many environmental and social problems. But, Mills argues, Victorian cities were more prosperous than ever before and were able to provide amenities such as lighting, water, sewerage, transport, dispensaries and universal schooling. New forms of transport within and outside the cities and towns encouraged the movement of people to and from the countryside, so that it became possible for rural workers to live in villages and travel to towns to work, and so for town dwellers who moved out to live in new suburbs and villages on the edge of towns. Mills reports that the inversion of the social composition of a rural population took no more than fifty years, as middle-class town dwellers replaced farm labourers and village craftsmen in the countryside. Alongside this shift, amenities and community welfare declined in inner-city areas, although in some cities this trend has since been halted by the upgrading ('gentrification') of some run-down areas to provide housing for single professional people. Mills concludes that community at the beginning of this period might be largely defined in terms of territory; today people live, shop, work and socialise in different territories and, he argues, in different communities (1996: 272–5).

This brief outline of social, economic and demographic change demonstrates that there has been a transformation in community as territory in Britain. But what can this tell us about the less tangible definitions of community; that is, about community as social networks or relationships? Dennis and Daniels (1996) indicate that because no agreement has been reached on the indices of community life, it is difficult to assess if and how community life has changed over time. The relative value placed on the notion of social mix in a community illustrates this point. Some writers assume that a degree of social mixing is a prerequisite of community, so that community life declines as segregation intensifies. Others believe that because community is based on class, it is more likely to develop as segregation increases. In reviewing the evidence from historical documents, Dennis and Daniels point out that nineteenth-century sources can tell us where people lived and near whom, how often they moved, where they worked, to whom they were related and whom they married. 'But', they ask critically, 'do these findings have any value as evidence of community life?' (1996: 203).

Oral histories and autobiographies give us further insight into community life in the past. Many of these accounts stress the quality of relationships between people, as poverty and hardship forced people to rely on each other for support. Many are also touched by the soft, rosy hues of nostalgia:

> In those days, too, there was real neighbourliness. You see, you might be four or five families in that house, and perhaps the one at the bottom would make some tea and she'd shout up the stairs 'I've just made a cup of tea – coming down?' And they'd more or less take it in turn each day, and if there was anyone in real dire straits, and couldn't pay their way, I've known a neighbour take their own sheets off the bed, wash 'em and pawn 'em to help them out. That's how it was in those days – real good neighbours. I mean they'd never let anyone starve. We never used to lock our front doors – not a bit of string or nothing, the house was open day and night . . . There were real criminals of course – but never against their own.
>
> (White 1988: 26)

Chapter 8

Research on crime, to be discussed in Chapter 8, will demonstrate that the last statement here, without a doubt, is an example of selective recall. Evidence suggests that crime has always been largely intra-class, not inter-class (Young 1999). The people most at risk of being attacked or burgled are working-class people, in crimes committed by working-class people. Moreover, community life is not always remembered so fondly. Dennis and Daniels report that 'close propinquity, together with cultural poverty, led as much to enmity as it did to friendship'. They assert that communities 'may be characterised as much by antagonism, jealousy, fear, and suspicion, as by more neighbourly attitudes and relationships' (1996: 222). Bornat *et al.* (1997) agrees. She points out that lack of privacy and physical space meant that community could be an oppressive experience, especially from the perspective of its more junior members who had less power and control over their lives. Community also brought with it discrimination and exclusion for some people, as demonstrated in the growing numbers of accounts of the experiences of minority ethnic groups in Britain. Bornat observes that in the memory of white working-class people, issues of 'race' and ethnicity are in the main absent. In contrast, the experience of members of minority ethnic groups was framed by 'the constraining force of an opposing community whose identity is delineated as other' (1997: 27). It is not only minority ethnic accounts, she continues, that have been largely missing from community history: the voices of disabled children and adults and stories of gay and lesbian life have also only emerged in recent years (1997: 28). This brings us to a consideration of anthropological writing on community.

Cross-cultural studies

Anthropology is, by definition, the study of the culture, practices and beliefs of different peoples, and hence, arguably, of communities. Early anthropologists were interested in finding out more about the culture and practices of those living in traditional, non-industrial, 'primitive' (less complex) communities, but defined their spheres of concern, Amit (2002) argues, as 'society', 'culture' or 'peoples' rather than 'community'. The term 'community', she continues, really only came into its own in anthropology as part of a shift of attention towards the cities and towards an exploration of the impact of urbanisation. Given their overlapping interests, sociological and anthropological contributions will be examined together in the rest of this chapter.

Implications for practice

- Historical evidence reminds us that our views about community are intimately connected with a rather rose-tinted perception of communities in the past. There is nothing which is necessarily positive and generous about any community, past or present.

- Anthropological approaches, as we will discuss in the next section, bring a new vocabulary and a new set of ideas of community as culture, symbol and boundary.

Traditional sociological approaches

Functionalist approaches

Conventional functionalist approaches stress that communities are necessary and important for the well-being of society as a whole. More than this, they assume that the processes of industrialisation and urbanisation damaged the 'ties that bind' communities together (Durkheim 1893), so that it is imperative that we find new ways to help communities regain their sense of shared identity and collaborative concern.

Gemeinschaft and Gesellschaft

A classic example of this viewpoint is found in the work of the nineteenth-century German sociologist Ferdinand Tönnies (1855–1936), who has had an enduring influence on sociological and everyday ideas about community, past and present. Writing in *Gemeinschaft and Gesellschaft*, first published in 1877 (and reprinted in 1955), Tönnies set out to make sense of the changes that he saw taking place in Europe as it was developing from a pre-industrial to an industrial society. Tönnies made a distinction between two ideal types: *Gemeinschaft* (community) and *Gesellschaft* (society or 'association'). He argued that industrialisation was transforming the quality and nature of social relationships from small-scale, personal, intimate and enduring *gemeinschaftlich* relationships to individualistic, large-scale, impersonal, calculative and contractual *gesellschaftlich* relationships. He writes:

> All intimate, private and exclusive living together . . . is . . . life in Gemeinschaft. Gesellschaft is public life – it is the world itself. In Gemeinschaft with one's family, one lives from birth on, bound to it in weal and woe. One goes into Gesellschaft as one goes into a strange country . . . Gemeinschaft is old; Gesellschaft is new . . . all praise of rural life has pointed out that the Gemeinschaft among people is stronger there and more alive; it is the lasting and genuine form of living together. In contrast to Gemeinschaft, Gesellschaft is transitory and superficial. Accordingly, Gemeinschaft should be understood as a living organism, Gesellschaft as a mechanical aggregate and artefact.
>
> (1955: 37–9)

The quotation makes it clear that Tönnies regretted what he saw as the passing of *gemeinschaftlich* relationships. In *Gemeinschaft*, people knew who they were: they knew their place in life; beliefs and values were clear and well internalised; and there was a high value placed on kinship, territory, and solidarity. Industrialisation was changing all this, Tönnies believed, and was bringing about the decline of community in the modern world. Significantly, Tönnies asserts that there are elements of *Gemeinschaft* and *Gesellschaft* in all social relationships and in all societies; they should not be understood as exclusive categories, but rather as tendencies or influences that pervade different societies in varying degrees. But he also admits that he sees a greater tendency towards *Gemeinschaft* in rural areas. This led some sociologists to equate *Gemeinschaft* with the countryside and *Gesellschaft* with the city; the city became the symbol of the breakdown of community in the modern world.

Tönnies's ideas are reflected in Durkheim's classic essay, *The Division of Labour in Society*, published sixteen years later in 1893 (reprinted in 1984), in which he distinguishes between the 'mechanical' solidarity of pre-industrial societies (that is, societies characterised by likeness and shared morality) and the 'organic' solidarity typical of industrial society (with its differences between people, specialisation and complex division of labour). Durkheim proposed that both types of solidarity could give rise to forms of community, either focused on similarity or interdependence. His concern was, however, that the excessive individualism of industrial society would lead to a breakdown in organic solidarity; 'instead of combining their efforts into a collective project, people would allow selfish interests and competitiveness to divide them' (Day 2006: 3). The end result would be social disorder and individual unhappiness or 'anomie', defined as a mismatch between individual circumstances and wider social mores. This vision of community has been central to the development of communitarian ideas.

Community as locality: urban studies

The first person to relate the ideas of *Gemeinschaft* and *Gesellschaft* to specific localities was Georg Simmel (1858–1918), a German contemporary of Tönnies and a friend of Max Weber. In his seminal essay *The Metropolis and Mental Life* (1971 [1903]), Simmel characterised urban life as a constantly changing series of encounters; this 'rapid crowding of changing images' encouraged people to deal with social situations at a rational, calculating, 'head' level, rather than at a more intuitive or habitual 'heart' level. At the same time, he argued that because the city was the centre of the money economy, social relationships had become impersonalised and standardised, untouched by the complications and involvement that personal relationships bring. Simmel believed that this had very negative consequences on the mental health of individuals. People became 'blasé' in outlook, reserved and estranged from one another, frantically searching for self-identity and individuality, and desperate to stand out from the crowd and be noticed. They experienced loneliness more in the city than anywhere else, he asserted, in spite of the 'metropolitan crush of persons' (Simmel 1971 [1903]). (There are, again, strong links with Durkheim's notion of 'anomie'.) The Italian novelist Italo Calvino expresses beautifully this vision of the city in his meditation, *Invisible Cities*. He writes:

> In Chloe, a great city, the people who move through the streets are all strangers. At each encounter, they imagine a thousand things about one another; meetings which could take place between them, conversations, surprises, caresses, bites. But no one greets anyone; eyes lock for a second, then dart away, seeking other eyes, never stopping.
>
> (1997: 51)

The principal site for the academic study of community in the early twentieth century was Chicago in the US, and its university's so-called Chicago School. Successive waves of immigrants had come to Chicago in search of work in the city's expanding manufacturing and retail sectors; the population of Chicago had exploded from being a small town of about 10,000 inhabitants in 1860 to becoming a city of over two million people by 1910 (Miller 1997). White immigrants from Europe (including thousands of Irish people and many others from Eastern Europe) competed with each other and with black African Americans from the Southern states for limited housing and jobs, and social (and racial) tensions erupted. Problems such as crime and delinquency, overcrowding and homelessness, poverty, racism and social exclusion were commonplace; this was a time of gangsters, prohibition and 'race' riots. Social researchers converged on Chicago and its neighbourhoods at this time, seeking to examine what was happening 'on the ground'. The city and its neighbourhoods offered ideal case-study material for an examination of the impact of locality on people's lives and behaviours, and more fundamentally, for providing an answer to the question, what influences human behaviour most: biology and genetics (as psychologists believed) or social environment and structure (as sociologists proposed)?

Robert Ezra Park (1864–1944) has been described as the greatest urban sociologist of all (Macionis and Plummer 2008: 789). Born in Pennsylvania in the US, Park worked as a journalist before going to study in Germany under Georg Simmel. He returned to the US to teach at Harvard, moving on to the Department of Sociology at the University of Chicago in 1914, where he remained until his retirement. Park urged his fellow sociologists to get out of their armchairs and onto the streets to see human life for themselves; he admitted that he had probably 'covered more ground, tramping about in cities in different parts of the world, than any other living man' (1950: viii). In his first published paper, Park noted that, contrary to the very negative portrayal by European sociologists, including Durkheim, Tönnies and Simmel, industrialisation and urbanisation had not destroyed either communities or community life. Instead, the city contained 'a mosaic of little worlds which touch but do not interpenetrate' (1967 [1915]: 608). Park argued that it was the variety which exists in cities that made them attractive to their inhabitants; diversity brought with it freedom and choice:

> The attraction of the metropolis is due in part to the fact that in the long run every individual finds somewhere among the varied manifestations of city life the sort of environment in which he expands and feels at ease; he finds, in short, the moral climate in which his particular nature obtains the stimulations that bring his innate dispositions to full and free expression.
>
> (Park 1967 [1915]: 41)

Park and his colleagues, Burgess and McKenzie, went on to compare the city with the natural world in which plants occupy particular habitats and compete with one another for space. They observed that 'natural areas' in the city had evolved alongside and in relation to one another, forming an urban ecology, a 'true human kaleidoscope' (Macionis and Plummer 2008: 790). Some of these areas were differentiated according to housing type; others were distinct ethnic communities within Chicago, such as 'Little Sicily', 'Chinatown' and what they described as 'the Black Belt'. There was also, they noted, a shopping district and a 'bright [red] light' area. Refining their ideas further, Park and his colleagues observed that as Chicago had grown, so land had come to be used in different ways. They saw this in terms of concentric zones radiating out from the city centre. Five concentric areas are identified in this model (Park et al. 1925):

1. the central business district;

2. the zone of transition (recent immigrant groups, deteriorated housing, abandoned buildings, light industry and factories);

3. the zone of working men's homes (working classes, single-family tenements);

4. the residential zone (middle classes, single-family homes, garages, yards);

5. the commuter zone (the outer suburbs).

Park *et al.* argued that successive generations of immigrants had displaced one another in the 'zone of transition' around the central business district. At the same time, those who were financially able to do so had gradually moved out towards the suburbs.

This model has been criticised for being too biological in its assumptions, and for failing to notice that vested interests could keep people out, just as local politicians and planners could (and did) at times intervene to change the situation (Fulcher and Scott 2007: 505). Moreover, the model may work for Chicago, but it is not known how far it makes equal sense for all cities, at all times. Macionis and Plummer argue that there is good reason to doubt that 'any single ecological model will account for the full range of urban diversity' (2008: 792).

Another prominent figure within the Chicago School was Louis Wirth (1897–1952), who, in his own words, was also concerned about the 'rise of the cities in the modern world' (1938). But Wirth was not interested in specific areas within the city; his aim was rather to create a sociology of the city. Wirth came to Chicago in the 1930s as a Jewish immigrant from a village in Germany. In his classic essay 'Urbanism as a way of life', published in the *American Journal of Sociology* (1938), he picked up and developed Simmel's ideas, arguing that urbanisation had had more impact on society than either industrialisation or capitalism, changing social relationships for ever, and leading to a state of 'anomie' (drawing on Durkheim's concept). He wrote:

> . . . the city is characterized by secondary rather than primary contacts. The contacts of the city may indeed be face-to-face, but they are nevertheless impersonal, superficial, transitory, and segmental. The reserve, the indifference, and the blasé outlook which urbanites manifest in their relationships may thus be regarded as devices for immunizing themselves against the personal claims and expectations of others . . . Nowhere has mankind been further removed from organic nature than under the conditions of life characteristic of great cities . . . [The city] wipes out completely the previously dominant modes of human association.
>
> (1938: 1–3)

Wirth presents the city and the countryside as two opposite poles: when we leave the countryside, we leave not only the physical environment of the countryside but we leave a rural way of life, taking on instead the values and behaviour of urbanism as a way of life. Urbanism is thus a cultural, as well as a physical phenomenon. It controls all economic, political and cultural life, drawing 'even the most remote parts of the world into its orbit' (1938: 2). Wirth goes on to identify what he sees as the defining characteristics of the city:

1. *The large size of its population*: Wirth argues that the increased population results in a high division of labour; people perform specialised roles. As a consequence, we cannot know each other

as whole, rounded individuals; our relationships tend to be segmental and 'secondary', related to a person's role as shop assistant, employer, etc. Bonds of kinship and neighbourliness are absent or, at the very least, weakened.

2. *A high population density*: Wirth suggests that the increased concentration of people in a limited space leads to a range of environmental and sociological problems, including competition for space, overcrowding and pollution. Different parts of the city 'acquire specialized functions', as Park *et al.* have also demonstrated. We are, Wirth argues, 'exposed to glaring contrasts between splendour and squalor, between riches and poverty, intelligence and ignorance, order and chaos' (1938: 3). There is, inevitably, a rise in social and interpersonal conflict in neighbourhoods as a result of this.

3. *Heterogeneity*: Wirth believes that the more diverse and specialised population may, on the one hand, allow for more personal freedom and greater choice; but it may also contribute to a sense of insecurity and instability, because we may be affiliated to many different interest groups, none of which allow us to express our personality as a whole. Wirth suggests that because of this, people living in cities were more likely than those in rural areas to suffer from mental breakdowns, commit suicide or become victims of crime. They were also, he argues, more susceptible to manipulation by politicians and the media, since they could no longer work out what was in their 'best interests'.

Commentators have argued that while presenting an extremely vivid characterisation of urban life, Wirth ignores the conflict that exists in the village as well as in the city, just as he underplays the capacity for mutual support within city neighbourhoods. There are, as the interpretive studies will demonstrate, very different kinds of urban dweller, just as villages are not always as comfortable as Wirth remembers them.

Community as locality: rural studies

While Wirth was investigating the defining characteristics of city life in Chicago, Robert Redfield studied rural communities in Mexico (Tepoztlán in Morelos and Chan Kom in Yucatán), seeking to identify the qualities of rural life. He described the way of life there as 'folk society'. As he explained:

> Such a society is small, isolated, non-literate and homogeneous, with a strong sense of group solidarity . . . Behaviour is traditional, spontaneous, uncritical and personal: there is no legislation or habit of experiment and reflection for intellectual ends. Kinship, its relations and institutions, are the type categories of experience and the familial group is the unit of action.
>
> (1947: 293)

Redfield's 'folk society' has strong connections with Tönnies's concept of *Gemeinschaft*. It is also very closely related to Wirth's belief that where we live has a profound impact on how we live; that locality determines lifestyle. Redfield's work has not gone unchallenged, however. Writing around the same time as Redfield, another anthropologist Oscar Lewis published (1949) a very different account of life in a Mexican village. Studying one of the same villages as Redfield (Tepoztlán), Lewis came up with very different results, finding individualism, lack of co-operation, tension, schisms, fear, envy and distrust amongst the inhabitants. Later studies of village life have stressed that there is a high degree of fluidity in relationships in country areas; that they were not necessarily as stable as presented. Others draw attention to the contractual employer–employee nature of rural relationships, which were much more characteristic of *Gesellschaft* than *Gemeinschaft* concepts.

Social class and community

Although not based at the University of Chicago, Herbert J. Gans came to the US in 1940 as a refugee from Nazism and studied sociology at the University of Chicago. He followed up Park and Burgess's earlier emphasis on community-based research, and developed their ideas about diversity in the city, but offers a more critical perspective on the reasons for this difference. His first book, *The Urban Villagers* (1962), describes Boston's West End neighbourhood, where he studied its Italian-American working-class community. His later book, *The Levittowners* (1967), explored New Jersey's Willingboro suburb. Here he examined the ways in which new home-owners came together to establish the community's formal and informal organisations.

Gans rejects Wirth's notion of a distinctively 'urban way of life'. He claims that Wirth concentrated too much on the inner city, and in doing so ignored the vast majority of city dwellers who lived in quite stable communities, offering them some protection from the worst consequences of urban living. Furthermore, he argues that even those who lived in the inner city were a mixed population, some of whom lived there by choice. Gans identifies five different ways of life in the inner city:

1. *The 'cosmopolites'*: students, writers, artists and intellectuals who live in the inner city to be close to educational and cultural facilities. Many are unmarried or childless. They have no wish to be integrated and have no connections with the neighbourhood in which they live; their social networks are elsewhere. Fulcher and Scott assert that global communications and extensive international migration have made this truer than ever before (2007: 497).

2. *The unmarried or childless*: Gans distinguishes two groups here; those who are temporarily childless and living in the inner city, and those who will permanently live there. They are geographically mobile workers who again have no interest in their local neighbourhood, and do not suffer from social isolation. They might be called 'yuppies' today; they live in gentrified flats in run-down parts of inner cities.

3. *The 'ethnic villagers'*: groups from a common ethnic background, living in a neighbourhood with strong family and kinship ties, but with little involvement in secondary relationships in the neighbourhood.

4. *The 'deprived'*: 'the very poor, emotionally disturbed or otherwise handicapped' (1980 [1968]: 400–2), single-parent families and those experiencing racial discrimination, forced to live in deprived areas with cheap housing and suffering from social isolation.

5. *The 'trapped' and downwardly mobile*: those who have no choice about where they live; they stay 'when a neighbourhood is invaded by non-residential land uses or lower status immigrants' or are older people on low incomes who have been left behind when others move out; they have lost their social ties and also experience social isolation (ibid.).

Gans concludes that ways of life have more to do with social class and family-cycle stage than with urban or rural location: some people are protected from the social consequences of living in a city by social class; the higher their income, the greater degree of choice people have over where they live. In addition, stage in the family cycle determines the area of choice within a social class, so that families with young children may only be able to afford to buy a new house on a modern estate. Any similarities between people living in the same area are not, he argues, to do with locality, but are instead the outcome of a series of constrained choices. This is echoed strongly in later analysis of social exclusion. Bill Jordan makes an important distinction between 'communities of choice' (among mainstream households) and 'communities of fate' (among the poor and excluded). He argues that the polarisation inherent in this has high social costs, not least in social problems associated with concentrations of deprivation and the expenditure on social control considered necessary to counter these problems (1996: 188).

While Gans was studying new and old communities in the US, sociologists in the UK were interested in what had been happening in their own cities and new towns. Studies of post-war working-class communities discovered that, contrary to widely held opinion, features of working-class life actively encouraged the growth of strong communities: workers lived and worked in one area, often for one employer; trade unions encouraged social solidarity, as did the need to rely on one another for support in times of deprivation (Fulcher and Scott 2007: 505). Once established, these communities were self-sustaining and able, to a degree, to resist external changes. For example, Young and Willmott's 1957 study of Bethnal Green in the East End of London uncovered a surprisingly homogeneous and stable

community, with strong kinship patterns still very much in evidence; although this depiction has been criticised for being overly romantic and ignoring the real hardships experienced by residents who lived in overcrowded, poor quality housing. (Their work is discussed more fully in Chapter 2.)

Chapter 2

Willmott and Young were also interested in middle-class communities, and in the UK context this meant the suburbs. In their 1960 study, they observed that family life had become more privatised in the suburbs; families were more likely to be in their homes than on the streets. The growth of the suburbs has been of continuing interest to sociologists, with many studies conducted; some emphasising the homogeneous nature of the suburbs, others their heterogeneity. Savage and Warde (2002) have gone so far as to argue that suburbanisation reinforced social inequality. Because the new residential areas were financed by the sale of houses to owner-occupiers, those on lower incomes were excluded. This, Fulcher and Scott argue, 'consolidated a distinctive middle-class culture and strengthened middle-class solidarity' (2007: 505). The process of suburbanisation can therefore be seen to contribute to class formation.

Marxist writers have further developed a structural analysis, arguing that lifestyle and community must be explained in terms of class and factors relating to class in a capitalist society. David Harvey, geographer and social theorist, is one of the most influential examples of this perspective. In his memorable text, *Social Justice and the City*, published in 1973, he says from the outset that he is not interested in describing how people live their lives in the city. Rather, he wishes to examine how power operates in the city, arguing that the city is a capitalist creation, built for the circulation of capital, whether that capital is human (that is, the workforce), commodities (goods and information) or abstract finance (credit for buying and selling property). Appositely, he draws attention to the fact that 'church and chapel spires dream over Oxford (a town created in the age of church power), whereas in the age of monopoly capitalism, it is the Chrysler building and the Chase-Manhattan Bank building which brood over Manhattan Island' (1973: 32). Harvey concludes that:

> Urbanism has to be regarded as a set of social relationships which reflect relationships established throughout society as a whole. Further, these relationships have to express the laws whereby urban phenomena are structured, regulated and constructed.
>
> (1973: 304)

From Harvey's perspective, problems such as poverty, housing and crime are not urban problems at all; they are societal problems revealed in an urban context, their causes related to capitalism and social and economic inequalities rather than to urbanisation. Giddens (2006) agrees, asserting that capitalism has transformed both urban and rural life; it is wage labour, not where people live, that shapes their lives.

Richard Sennett (1992 [1977]) picks up this theme. He argues that people have been diverted from the realities of power by an emphasis on community. He is concerned that by always looking inward, and by placing all our faith in personal, intimate relationships within the family (he calls this 'destructive *Gemeinschaft*'), we fail to give attention to the large-scale forces in society. He expresses this powerfully:

> Localism and local autonomy are becoming widespread political creeds, as though the experi-ence of power relations will have more human meaning the more intimate the scale – even though the actual structures of power grow ever more into an international system. Community becomes a weapon against society, whose great vice is now seen to be its impersonality. But a community of power can only be an illusion in a society like that of the industrial West, one in which stability has been achieved by the progressive extension of the international scale of structures of economic control. In sum, the belief in direct human relations on an intimate scale has seduced us from converting our understanding of the realities of power into guides for our own political behaviour. The result is that the forces of domination or inequity remain unchallenged.
>
> (1992 [1977]: 339)

Interpretive approaches

In the 1960s and 1970s another 'Chicago School' emerged at the University of Chicago, this time focused on symbolic interactionism and the study of culture; the work of Clifford Geertz is central here. Geertz defines culture as 'an historically transmitted pattern of meanings embodied in symbols, a system of inherited conceptions expressed in symbolic forms by means of which men communicate, perpetuate, and develop their knowledge about and their attitudes toward life' (Geertz 1973: 89).

The UK anthropologist Anthony Cohen takes up this idea in his exploration of community. He argues that:

> The quintessential referent of community is that its members make, or believe they make, a similar sense of things either generally or with respect to specific and significant interests, and, further, that they think that that sense may differ from one made elsewhere.
>
> (1985: 16)

The purpose of symbols (football teams, war memorials, etc.), according to this perspective, is to construct difference as well as meaning within a community. This introduces a new dimension to the study of community. Community is not only symbolic; it is constructed by people themselves, in such a way that they can express their difference from other communities. It is therefore fundamentally about the creation and maintenance of boundaries:

> The boundary thus symbolizes the community to its members in two quite different ways: it is the sense they have of its perception by people on the other side – the public face and 'typical' mode – and it is *their* sense of the community as refracted through all the complexities of their lives and experience – the private face and idiosyncratic mode.
>
> (1985: 74)

It is in the 'private mode', Cohen continues, that we encounter people thinking about and symbolising community. This suggests that community is a highly complex, personal relationship between ourselves and others; between how we see and think about ourselves and how we think others see us. This notion of community as boundary is central to later anthropological and sociological writing on community, as will be demonstrated.

Implications for practice

• Traditional sociological representations of community (community as a rural *Gemeinschaft* or community as a tight-knit, post-war working-class neighbourhood) have had a major influence on social work practice. This creates a problem because the notions and the worlds on which policies are built simply do not exist any more, if they ever did. We cannot rely on either the existence or the continuing survival of reciprocal, supportive relationships between family and neighbours. People's social networks are now more widely spread geographically, and at the same time are more focused within the private, nuclear family. Hence an attempt to foster local attachment is not in any way 'natural', as is demonstrated by a long line of 'not in my backyard' (NIMBY) campaigns waged at community level.

- Bulmer argues that we should not be thinking in terms of drawing out attachment which is already there waiting to be used, but instead we must create it through 'new mediating structures' (1987: 70). This takes us in new directions.

New directions

We have already drawn attention to the growing criticisms of the idea that *where* we live determines *how* we live – that locality determines lifestyle – and criticisms too of the romanticism implicit in the earlier studies. An alternative approach argues that the community is not about the city, nor about the rural–urban dichotomy, nor about locality, nor even about social networks, but is, as we will discuss, about wider structural issues.

Structural issues and communities of difference

Sociologists have demonstrated that a range of structural factors have an impact on our communities: social class (as previously discussed), and also 'race' and ethnicity, gender and sexuality, age and disability.

'Race', ethnicity and community
The existence of diverse ethnic communities was first identified by Chicago School sociologists as early as the 1920s, in the work of Park, Burgess and McKenzie, and was later developed in Gans's research. One of the most well-known UK studies of 'race' and community is Rex and Moore's (1967) study of Sparkbrook, a district in the south-east of Birmingham. Rex and Moore built on the work of the Chicago School, and in particular, the idea of concentric zones. Rex and Moore used an ecological approach to chart the distribution of housing use within Sparkbrook, describing the various movements in and out of the district from the 1930s onwards, as well as describing the inhabitants themselves. They noted that different types of housing were used by different groups of people. For example, the large houses in the 'zone of transition' vacated by the middle classes on their progress out to the more desirable suburbs had been turned into lodging houses and occupied by incoming immigrants: first Irish, then European and, increasingly in the early 1960s, 'coloured' (*sic*) immigrants.

Rex and Moore distinguish six different housing situations, also referred to as 'housing classes' (1967: 274):

1. The outright owner-occupier of a whole house.

2. The owner of a mortgaged whole house.

3. The council tenant: a) in a house with a long life; b) in a house awaiting demolition.

4. The tenant of a whole house owned by a private landlord.

5. The owner of a house bought with short-term loans who is compelled to let rooms in order to meet his repayment obligations.

6. The tenant of rooms in a lodging house.

They make an important point here. Not only were different groups of people inhabiting different types of housing; the demarcation was not accidental. It was caused, in part, by local authority housing policies. Criteria such as the 'residence rule' which stated that applicants for council housing must have lived in the area for five years effectively excluded minority ethnic people from council housing. This 'left them to the mercy of the free market' (1967: 260), forcing them into lodging houses and poor-quality accommodation in run-down areas. Rex and Moore assert that the consequences were damaging for 'race relations' and for the city itself (1967: 265).

Rex and Moore's study is significant because it demonstrates that structured inequality is what determines an individual's housing and neighbourhood; not personal choice or lifestyle. Their work has been criticised, however, for being too geographically and historically specific, and for misunderstanding some of the issues for black people, including the reality that large numbers of Indian and Pakistani immigrants actually chose to buy larger property in city centres because it suited their requirements, rather than because they were passive victims of housing policy. More recent studies of ethnic communities have described the complex interplay of 'push' and 'pull' factors in community formation. Fulcher and Scott (2007) argue that various aspects of the situation of ethnic minorities facilitate community formation: they tend to be geographically concentrated in one area; they have distinctive cultural, linguistic and religious traditions that bind them together; and, crucially, this is 'reinforced by ethnic conflicts and racism that commonly accompany ethnic diversity'. They continue:

> Ethnic communities are not just the product of shared customs and beliefs. They are also the result of common experiences of exclusion and discrimination, and the creation of organizations for mutual support and protection.

> (2007: 517)

Of course, white people also have ethnic identities; ethnicity, as Fulcher and Scott argue, has provided a basis for white communities as well. They describe the emergence of 'defended communities' amongst white people in the East End of London and in the Beaumont Leys estate in Leicester, as a result of competition for local jobs and housing. In an illustration of this, Foster (1996) tells the story of the Isle of Dogs in London's Docklands, where the white working-class residents united against the predominantly Bengali population who had been forced to move into the area because of changes in local authority housing allocation. Foster records that her sympathies initially lay with the indigenous population, but that she had changed her mind:

> The positive sense of 'belonging', community and traditional attachment to a way of life valued by some of the indigenous residents had to be weighed against the negativity of a culture which by definition stigmatised, marginalised and was hostile to those who did not 'belong'.
>
> (1996: 151)

Interestingly, in a postscript to our earlier analysis of Young and Willmott's 1960s work on Bethnal Green, Young returned to the area with new researchers in 1992 to conduct a follow-up study, finally published in 2006 (Dench, Gavron and Young 2006). Here it is argued, controversially, that the administration of local housing policy had benefitted Bangladeshis, leaving the white working-class community resentful, and thus contributing to the rise of racism in Tower Hamlets through the 1980s and 1990s. The findings have led to disagreement amongst sociologists, some of whom feel that the study justifies, at the same time as it presents, racist views. This is a crucial issue for sociologists: how far should they/we give voice to what might be seen as potentially harmful views?

Fulcher and Scott (2007) present a more optimistic view of the capacity for communities to support ethnic difference. They discuss successful attempts to reduce ethnic and racial conflict by fostering interdependence between groups, through an organised, multi-ethnic initiative such as a sporting activity or improvements in a housing estate. These initiatives have sought to establish communities on a residential, rather than an ethnic, basis, taking us directly back to the idea of community as locality.

Gender and community

One of the most common statements made in relation to gender and community is that men and women have different understandings and experiences of community, in terms of location, social relationships and a sense of identity. While other factors such as class, age, disability, 'race' and ethnicity also have an impact on men's mobility and resources, men's communities are said to be broader and more diverse than those of women. Men, it is argued, are more likely than women to live and work in different areas, and can choose to socialise and take part in leisure and sport activities across community boundaries; at the same time, public spaces (particularly sporting facilities and bars) are largely dominated by men. Women, on the other hand, are said to be more neighbourhood based, and said to invest more care and attention in building and sustaining social contacts in the locality. But how far is this characterisation still relevant today?

Histories of social work have demonstrated that middle-class women in the nineteenth and early twentieth centuries fought to be allowed freedom of movement beyond the confinement of their homes and families (Cree 1995); the presence of working-class women on the streets was often associated with prostitution (hence the term 'street-walker') (Fulcher and Scott 2007: 506). As industrialisation and urbanisation progressed, so men were more likely to travel outside their locality to work. Women, on the other hand, were more likely to make more use of their local communities, as Cornwell's (1984) study in East London demonstrates. Women here occupied a much wider range of communal spaces than men: 'the shops, the street, the school gates, their relatives' houses'; and they had a much wider variety of contacts, 'not only with shopkeepers and other mothers, but also in the schools, pubs and blocks of flats where many of them are employed as cleaners' (1984: 50).

Campbell (1993) also highlights the importance of gender differences in an analysis of community in her account of the riots in the early 1990s in the working-class housing estates on the outskirts of Newcastle, Oxford and Cardiff. She conceptualises the destructiveness and brutal behaviour of young men as an attempt to reassert the power and privilege that had been lost along with the 'respectable' working-class neighbourhood, with its community facilities, clubs and employment. She contrasts the behaviour of the young men and young women as follows:

> The angry young men victimised the women, the neighbours, the community . . . The unruly women . . . had babies, made relationships, put food on the table, they cooperated and organised and created community politics.
>
> (1993: 244–5)

More recent analyses suggest that the question of men's and women's communities may be less stark and may, in reality, be changing. For example, Williams (1997) challenges the idea that women's centredness in their locality represents an exclusion from the outside world. She agrees that factors such as poverty, lack of time and independent transport, the identification of leisure facilities (pubs, clubs and playing fields) as 'men's spaces', and fear of violence or racial or sexual assault can confine women to their local neighbourhoods. Yet, she argues, women turn this confinement to their own ends, developing supportive relationships or getting involved in community action to fight for safer roads, for nursery provision, etc. Williams suggests that community has particular significance for many women: 'It is the point of negotiation over public provision; it is a site of organisation and struggle over welfare issues; and it is the arena of paid, unpaid and low-paid work' (1997: 34). Community, she continues, marks the overlap for women between private and public issues, between the personal and the political. Women as a result have a contradictory relationship with community: community as the 'space that women struggle to define as theirs', and community as the 'place to which women are confined' (1997: 42–3).

Other accounts of women's communities stress the shifts that have taken place over the last twenty years or so, as well as the different communities of which women are now a part. Wilson (1995) argues that, overall, the city has been a place of opportunity for women, as well as for men. Employment in the city brought women the chance of escaping the drudgery of unpaid labour in the household, and shopping became one of women's legitimate public activities. Of course, this is not to ignore the reality that occupational segregation still exists in employment, or that women continue to experience marginalisation, if not downright exclusion, from key areas of public life. Women, for example, made up only 19 per cent of UK Members of Parliament in 2009. Current sociological research shows much

Chapter 8

preoccupation with new communities of women, particularly those of young women, who can be seen testing both real and imagined boundaries any Saturday night across the cities of the UK. This will be explored further when we consider crime and deviance in Chapter 8.

Sexuality and community

Fulcher and Scott suggest that the 'hollowing out' of the city (the loss of economic activity, employment and population from the city centre) provided the space for another kind of community to emerge, one based on sexual orientation (2007: 517). The appearance of 'gay villages' in cities across the UK and US has been of considerable interest to sociologists. In an early example, Castells (1983) examined the ways in which gay men and some women came together in San Francisco to campaign for a space where they could feel safe from harassment and express their sexuality openly. This was, he argues, a very positive experience for those who subsequently chose to live or socialise in Castro Valley. But he acknowledges that within the community, class and political differences remained, just as competition remained between different oppressed groups in the city.

Taylor *et al.* are also interested in sexuality and community, this time focusing on two English cities, Manchester and Sheffield. In their 1996 study, they highlight four very different populations who make use of the town centres, shopping malls and major thoroughfares in these cities during the daytime and in the evenings: youth, gay men, shoppers and women. Of the four groups, only two (youth and gay men) had developed their own spaces within the public arena, creating their own safe areas. They highlight Manchester's gay village, with its own gay bars, clubs and shops: '. . . rather than being seen as a "gay ghetto", it is seen as a gay developed space, a place of ownership, a place of which to be proud' (Taylor *et al.* 1996: 117). Although used by some lesbian women, they note that this area has developed mainly as a space for gay men. The other two groups (shoppers and women) have not been able to create their own spaces in the same way. The shoppers are split between those who can afford to shop at the upmarket, American-style malls and those who are forced to use the declining city centres. Women's use of public space varies considerably according to the time of day. While almost half of those using the public spaces during the daytime are women, they constitute less than one-third of those using these areas in the evenings.

Taylor *et al.* (1996) argue that the sheer size of the city of Manchester meant that there were enough gay people to sustain an openly gay area. Furthermore, the existence of various ethnic communities (including a Chinatown and distinct Indian and Jewish areas) 'facilitated the tolerance of a gay village as just one more minority culture' (Fulcher and Scott 2007: 518). But their research highlights that sexuality was not the only structural factor to influence the creation of Manchester's gay village. Instead, gender remained an important subject in the equation.

Age and community

We have already noted that community is about keeping people out, as well as keeping people in. As the anthropologist James Brow notes: 'Differences among those who are incorporated within a community are often muted or obscured, while differences between insiders and outsiders are loudly affirmed' (1990: 3). This point is well made by Dawson (2002) in his study of older people and leisure clubs in Ashington, a former mining town in the north-east of England. Dawson found that the older people who used the clubs distinguished themselves from their more middle-class 'incomer' neighbours at many different levels, through use of local language and culture. But there were, significantly, generational differences too. The older people saw themselves as in a similar position to each other and different to the younger people of the area. What united them, Dawson argues, was their shared experience of bodily ageing, and they built a sense of community around this:

> The end of mining, the community's central referent was bound to threaten the end of community. Having said this, sameness and, in turn, community, is also represented as a consequence of bodily ageing. Most straightforwardly, talk amongst the elderly about bodily ageing leads to their self-identification as a common interest group. Similarly, their mutual participation in the activities surrounding management of bodily ageing, visiting clinics, picking-up prescriptions and so on, yields new social contacts.
>
> (2002: 31)

Disability and community

We cannot leave a discussion about community without considering the position of people with disabilities in relation to community. Two different issues come to the surface here: firstly, the systematic exclusion of disabled people from public spaces across our towns, cities and countryside; and secondly, the creation of a community of people with disabilities by disabled people themselves in reaction to this exclusion. In the introduction to a second edition of a classic text on disability, Swain *et al.* argue that the social model of disability (which locates disability within barriers and structures in society, not individuals) 'remains the fundamental stance for the critique of changing theory, policy and practice' (2004: 2). They point out that despite significant changes in legislation, disappointingly the dominant picture 'remains one of discrimination, prejudice, injustice and poverty, often rationalised on the grounds of supposed progress for disabled people' (2004: 1). Any improvements, they assert, have come as a direct result of action by disabled people themselves, either collectively or individually, rather than by a democratic impulse from government.

It is the concerted efforts of disabled people that Mayo (2000) is interested in exploring. She suggests that the Disabled People's Movement, which emerged in the UK in the 1960s, was initially focused on issues such as inadequate services and benefits. Since then, it has broadened its agenda to tackle the exclusion of disabled people from all areas of community life, arguing that changes are needed in attitude as well as environment. The Disabled People's Movement is now a worldwide organisation, with representation from over 100 countries; Disabled Peoples' International has its headquarters in Canada. But in spite of its successes, it has not, Mayo suggests, been 'any more free from internal tensions and conflicts than other parallel organisations' (2000: 58). Sometimes disagreement surfaces within countries, as seen, for example, in the debates in the UK about the special position of disabled women. At other times, conflict has arisen at international level, as different priorities and different issues come to the surface in relation to disabled people in the North (developed countries) and the South (developing countries).

Summary

In each of the discussions in this section, we have seen that community is positive and life affirming for its members and at the same time, reactive, negative and oppositional, both to other community groups and to individuals. We have also seen that there are complex interconnections between structural issues: people are likely to be excluded and oppressed on the basis of gender *and* disability, class *and* ethnicity. They also likely to gain by being a member of more than one powerful group: for example, by being white *and* middle class, or by being male *and* able bodied. But these groups are themselves changing; communities develop as they interact with each other and with their members. This takes us into post-modern perspectives.

Post-modern approaches to communities

Post-modern perspectives accept that we each participate in a range of different communities, and may identify ourselves as having 'multiple identities' and memberships; as people who are black and gay, white and working class, or female with a disability. Furthermore, some communities, as we will now explore, intentionally cross community groupings, while others have no physical presence at all, but exist in the 'virtual' world.

New social movements and community

One of the interesting features of community life over the last twenty years or so has been the emergence of 'new social movements', bringing together everyone from feminists and anti-racists to punks, gays and churchgoers, as seen in the creation of a number of groups which have developed to fight climate change, to campaign against the war in Iraq or to express concern about the global financial crisis. Castells sees these movements as largely positive, describing them as 'live schools' which produce new historical meanings, addressing real issues even if, as he argues, they lack the resources (financial and political) to actually resolve them (1983: 331).

The formation in social work of the Social Work Action Network (SWAN) in 2004 demonstrates another such grouping. As its website tells us, SWAN is a 'loose network of social work practitioners, academics, students and social welfare service users united in their concern that social work activity is being undermined by managerialism and marketisation, by the stigmatisation of service users and by welfare cuts and restrictions' (www.socialworkfuture.org/). SWAN organises national conferences and local events, bringing people together under the shared belief that social work is 'a profession worth fighting for'. It is too early to see whether SWAN will have a lasting impact on social work as a professional community. However, in bringing together students and academics with service users and practitioners, it is both reflecting and spearheading a wider drive towards collaboration and partnership in the social work enterprise. It is also acting as a driving force for change, reinvigorating a radical voice within social work.

Virtual communities

We acknowledged at the start of this chapter that communities do not need to be locality-based to survive; that communities can survive and even thrive across long distances. From as early as the 1960s, studies have demonstrated that social relationships do not need to be located in one geographical place in order to survive. Colin Bell's much acclaimed research into a middle-class housing estate in Swansea demonstrated that kinship ties and social networks could be maintained over long distances (Bell 1968). This is, of course, no longer just a middle-class phenomenon. Increasingly, working-class people live at some distance from their extended family; meanwhile friendship groups become more important on a day-to-day basis (Bulmer 1987: 55). Fulcher and Scott assert that while older communications technologies such as national postal systems and the telephone allowed for the extension of communities, it is the Internet that has enabled the creation of the 'virtual community'. Mobile phones, they continue, may allow us to carry our community around with us, but

> do not provide the independent basis for community in the way that the Net does. The bulletin boards, chat rooms, and multi-user domains of the Net escape the one-to-one limitations of the phone and make it possible for whole groups of people to interact electronically.
>
> (2007: 518)

In an analysis of what they call 'communities in cyberspace', Smith and Kollock note that there are two alternative visions about these virtual communities. The first highlights the positive effects of networks and their benefits for democracy and prosperity, arguing that they will

> generate opportunities for employment, political participation, social contact and enter-tainment. At their best, networks are said to renew community by strengthening the bonds that connect us to the wider social world while simultaneously increasing our power in that world.
>
> (1999: 4)

The alternative view is that the Internet has a darker side and offers new opportunities for surveillance and social control; it has the capacity to concentrate political power, and to create new forms of domination. Smith and Kollock do not express their own view about this debate; they sit on the fence, as I do, arguing that the outcomes of the changes that have taken and are taking place are not uniformly positive or negative. They put this succinctly: 'The new opportunities and constraints online interaction creates are double-edged, leading to results that can amplify both beneficial and noxious social processes' (ibid.).

This is very much the position adopted by Fulcher and Scott. They point out that some online communities are, more or less, 'disguised commercial operations', providing 'yet another means of targeting people with advertisements and selling them goods and services' (2007: 519). In addition, participation in a virtual community may take a person away from spending time in their 'real' communities. Yet virtual communities can, and do, offer support to their members. Slevin argues that we need to realise that when individuals use the Internet to establish and sustain communal relationships, they do as 'intelligent agents': they know a lot about the constraints and capabilities in this, but their knowledge is, essentially, 'always bounded' (2000: 109–10), as is knowledge in any other context. He challenges us not to ignore the structured social relations and contexts within which information is produced and received. Furthermore, he asserts that people do not build relationships out of nothing. What this suggests is that the communities that we build online may be no more or less 'real', intermittent or superficial than any of our other communities; that it is up to us to manage the complexities within this. Wall and Williams (2007) offer an interesting angle on this in their exploration of the ways in which virtual communities are controlled and regulated. They argue that online communities are surprisingly well ordered; that they employ

> [a] form of online community policing which exploits the 'natural surveillance' of networked technologies to facilitate both primary and secondary social control functions, while also mediating, where they arise, any disparities arising from national or jurisdictional legal differences in definition.
>
> (2007: 410)

The global village

But what of community in its broadest sense? It is a truism that in the twenty-first century,

globalisation embraces all aspects of our lives. As outlined in Chapter 1, Fulcher and Scott define globalisation as: 'a complex of interrelated processes, which have in common the idea that relationships and organisations have increasingly spread across the world, bringing about a growing awareness of the world as a whole' (2007: 623).

Chapter 1

Reviewing the impact of globalisation, some sociologists believe that it has led to the decline of the nation-state, with its separate territory, citizens and administration. Others dispute this, arguing that global organisations will continue to be dependent on nation-states in order to function. Furthermore, it is argued that local communities modify global cultures into something that fits their own culture, in a process known as 'glocalisation' (Robertson 1992). Looking ahead, it seems likely that as the world gets smaller and the power of multinational companies grows, so people will wish to look for meaning in their lives through the stories and traditions that are at the heart of imagined community. This means that in the future, while seeing ourselves as part of a worldwide social network (a 'global village'), we may also develop stronger ties with those around us; our sense of shared identity may be consolidated on a more local basis.

Nation and community

We began this chapter with the idea of the 'dream world' of community. It is appropriate to end with Benedict Anderson's (1991) definition of the nation as an 'imagined community': '*imagined* because the members of even the smallest nation will never know most of their fellow-members, meet them, or even hear of them, yet in the minds of each lives the image of their communion' (1991: 6). Anderson argues that all communities larger than primordial villages of exclusively face-to-face contact (and perhaps even these) are imagined; what distinguishes one community from another is the style in which they are imagined (ibid.). He continues:

> The nation is imagined as *limited* because even the largest of them . . . has finite, if elastic, boundaries, beyond which lie other nations . . . It is imagined as *sovereign* because the concept was born in an age in which Enlightenment and Revolution were destroying the legitimacy of the divinely-ordained, hierarchical dynastic realm . . . nations dream of being free, and, if under God, directly so . . . Finally, it is imagined as a *community* because, regardless of the actual inequality and exploitation that may prevail in each, the nation is always conceived as a deep, horizontal comradeship. Ultimately it is this fraternity that makes it possible, over the past two centuries, for so many millions of people, not so much to kill, as willingly to die for such limited imaginings.
>
> (1991: 7)

This, then, is the main focus of Anderson's enquiry: to reflect on why so many people have been willing to make the sacrifice of dying for their 'imagined community'. McCrone's (2001) study of Scotland provides further insight. He calls Scotland a nation without a state, or a 'stateless nation'; it lacks the political and economic control over its own affairs that is normally associated with nationhood. But Scotland is more than simply a geographical place. It is 'a landscape of the mind, a place of the imagination'. As Scotland lost its identity politically, culturally and economically, so it appropriated another vision, 'the Gaelic vision', further appropriated and incorporated into the twentieth-century tourist vision of Scotland. McCrone argues that the inventing of traditions and the creation of myths is not peculiar only to Scotland: 'myth-history' is a vital part of the storytelling of any country, and traditions themselves serve a positive function in legitimising institutions, symbolising group cohesion and socialising others into values and beliefs. McCrone rejects the idea that nationalism is always reactionary or atavistic. He argues that there is neither a 'single' explanation of nationalism, nor one single type. Above all, he writes in the first edition of his book, 'nationalism, or national identity, is not a characteristic, but imputes a relationship between different identities. To be Scottish, for example, is to be not English' (1992: 207).

This demonstrates that community is about creating and maintaining the boundary between 'us' and 'them', as much as about a specific quality or sentiment shared by 'us'. Territory and boundaries are not real in themselves, but are socially created and recreated in our encounters with those on the other side of the divide. So how are we, finally, to view this? Bauman (2001) seems pessimistic. He argues that it is in the search for community, real or fabricated, that some of the worst aspects of social exclusion, racism and fascism are brought into being. And yet he ends his discussion on community with the thought that: 'If there is to be a community in the world of [the] individuals, it can only be (and it needs to be) a community woven together from sharing and mutual care; a community of concern and responsibility for the equal right to be human and the equal ability to act on that right' (2001: 149–50). This is very much the community envisioned by Bob Holman (1997), radical social worker and neighbourhood activist, and one which he challenges us to play a part in supporting. It is also the community outlined in more recent textbooks on community social work (see Butcher *et al.* 2007, Pierson 2008).

Implications for practice

- In attempting to build community solidarity, we need to be aware of the dangers within this, since it is the perceived differences between 'us' and 'them' that strengthen our sense of 'us'.

- We also need to remember that people are part of different communities and that our communities are often contradictory and fluid. This will have an impact on how we work with both individuals and communities.

Conclusion

I have argued that although it is easy to be in favour of the idea of community, community is, in practice, a highly problematic concept. Community is as much about social polarisation and exclusion as it is about mutuality and neighbourliness. Whether we understand community as a geographical locality, social network or sense of identity, it has the capacity to be used both positively and negatively: 'community can serve to integrate membership groups with antagonistic interests, and to mobilize them for conflict, rather than sustain programmes for harmonization and inclusion' (Jordan 1996: 164). What this suggests is the need for a critical community practice, as outlined by Sarah Banks. She admits that there is 'no single recipe for developing the qualities of the critical practitioner' (2007: 145), but nevertheless, she proposes that we should work towards the following:

- Clarifying and questioning personal, professional, organisational and political values;

- Identifying underlying assumptions or dominant narratives in the discourses of practitioners and others;

- Challenging dominant discourses that are disempowering;

- Being honest about the power relations in situations, while working towards greater equality;

- Paying attention to the whole context in which the practice takes place.

(Banks 2007: 146)

Recommended reading

Bauman, Z. (2001) *Community: Seeking Safety in an Insecure World*, Cambridge: Polity Press. A challenging, inspirational, short book.

Butcher, H., Banks, S., Henderson, P. and Robertson, R. (eds) (2007) *Critical Community Practice*, Bristol: The Policy Press. An edited collection which will be very useful in practice settings and includes Banks's chapter discussed above.

Day, G. (2006) *Community and Everyday Life*, London: Routledge. A good overview of the issues discussed in this chapter.

6 Care and caring

Introduction

The focus of this chapter is a sociological examination of the concepts of care and caring. As we will discover, care and caring have been largely unproblematised in sociology, invisible in normative, functionalist notions about women and women's role in the family and society. Disappointingly, care and caring still struggle for attention in sociological textbooks. There is only a brief mention of both

Chapter 1

in the reference books recommended at the end of Chapter 1, and always in a broader analysis of something else, often the family or gender issues or, in the case of Macionis and Plummer (2008), a discussion about disability. The lack of attention to care and caring in conventional sociological writing should not, however, let the reader think that these topics have been under-researched, or that there is little to say about them. On the

contrary, there has been a huge amount of empirical research and theorising about care and caring over the last thirty years or so. More recently, analysis has taken on board insights from care recipients as well as care givers, and a wider structural perspective has emerged highlighting the importance of 'race', class, age and disability, as well as issues of gender and sexuality. The twenty-first century has also brought new challenges, as the information revolution and 'telecare' change the ways in which care is conceptualised, delivered and received.

This chapter will discuss care and caring together, not least because the terms are used inter-changeably in much of the literature. The context in which the discussion is set in this chapter will be largely a developed world, UK/US context, although it will be acknowledged that care and caring are conceptualised and delivered in very different ways in the developing world. We begin, as always, by exploring definitions.

Definitions

The concept of 'care' is extremely diverse, and this can lead to some confusion, as academics and researchers, politicians, policy makers and practitioners, user groups and members of the public all make claims about 'care' as if they were all talking about the same thing, when often, in reality, they are not. Care can be paid or unpaid, carried out by oneself, by family members or non-relatives, carried out in institutional settings or in one's own home, conducted as part of a loving or a professional relationship. The different aspects of care can be outlined as follows (adapted from Brechin *et al.* 1998).

But is it as simple as this might seem to suggest? For example, where is foster care located here? It is, in many ways, a kind of informal care at home, but it is also increasingly being treated as a professional job comparable to that of a child care worker in any other setting. This is necessary, given the ever more complex backgrounds of many fostered children. Similarly, what happens when a friend or partner becomes the paid carer of a person with a disability or dementia? What is the dividing line between this and professional care? Should we, as members of society, expect different things of people, depending on whether they have a professional or loving relationship with a person who requires support services? What is the difference, if any, between care and caring? And where does parenting fit? Would it be desirable (if affordable) for parents to be paid to look after their own children at home, as early feminist campaigns urged, or would this change the very nature of that caring?

Defining care and caring is made all the more difficult because of the value judgements at the heart of our understandings of care. Brechin *et al.* identify four key assumptions at work in this. Firstly, there is the idea that the impulse to care occurs 'spontaneously within families and kinship systems', that families 'look after their own', and that this is 'the primary, everyday route by which care is made

Table 6.1
What is care?

	Formal	Informal
Paid	Paid care by non-relatives (social care, social work or health practitioners), likely to be in an institutional setting, which may be day care or residential	Paid domestic help, or paid care by family members or partners, often at home or in the carer's home
Unpaid	Volunteer carers trained to work with those in institutional settings	Unpaid care by family members, friends or neighbours of someone in their own home

available' (Brechin *et al.* 1998: 2). Running alongside this is the notion that paid and regulated care 'do not arise spontaneously as a result of a naturally-occurring, affectional relationship' (ibid.). The third assumption, leading on from the first and second, is that family care is the ideal; paid care, in contrast, is always understood to be 'a second best – a substitute, as it were, for the genuine article' (1998: 3). Research on the positive value of residential childcare for some children would suggest that this claim is far from incontrovertible (Smith 2009). This takes us to the fourth assumption: that community care should either sustain family-based care or be modelled on a notion of family care. This is highly problematic, argues Brechin, not least because it is 'an idealised western version of family and home' which is presenting the model for 'good care' (ibid.)

There is one final issue about definitions. Care, as we will see, might mean a small amount of help which allows a person to remain independent at home, or it may mean the round-the-clock physical care of someone who is unable to feed themselves or manage their personal care. This tells us nothing, however, about either the feelings that care generates or the quality of the caring relationship. Care has the potential to be, in Brechin's words, 'a disempowering and dependency-inducing process' or 'a wholly enabling, non-possessive form of assistance (ibid.). There are a great many influences on how care is given and received, as this chapter will demonstrate. There are also many different perspectives to be considered, including those of service users, carers, practitioners from different fields (social work, health and education), academics, researchers and social policy analysts.

Implications for practice

- As always, we must be careful about what is meant when we come across the terms 'care' and 'caring' in social work. We must question the assumptions behind what is being said, as well as our own, often unexamined, assumptions.

- Ideas about 'good care' are intimately linked with Western notions about families; this might not fit in different contexts. Moreover, the reality of care might be quite different to the idealised picture.

Historical accounts

To understand where our ideas about care and caring come from, we need to go back in time (see Cree and Myers 2008 for a fuller account). In pre-industrial Britain, all family members were expected to contribute to the family's livelihood, and in return, they were cared for by, and in, the family. Over and above this, landlords gave some support to their tenants (this might have been financial and/or practical help) in times of short-term need while voluntary collections were made and distributed by churches to those in need, and monasteries provided residential and hospital care (almshouses) for some sick and elderly people. With the decline of the monasteries and their subsequent dissolution in 1536, an important avenue of care disappeared from the social landscape. In 1601, the Elizabethan Poor Law Act (England & Wales) confirmed the principle that family duty in welfare was paramount:

> It should be the duty of the father, grandfather, mother, grandmother, husband or child of a poor, old, blind, lame or impotent person, or other poor person, not able to work, if possessed of sufficient means, to relieve and maintain that person.
>
> (Section 6 of the Poor Law Act 1601, referenced in Thane 1996: 205)

The 1601 Act, mirrored by legislation in Scotland, authorised parishes to raise income through a tax on property to pay for help for those who had no family support. It also determined for whom help should be provided (Fraser 2003):

- The 'impotent poor' (the aged, chronic sick, blind and mentally ill who needed residential care) were to be accommodated in voluntary almshouses.

- The 'able-bodied poor' were to be set to work in a workhouse (they were felt to be able to work but were lazy).

- The 'able-bodied poor' who absconded or 'persistent idlers' who refused work were to be punished in a 'house of correction'.

Industrialisation and urbanisation put new pressures on families and parishes alike. As the young and mobile left the countryside in search of work, so older people, sick and disabled people and children were left without a family member to care for them. At the same time, as production shifted to factories, shops and offices, 'this separation of work from home signalled a profound change in gender relations' (Bilton et al. 2002: 142). Traditional systems of care broke down, and increasing numbers of people were forced to seek help from voluntary and public agencies (Fraser 2003). In 1834, a new Poor Law Amendment Act was passed in an attempt to stem the flood of need and demand. This Act reaffirmed that there should be no poor relief for the able-bodied unemployed outside the workhouse, and divided the poor into two groups (Mooney 1998):

1. the 'deserving poor' (e.g. elderly, sick or disabled people, orphans and widows) who were to receive financial and practical support (often home based) from charitable or voluntary organisations;

2. the 'undeserving poor' (e.g. able-bodied unemployed men, single mothers, prostitutes) who were forced to turn to the state, and thus to the workhouse.

The late eighteenth and nineteenth centuries saw the introduction of a great many initiatives which might be described as public care: schemes for sanitation, education, hospitals and clinics, policing and prisons, juvenile correction, workhouses and mental asylums. New laws governing working conditions and the treatment of children were introduced, as well as new mechanisms for recording population change (Cree 2008). On the voluntary front, there was an explosion in philanthropic activity, with the emergence of visiting societies and charities dedicated to treating every conceivable social ill. The underlying idea behind these efforts was the same. Those who were seen as 'deserving' were to be helped to help themselves; care would always be limited, so as to encourage self-reliance and independence. At the same time, the 'undeserving poor' were to be deterred from seeking help, by their separation from family and friends and by the harshness of the institutional regime (see Cree and Myers 2008).

By the end of the nineteenth century, social and economic problems had increased to such an extent that the old principles that had defined the Poor Law were glaringly no longer fit for purpose (if they had ever been). Voluntary measures of care could no longer meet the growing needs, and neither could the workhouses and poorhouses, which were full to overflowing at the end of the nineteenth century (Fraser 2003). In the twentieth century, new, more egalitarian, ideas came to the fore, as demonstrated in the provision of universal services in education and health, as well as the 'safety net' of social services. Care became increasingly incorporated into the state, either carried out directly by the state, or by the voluntary sector on its behalf, and statutory agencies became responsible for controlling the voluntary sector (and more recently the private sector) through funding and inspection arrangements. At the same time, care work became progressively conceptualised as a professional activity, not something which could simply be left either to the untrained relative or the 'do-gooding' amateur without guidance and supervision.

Reviewing the historical narrative, it is clear that the idea that the family should be the main provider of care is deeply rooted in the UK psyche. However, it is also accepted today that this care should be regulated and monitored by the state, through the provision of a host of professionals whose job is, in Donzelot's words (1980), to 'police' families. Beyond this, there is the ever-present notion that those in need should be deterred from asking for support, and that any help that is provided should always be at a minimum level. Cross-cultural evidence reminds us that these ideas are culturally specific, not universally held by all.

Cross-cultural studies

Oakley's 1974 study of housework identified that in non-industrialised societies there was no division between work and family life, or between something that was done to earn a living (called 'work') and what was done the rest of the time. She cites the work of Rapoport and Rapoport, who argued that in traditional societies, work and family structures tended to be linked as 'parts of an integrated cultural whole sustained by a complex web of social controls' (1965: 831). Oakley provides two examples of African societies to illustrate this point. In one, there was a minimal division of labour by sex, and work relationships coincided with kin relationships. In the other, a relatively rigid system of rules for the division of labour by sex was applied, but even here the distinction was not between home, domestic work and family life on the one hand and non-family work outside the home on the

Chapter 3

other. Instead, work tasks were divided by gender, in much the same way as we have already discussed in Chapter 3 in relation to the work of Scottish crofter families in the early years of the twentieth century. Oakley concludes that the separation between home and work is not a universal feature of human society, but rather an aspect of industrialised society (1974: 13).

More recent anthropological studies of welfare suggest that this might be overly simplistic; that communities where there is little separation between home and work continue to exist within industrialised societies. For example, in writing about their research in an agricultural community in the north of England, Christensen *et al.* (1998) point out that here family relationships are also work relationships, 'mapped onto the land and patterning the local community' (1998: 20). This means that when someone becomes ill and needs care, it is the family and the community (some of whom are relatives) who step in to give support, until the sick person is able to ease himself or herself back into work again. Christensen *et al.* identify a continuum between sickness and well-being within the farming community, in contrast to 'the urban polarization of illness and health which is marked by receipt of "sick pay"' (1998: 24). They conclude that distinctions between 'client' and 'carer' and between 'self' and 'family' may not be appropriate in some cultural contexts; that a model of care which privileges the individual cannot accommodate the interdependence that is at the heart of the experience of farming communities.

Cross-cultural evidence confirms that understandings of care are inevitably rooted in cultural and social contexts. The organisation and delivery of childcare is a good case in point here, illustrated in two very different examples. In the first, let us consider the 'children's societies' which were the traditional pattern in the kibbutz in Israel. Children were raised in common dormitories and stayed at their parents' homes for only a few hours each day, allowing the adults to engage in work and leisure while the children were being educated by others (Gavron 2000). The second example concerns Nigeria's customary practice of fostering children out to a senior member of the extended family who took on the responsibility to care for the child. Fostering was seen as a positive choice for children, strengthening their relationships and their socialisation (Oyemade 1980). In more recent years, this practice has been extended to non-family members. Oni (1995) suggests that child fostering demonstrates the Nigerian view that a child does not belong only to his or her biological parents, but rather to both the immediate and the whole extended family. Not only this, it is viewed as having both social and economic benefits, since it enables children from rural families to attend school in towns and, at the same time, to make a contribution to the family's income through paid work as 'house helps'. It is not my intention to comment on either of these examples as illustrations of 'good' or 'bad' childcare. Instead, the fact that such different patterns exist at all reminds us that our own ways of thinking about childcare are just that: they are our own ways of thinking.

> **Implications for practice**
>
> • Historical evidence demonstrates that the underlying assumption about care and caring is that it is provided in, and by, the family. How then, do we as social workers judge those who feel unable to care for their family members?
>
> • Cross-cultural studies show that UK patterns of care and caring are culturally, as well as historically, specific.

Traditional sociological approaches

As already stated at the beginning of this chapter, conventional sociological approaches did not see the topic of care and caring as worthy of investigation in its own right, unlike employment, which has generated extensive sociological attention over the years. Caring was invisible in the family; something which women did (predominantly), and which was only carried out by other people when 'normal' family care systems failed, for one reason or another. If functionalist sociology had anything to say about caring, it was to affirm that the sexual division of labour (with men working in a paid capacity outside the home and women working unpaid inside the family) was desirable for individual family members, and an important part of the socialisation of children. It was also seen as being useful ('functional') for the well-being of society as a whole (see, for example, Parsons 1964).

Marxist accounts, as discussed in Chapter 2, drew attention to the inaccuracy of this narrow representation of women as homemakers. It was noted that women performed a dual role in society, at home and in the workplace, sometimes at times of labour shortage – for example, during the Second World War – at other times as part of the regular workforce (Knuttila 2005). It was women's paid work that was the object of scrutiny here; their caring work in the family merited little notice.

The emergence of caring as a subject of sociological interest in the mid-1970s both reflected and anticipated wider political, social and economic changes. From the 1960s onwards, feminist sociologists and psychologists had been asking fundamental questions about the relationship between women's private and public lives, seeking to challenge the sexual division of labour in the home and in society. One of the first sociological studies to focus directly on women's home-working was Ann Oakley's groundbreaking *Housewife*, published in 1974. In this book, she highlights the ways in which women's work at home is concealed. She identifies that it is physically isolating and totally self-defined, with a role that she describes as infinitely variable and personal. The fact that housewives were often also engaged in paid employment outside the home does not escape her attention. She reports that while nine out of ten women who were not employed were housewives, so were seven out of ten of those with a job outside the home (1974: 6). She concludes that the trivialisation of housework was intimately connected to the fact that it was work which was largely carried out by women. Two US psychological texts published in the late 1970s and early 1980s have been similarly influential in helping to challenge conventional ideas about women, men and human agency. In *The Reproduction of Mothering*, Nancy Chodorow (1978) observed that girls grow up to be more involved in care than boys because it is mothers, not fathers, who are mainly involved in their upbringing; they learn to be good at relationships and to care for others through their own experience of being cared for by their mothers. Women's connectedness to others was also the central theme in Carol Gilligan's 1982 book, *In a Different Voice*, in which she criticised Lawrence Kolhlberg's six-stage model of human development (1981), arguing that this model had been created on the basis of men and men's way of thinking about the world (all Kohlberg's subjects were men). Gilligan asserted that an ethic of care that is built on relationships (that is, a woman's perspective) is just as important as an ethic of justice (which was identified as a male world-view). Much of the subsequent literature on caring explicitly, and sometimes implicitly, engages with and builds on these ideas.

Sociological research has also been hugely influenced by the emergence of the Disabled People's Movement. It was the Union of the Physically Impaired against Segregation, set up in the United States in 1974, that first defined disability as being socially caused, and acted to spearhead a collective struggle for change (Davis 1996: 126–7). The disability rights movement subsequently challenged the 'personal tragedy theory of disability' (Oliver 1990) and put in its place a campaign for civil rights for people with disabilities.

Demographic changes forced the issue of caring onto the academic and government agenda. While women's rights and the rights of disabled people were being championed, so forecasts of escalating costs of meeting the health and welfare needs of older people strengthened the UK government's preference for community care (Arber and Ginn 1992b: 86). Henwood (1990) reports that the total population of disabled and older people increased by nearly one-third between 1961 and 1981. Although the overall increase was expected to slow down between 1981 and 2001, the proportion of very elderly people (and hence those most likely to need some form of assistance and care) was expected to more than double. As older people were living longer (and, it was suggested, living longer with increasing ill health), so divorce and women's employment outside the home were increasing, raising fears about how care needs might be met in the future. In consequence, there was a qualitative shift in the meaning of community care during the 1970s, from care 'in' the community to care 'by' the community.

New directions

Three interrelated questions were addressed in the 1980s' sociological literature on caring: Who cares? What is caring? Why do people care? Much of this research was grounded in feminist theory and practice. The methodology used was predominantly interpretive, seeking to understand what care means to those who provide it.

Who cares?

The starting point for the problematisation of caring lies in an Equal Opportunities Commission (EOC) research study and a polemical article by Finch and Groves, both published in 1980 and both drawing attention to the fact that caring was something which was done mainly by women. The EOC study was based on a postal questionnaire to 2,500 randomly selected households in West Yorkshire. The study found that of the 116 people identified as carers, 75 per cent were women and 25 per cent were men. An EOC report, published two years later, estimated from this that there were 1.25 million female carers in Britain. Finch and Groves's (1980) article is scathing about what they identify as a discrepancy between the government's commitment to equal opportunities for women and men (as evidenced by legislation) and community care policies that relied on women's unpaid domestic labour. They argue that the two cannot go together: policies for community care were, within a context of public expenditure cuts, incompatible with policies for equal opportunities for women. They summarise with what became a much-quoted equation: 'that in practice, community care equals care by the family, and in practice care by the family equals care by women' (1980: 494). (A *Women and Employment Survey* (Martin and Roberts 1984) provided further evidence, stating that 13 per cent of all women had caring responsibilities for sick or elderly dependants.) A number of studies of women carers confirm that it is women who are carers, including Brody (1981) on 'women in the middle', caught at a time in their lives between caring for children and parents at the same time; Lewis and Meredith (1988) on daughters who care; Glendinning (1992) on the costs of care giving; and Nissel and Bonnerjea (1982) on caring for older relatives.

Although the EOC research has subsequently been severely criticised for its overly simplistic methodology and analysis (see Fisher 1994), this study and Finch and Groves's article set the parameters for the feminist critique of caring in the 1980s. Elizabeth Wilson (1982), for example, argues that older people were not being cared for by the 'community': 'They are being cared for exclusively and predominantly by their daughters and daughters-in-law'. She urges that the term 'community' be abandoned altogether as a 'veil of illusion' which cocoons and oppresses women (1982: 55). Janet Finch, provocatively, goes on to propose that in order to safeguard the position of women, residential and institutional care should be extended as an alternative to community care. She asserts that there can be no non-sexist version of community care; informal care inevitably falls on women and women's networks. Because of this, 'the residential route is the only one which ultimately will offer us a way out of the impasse of caring' (1984: 16). Gillian Dalley (1988) agrees with this position. She asserts that social policy must develop along collectivist principles, in place of the familist and individualist principles that motivated community care policies at that time.

What is caring?

An important issue for the unfolding sociological analysis of caring has been the exploration of the nature of caring itself; that is, what is caring? Sociologists have drawn attention to the fact that caring is work, although often unseen and unrecognised as such. This subject was first exposed in Ann Oakley's 1974 classic investigation of housework. It was then developed by Roy Parker (1981), who makes the distinction between caring *for* and caring *about* someone: while friendship typically involves the latter, it does not usually involve the former. Caring *for* someone, he suggests, 'comprises such things as feeding, washing, lifting, protecting, representing and comforting' (1981: 3). All these tasks take time, and the time cannot be used for anything else. Caring *about* someone, in contrast, does not use up time in this way. Thus caring for someone, he argues, should be re-named 'tending' a person, since it is a time-consuming activity that takes place in the context of obligations that are socially, not affectively, constructed. The idea of caring as 'tending' was subsequently taken up by feminist writers including Ungerson (1983).

Hilary Graham takes issue with Parker's conceptualisation. For Graham, caring is more than 'a kind of domestic labour performed on people . . . Caring cannot be understood objectively and abstractly, but only as a subjective experience in which we are all, for better or worse involved' (1983: 27–8). Drawing on the earlier feminist analysis, Graham considers the ways in which caring is a fundamental part of female self-identity. The caring role, she advises, is reproduced in women themselves through the dynamics of the mother-daughter relationship. It is also linked to the wider sexual division of labour in society:

> [It is] constructed through a network of social and economic relations, both within the home and the workplace, in which women take responsibility for meeting the emotional and material needs not only of husbands and children, but of the elderly, the handicapped, the sick and the unhappy.
>
> (1983: 22)

Graham argues for a re-conception of caring, one that takes on board 'both love and labour, both identity and activity' (1983: 13). Caring, she suggests, is a work-role 'whose form and content is shaped (and continually reshaped) by our intimate, social and sexual relationships' (1983: 29). It is also the medium through which women gain access to both the private and the public world, as wives and mothers, secretaries and social workers. She concludes:

> . . . caring defines both the identity and the activity of women in Western society. It defines what it feels like to be a woman in a male-dominated and capitalist social order . . . Thus, caring is not something on the periphery of our social order; it marks the point at which the relations of capital and gender intersect.
>
> (1983: 30)

Graham's article has proved to be extremely influential, and also controversial, for feminists and sociologists alike. Conflict between the idea of caring as work and caring as identity has remained a live issue in the caring literature. Graham has herself shifted her position considerably in recent years, as we will discuss later in this chapter.

Why do people care?

Sociological studies conducted in the 1980s offer a range of explanations for why people care, many of them overlapping with each other.

Practical considerations

Some research has focused on the impact of practical exigencies in determining whether or not people care for others. For example, studies have considered the number of people in the household ('is there space for granny?') and geographical proximity (is daily or weekly care feasible and possible?). Research has shown that physical proximity is not the only reason for caring. Abrams et al. (1989 [1978]) in a study of neighbourhood care found that although living near someone may facilitate the giving of help, it does not determine that help will be given. They argue that informal neighbourhood caring is activated primarily as a result of an existing social context, within which resources, relationships and culture enable or impede help. In addition, physical space (or the lack of it) seems to bear little relation to whether or not care is given.

Time and opportunity

Another way of answering this question might be to think about which family members actually have the time or opportunity to care. Ungerson (1983) demonstrates that this issue is fundamentally connected with women and women's place at home and in the labour market. She argues that women's unequal position in the labour market makes it likely that for a married couple the most 'rational' decision is usually that the women should give up work to look after a relative in need of care. This in turn reinforces the general belief that caring is women's work. She writes: 'The ideology of housework and women's place within it has a material impact on women's paid work which in turn serves to reinforce that very ideology' (1983: 38).

Researchers were also interested to see what impact, if any, unemployment had on people's caring. Nissel and Bonnerjea's (1982) study used time diaries with forty-four married-couple households caring for an older dependent relative. They found that wives spent on average between two and three hours every day undertaking essential care for the relative, irrespective of whether or not they were in paid employment. The husbands, in contrast, spent only eight minutes. This finding is reflected in studies of men's and women's involvement in housework in dual income families. Hochschild (1990) observes that it is women who are most likely to do 'the second shift' – preparing the evening meal, loading the washing machine and getting up in the night for a sick child. Interestingly, Qureshi and Walker's study of fifty-eight carers found that working sons were more likely to provide assistance to elderly parents than unemployed sons: nearly two in five did so, as compared with only one in five unemployed sons (1989: 115). More recent research confirms that being unemployed does not make a person more likely to care, as cited at the end of this chapter.

By accident

Some people (men and women) find themselves caring for someone by accident. They may never have left home, and find themselves in adulthood caring for an elderly or sick parent. Many others find themselves in a caring role when a partner (or parent) becomes sick or disabled. Fay Wright's (1986) research into single people caring for relatives found that whilst women and men both cared for their relatives in this situation, gender played a significant part in determining the kind of care that was sought and given. In her study, mothers living with sons were less dependent than were those living with daughters. She also established that caring for a parent affected women's employment far more than men's; they were more likely to go part time and even give up work completely to care for a relative. Perhaps surprisingly, she discovered that sons received less help from kin and neighbours, because they were less likely to be plugged into informal caring networks and exchanges.

For money

Some people care for others for money. It is the decrease in availability of women to carry out unpaid caring which has forced the government to look at ways of encouraging women back into caring through financial inducements. More women are working, full and part time; less women are at home caring for children and dependent relatives (and so available for volunteering); more women are married (so there are less single daughters around); and more women are living too far away to provide daily or even weekly care. The family may not be able to continue to meet its own needs for care, never mind take on caring for others. As a consequence, there has been a steady expansion in new schemes to pay carers, such as community care schemes which pay relatives for expenses only, and schemes in which 'ordinary people' provide live-in and foster care situations for an increasingly wide range of client groups (Leat and Gay 1987).

Affect and reciprocity

In an early study, Abrams (1978) suggests that affect and reciprocity are important determinants of informal helping; in other words, we care for those we like, and those who we feel a debt of gratitude towards. Qureshi and Walker (1989) surveyed three hundred people aged seventy-five or over living in Sheffield in 1982 and 1983, and conducted follow-up interviews with fifty-eight informal carers. They investigated both affect and reciprocity: firstly, in questions about emotional closeness and shared interests between the older person and their helper; and secondly, in questions about past and present help given by the older person to the helper. Their findings suggest that neither affect nor reciprocity is essential for the provision of practical care or tending. Although affect and reciprocity are extremely important in determining the nature of the caring experience, they do not determine the actual supply of practical assistance.

Duty and obligation

Duty and obligation are closely linked to the idea of reciprocity, and are rooted in societal and kinship norms. In Qureshi and Walker's 1989 study, both care givers and care recipients agreed that caring needs should be met first and foremost in the family. They went on to identify a hierarchy in decision making about who the carer should be, based firmly on traditional (and Western), normative expectations of kinship obligations. Perhaps surprisingly, gender was not the most important determinant of the obligation to care. Instead, marital relationship and long-term co-residence took precedence over gender. Although the hierarchical principles could be overruled by the ill health of prospective helpers, they suggest that the following model largely holds true (1989: 126):

1. spouse (or relative in a lifelong joint household);

2. daughter;

3. daughter-in-law;

4. son;

5. other relative;

6. non-relative.

Challenges to the feminist orthodoxy

Although the 1980s' studies made a significant contribution to an understanding of care and caring, there have been a number of fundamental objections to the studies. These have centred on three main criticisms: that the studies largely ignored the perspectives of those who were cared for; that care givers were too narrowly defined in the studies; and, leading on from this, that the studies failed to realise that the experience of caring, whether from the perspective of the 'service user' or 'carer', must be located in wider structural issues, including class, 'race' and ethnicity, gender, age and disability, etc.

Perspectives of those who receive care

Critics argue that by focusing on the experiences of care givers and the perceived 'burden' of care, many of the feminist studies from the 1980s ignored the perspectives of care recipients, and the importance of the two-way relationship between carer and recipient (for example, Fisher 1997, Morris 1991, 1995 and 1997). Research demonstrates that many of those who receive care (for example, older people and those with physical disabilities and mental health problems) also continue to care for others in spite of their disabilities; caring for a child, grandchild or older person, preparing meals, doing housework, etc. (for example, Clarke 1995, Widdowson 2004). In consequence, there is a much less clear division between care giver and care recipient, or to use more emotive language, between 'carer' and 'dependant'. Morris observes that none of the disabled people whom she interviewed for her study referred to the family members who helped them as 'carers': they talked about their relationships with their partners, children, parents and friends, not their 'carers' (1995: 90). Caring is not a 'one-way street': people care for each other in what is frequently a shared, reciprocal relationship. Morris goes as far as to assert that the ideology of 'care' and 'carers' is itself a form of oppression (1997).

Research studies also show that people who may require care hold onto their independence for as long as they can, struggling alone at home, or in the marital relationship, before admitting that they need help. The older people surveyed by Qureshi and Walker (1989) felt strongly that they did not wish to become a burden to their children. They write: 'Elderly people do not give up their independence easily; with few exceptions they are reluctant subjects in caring and dependency' (1989: 18–19). When care was inevitable, they preferred their care needs to be met in the family, first and foremost by their spouse or an adult who shared their household. Arber and Ginn (1992b: 93), drawing on their own earlier research and on wider literature, offer a revised hierarchy of older people's preferences for care contexts:

1. In elderly person's own home – self care.

2. In elderly person's own home – care provided by co-resident:

    (i)   Spouse.
    (ii) Other same-generation relative.
    (iii) Child or non-kin.

3. In elderly person's own home – care provided by extra-resident:

    (iv) Child.
    (v)   Other relative.
    (vi) Neighbour, friend, volunteer.

4. In care-giver's own home:

    (vii) Unmarried child.
    (viii) Married child.

This model confirms Qureshi and Walker's broad findings, but provides new insight into the experience of receiving care. Care preferences can be understood as being based largely on a context of care where the older person feels that they can hold onto the freedom and integrity that they enjoyed in the past. Studies of care preferences of people with disabilities shed further light on this issue. This literature suggests that some care recipients may prefer to receive at least some of their care from a person outside their family; for example, a volunteer or a paid professional (Clarke 1995: 30). This allows them to feel more independence and autonomy, and enables them to protect the balance of their personal relationships. Morris (1995) cites the views of one disabled care recipient, Catherine:

> It's very difficult to ask somebody that you're also in a loving relationship with, it's very difficult to constantly ask them for the basic things you need. I find it's a sort of breath of fresh air in a way when my helper comes in and I have loads and loads of different things that I couldn't ask Robert to do . . . I know that there'll be no strings, no other strings attached to the asking, it's just a straight can you do that.
>
> (1995: 86)

This quotation clearly refutes the notion that unpaid 'family' care is always somehow superior to professional or unpaid care. It also resonates strongly with Parker's early (1981) conceptualisation of caring as 'work'.

Perspectives of those who give care

Critics argue that by concentrating on the kin care provided by women carers, (specifically, Brody's (1981) 'women in the middle'), many of the 1980s studies lost sight of other people who care; notably male spouses, sons, children and other older people, as well as the paid carers who work in different settings. In reviewing the early studies, Thomas concludes that the very narrow characterisation of caring led to a 'partial and fragmented understanding of society's caring activity' (1993: 667).

Recent research on those who care for others demonstrates that four in ten carers are spouses, mainly older people, and half of these are men (Fink 2004). Many men (just like women) become carers 'by default', either because their partner becomes ill and is in need of care or because they never left the parental home and a parent becomes unwell. This does not imply that they are unhappy with this, however. Fisher (1994) criticises the idea of caring as a 'burden' for three main reasons. Firstly, he points out that many carers, both men and women, feel that they have 'chosen' their role; as they say, 'they would not have it any other way' (1994: 668). Secondly, studies demonstrate that caring may be a rewarding experience for carers, when it takes place in the context of an enduring and mutually satisfying relationship. Thirdly, there is no absolute 'burden' experienced by all. Instead, there are moments when the caring burden seems greatest, at different stages in the caring relationship, and in different ways with different people. This reflects Lewis and Meredith's (1988) observation that caring is best understood as a sequence, not a fixed entity. In their study of daughters who care, they argue that just as a person's need for care is likely to move along a continuum from needing a little care to needing a lot, likewise a carer's need for support will change. They urge that care professionals take this into account in making assessments, instead of waiting for support systems to break down before intervening.

Fisher concludes that men's feelings about taking on caring responsibilities differ little to those of women: men discuss a sense of love and duty, a desire to 'pay back' the care that they have received from their wives, and to protect their children from the demands of caring. Men also report an increased closeness to their partners, and a feeling of satisfaction in 'doing what is right' (1994: 669). An excerpt from Bytheway's 1987 transcript of an interview with a male carer expresses this well:

Interviewer: . . . I'm just wondering if [the nursing] came easily to you?

Steelworker: It did. It astonished me. It really astonished me because I found I've got an enormous amount of patience . . . She was a marvellous housekeeper. She could whip up a meal in ten minutes flat honestly, if people called to the house, and that's happened on more than one occasion . . . But then, when it came to be my turn, when I had to do it, I had no regrets because she had looked after me for over thirty years and I thought well she can't do it now,

I have to do my best. I didn't prevaricate, I didn't think it was the wrong thing to do. I was glad of the opportunity to pay her back ... I accepted that. Put it as a labour of love more than anything else.

(1987: 56)

This is precisely the language that Graham used in 1983 to describe women and caring. It makes it clear that the ability to 'recognise the need for care, and prioritise social relationships above personal gratification' (Fisher 1994: 670) is a quality that is not owned solely by women. This is important for social work and for society more generally, as I have argued previously (Cree 1996). Ideas of women's 'natural' or 'essential' capacity to care lead to harsh judgements of women who do not live up to this stereotypical picture. They also seem pessimistic about the possibility of change; of greater equality between men and women (1996: 66).

'Doing what is right' is a central concern of Finch and Mason's (1993) study of family obligations. They interviewed 978 adults of all ages living in Greater Manchester, seeking to answer three key questions:

1. Do people acknowledge that parent–child relations are founded upon norms of obligation?

2. What is the substance of these norms?

3. How do norms operate in practice?

Finch and Mason found that at the most general level, the majority did assent to the idea of filial obligations, but that this assent was by no means either universal or unconditional. Although there was broad agreement that an adult should 'do something' to support their parents, there was less broad agreement about what exactly that 'something' should be. In reality, people expected to negotiate their obligations; to work out their own responsibilities in a given set of circumstances. Finch and Mason conclude that there may be different ways of fulfilling obligations legitimately: 'People do have an understanding of what would be generally accepted as proper, but they use it as a resource with which to negotiate rather than as a rule to follow' (1993: 105).

Finch (1995) extends this analysis. She suggests that there are different, at times competing expectations of British family life. The idea that 'adult children should be able to live lives independently of their parents and vice-versa' may be just as strong as the notion that children should look after their parents when they become ill or frail. Responsibilities are therefore likely to be tempered on both sides with the desire to retain mutual independence (1995: 51). She proposes an alternative 'commitments' model as a better way of understanding how family responsibilities operate in practice: commitments are built up over time between specific individuals, through contact, shared activities and giving help when it is needed. She states that the process of reciprocity 'is the engine which drives the process of developing commitments' (1995: 54). She ends by suggesting that the idea of fixed obligations may be more meaningful in the relationship between spouses. Most critically, she observes that there may be little room for a spouse to decline to offer care (ibid.).

Alongside the scholarly and academic research, there has been an upsurge in what might be broadly termed 'self-help' literature on caring. Marriott's (2003) book, lent to me by a member of the University of Edinburgh User and Carer Forum, is a good example of this tradition. Marriott dedicates his book, not to the people whom he categorises as 'saints' nor to paid carers, but to those 'who have come reluctantly to caring. We feel bad about our unwillingness, and secretly think of ourselves as selfish pigs'. Over the next 300 pages, he takes readers through the highs and lows and, most critically, the ambivalence he feels in caring for his partner who has Huntingdon's Disease. The book deliberately takes the carer's viewpoint, and even has a chapter provocatively entitled 'Pushing them down the stairs'. Yet the book illustrates the complexities and the humanity at the heart of caring.

Joan Tronto's 'ethic of care' brings a new slant to the discussion (1993). Tronto, a US feminist and political theorist, argues that 'we need to stop talking about "women's morality" and start talking about a care ethic that includes the values traditionally associated with women' (1993: 3). She goes on in her seminal book to spell out what this might look like, quoting a definition devised by herself and Berenice Fisher:

> On the most general level, we suggest that caring be viewed as a species activity that includes everything that we do to maintain, continue and repair our 'world' so that we can live in it as well as possible. That world includes our bodies, our selves, and our environment, all of which we seek to interweave in a complex, life-sustaining web.
>
> (1993: 103)

Care, from this perspective, is political as well as individual. It is about looking after each other and the planet. It varies from culture to culture. It can be a single action or a process. She continues: 'caring is not simply a cerebral concern, or a character trait, but the concern of living, active humans engaged in the processes of everyday living. Care is both a practice and a disposition' (1993: 104). Tronto makes an important distinction between care and protection. Although they may seem to share certain aspects, protection is self-serving; it presumes that something bad will happen and sets out to protect against that, whereas care is about 'taking the other's needs as the starting point for what must be done' (1993: 105). She identifies four analytically separate but interconnected phases in caring: caring about; taking care of; care giving; and care receiving. She also outlines four moral principles of care: attentiveness, responsibility, competence and responsiveness. This takes us a long way from the very sterile, polarised debates about care towards a much more rounded, holistic understanding of caring.

Structural constraints on caring

The third criticism of the 1980s research is that by creating an analytical framework that was premised largely on the accounts of white, middle-aged women, the studies failed to take account of the importance of social class, 'race' and ethnicity, gender and sexuality, age, disability and mental health in structuring experiences of caring. Moreover, by focusing on the caring dyad, that is, on the relationship between two individuals, the early studies presented care as individualistic, and failed to see how it functions socially and politically (Tronto 1993).

Social class

Studies suggest that interrelated factors such as class, income, health and housing play a key part in determining experiences of care and caring. Importantly, while working-class people are likely to have fewer resources and poorer health than middle-class people, research demonstrates that it is working-class families who are more likely to take in an older relative who needs care. It is suggested that this reflects both the lack of viable alternatives (in terms of paying for care) as well as specific ideas about family responsibilities and about the value of independence (Arber and Ginn 1992a). There are age differences here too, in that working-class people are more likely to need care at an earlier age than middle-class people, because of inequalities in health, housing, diet, etc., as will be discussed more

Chapter 7

fully in Chapter 7. In addition, it is known that informal caring has a significant impact on household income (see Parker and Lawton 1994). Caring can be expensive, and while the person who is cared for may contribute financially to the costs of their care, this may not cover all the necessary extras, such as household adaptations, extra heating, additional laundry, etc. (Glendinning 1992). Parker and Lawton conclude that the impact of caring on the income and savings of carers may be such that this has serious consequences for their own standard of living in old age.

If we widen the concept of care to include paid care, and specifically waged domestic labour, issues of class again come to the fore. Graham (1991 and 1997) argues that care cannot be understood without reference to social divisions constructed around 'race' and class as well as gender. Her study of domestic service points out that the burden of low-paid domestic service has always been carried by working-class, often black or immigrant women. In the seventeenth and eighteenth centuries, black slaves were brought to Britain from Africa and the West Indies to work as personal and household servants, as cooks, maids and valets. In the nineteenth century, African Caribbean women continued to be employed as domestic servants in middle-class households, as well as white working-class women and Irish and other minority ethnic groups who entered domestic service in large numbers. Today domestic service continues to characterise the labour market for many black and white working-class women, who are engaged in low-paid, low-status jobs in households, in the health and social services sector and in private care homes (1997: 130).

Gregson and Lowe's (1994) investigation of waged domestic labour (nannies and cleaners) in contemporary Britain adds to this analysis. Gregson and Lowe argue that the resurgence of waged domestic labour in the 1980s and 1990s is indicative of 'a breakdown in the post-war cross-class identification of women with all forms of reproductive work' (1994: 233). As women have entered the paid workforce in greater numbers, so they have relinquished part of their traditional reproductive labour to others; that is, to lower middle-class and working-class women. Gregson and Lowe assert that a 'class-mediated hierarchy of domestic tasks' is once more being constructed. At the top are the tasks that middle-class partners (women and men) are more or less happy to share, and these tasks remain unwaged; for example, some childcare activities, shopping and cooking. Below this are the routine, day-to-day domestic tasks such as daily childcare and feeding. These are largely shared by middle-class women and waged domestic labour. At the bottom are the labour-intensive activities (notably cleaning and ironing) that are increasingly being identified with waged domestic labour from the working class. The consequence of this is that working-class women, as well as carrying the burden of reproductive work in their own households, are increasingly assuming part of the same responsibility within middle-class households (1994: 234). This has major implications for our discussion of women and caring. Graham (1997: 130) states that many white working-class women and black and ethnic minority women have found that their care arrangements are structured by employment opportunities and immigration restrictions in ways that restrict their opportunity to receive and give care within their families. It is therefore white middle-class women who have greater access to a family life, sustained by the care of other women from other groups.

'Race'/ethnicity

We have already explored some of the important issues in relation to caring and the use of black women's labour in domestic care. There are, however, other important ways in which 'race' and ethnicity structure care and caring. While some may be seen as pertaining to culture and tradition, others are related to the impact of discrimination, racism and exclusion.

Housing patterns and age structures inevitably affect whether care is available and the nature of that care, in both majority and minority ethnic communities. In a study reported in 1994, Fisher found that 25 per cent of Asian elders had no close relative living in Britain; the setting up of an Asian elders' support scheme in London in 1992 reflected the need for support amongst this group. Graham (1997) substantiates this, indicating that in one study of 400 older people, one-third of the Asian respondents and half of the African Caribbean respondents had no family in Britain. She describes the isolation experienced by those who have no family here, and no hope of family reunification (1997: 129). Tester (1996) concludes that immigration controls and employment patterns have restricted opportunities both for black people to live with their families and to care for one another.

For those in minority ethnic communities who do have family members in the UK, additional issues pertain. Fisher (1994) noted that Asian people who were caring for other family members were unlikely to be doing so on their own, in the one-to-one dyad which characterises much of the caring literature. Instead, care was much more likely to be shared in the community, by relatives and friends. Furthermore, it was seen as culturally appropriate for sons to take the lead in caring for their Asian mothers. This suggests that Qureshi and Walker's (1989) much-quoted 'hierarchy of care' did not fit this minority ethnic community.

Gunaratnam (1997) reminds us that even within ethnic communities, there are significant differences, influenced by factors such as class, migration history, gender and the disability of the person requiring care (1997: 115). The popular image of a black family, irrespective of ethnicity, is one of the extended family network: 'families within families, providers of care and social and psychological support' (Patel 1990: 36). Gunaratnam states that the most dominant stereotype of black and ethnic minority communities, and particularly Asian communities, is that they do not make use of support services because 'they prefer to look after their own' (1997: 116). His study of thirty-three carers indicates a high level of diversity in the caring contexts of older Asian people. Some elderly couples lived alone in reciprocal caring relationships, while others lived apart from their carers; only eight of the thirty-three carers lived in extended, multi-generational families (ibid.). Gunaratnam argues that more research is needed to explore the nature and meanings of care within black and minority ethnic families, specifically the ways in which caring relationships can be influenced by individual identity, cultural prescriptions and wider socio-economic conditions (1997: 117).

Gunaratnam illustrates this by considering the low take-up of services (such as home help, day centres, meals on wheels) by black and minority ethnic people. Low take-up, he suggests, is not just about lack of information or lack of accessibility of services. It is also about culture and tradition; for Asian carers, the concepts of 'care' and 'caring' are, Gunaratnam asserts, highly ethnocentric. One carer in his study expressed this simply: 'I think that it is difficult for us Asian people to see ourselves as "carers" . . . the idea is not something that is a part of our culture or language, it is just another part of family life' (1997: 119). There is, however, a second issue in relation to black and Asian carers, and that is how far services are inappropriate and fail to meet their specific and different needs. Most of all, Gunaratnam argues that service providers fail to acknowledge the impact of poverty, poor housing and racial harassment on the lives of black and minority ethnic service users (1997: 120). Similar issues are taken up by Vernon (2002) in her study of Asian people with disabilities. She again challenges the myth that low take-up of services among minority ethnic communities is due to poor language and the belief that 'they prefer to look after their own'. She argues that even those who are fluent in English struggle to access services. Moreover, the idea that 'they prefer to look after their own' is a self-fulfilling prophecy which discourages people from asking for help.

There is, of course, a bigger question to be addressed here. The models of care that emerged in the 1980s' literature were built on an assumption of a white, majority community perspective; where other communities were mentioned it was usually as a colourful (literally) exception to the 'norm'. This 'deficit model' (Graham 2007) is deeply racist and leads to incomplete theorising. It is also damaging to minority and majority ethnic community members alike.

Gender revisited

The notion that it is only women who care has been challenged by evidence from large-scale quantitative surveys and by more localised, qualitative studies. The 1985 General Household Survey (GHS) identified that of the 6 million carers overall, 3.5 million were women and 2.5 million were men. This figure has been replicated in subsequent research, as the presentation of current statistics at the end of this chapter demonstrates. Research also identifies that men (particularly older men) have always been carers of their wives and elderly parents (see Arber and Gilbert 1989, Fisher 1994, Qureshi and Walker 1989). In addition, men play an increasing role in childcare and in professional caring capacities, working as social workers, nurses and primary school teachers (see Christie 2001, Cree 1996, Popay et al. 1998). There is also increasing interest in the research literature on men as fathers (see Daniel and Taylor 2001, Featherstone 2009).

There has, however, been some debate about what these findings actually tell us. Most critically, the question is posed as to how far an overall figure like this can differentiate adequately between the known differences in the amount and nature of caring provided? Parker and Lawton (1994) distinguish between personal and physical care, and between 'caring' and 'informal helping'. They estimate that only 1.7 million carers are heavily involved in 'hands-on' care, and point out that women are more likely to provide both personal and physical care, whereas men are more likely to provide physical care and/or practical help, and are less likely to provide personal care. This fits with what we know about women and paid work. Women are still more likely than men to work part time or take advantage of flexible working arrangements in order to facilitate their caring responsibilities (Office of National Statistics (ONS) 2 December 2009 update, www.statistics.gov.uk/). Although there has been movement towards greater equality for women and men at work and at home, the expectation remains that women should be the 'primary carers', and all the systems for providing social support in the UK continue to support this assumption.

Sexuality

There is another important consideration here. I have asserted that models of care tend to presume a white, Western model; they also assume a heterosexual model. Studies of the experiences of people who have HIV and AIDS have found that for a significant number of gay men, support from parents is not readily available. Instead, care is often provided by partners, friends and the gay community, through 'buddy' schemes and drop-in centres (Brown and Powell-Cope 1992). Tester (1996) makes a similar point in relation to lesbian women who seek and provide care outside the nuclear family. Tester suggests that care services are based on familist norms that promote the heterosexual nuclear family and stigmatise other family forms and living arrangements. She reminds us that older or disabled lesbian women may not have daughters to care for them, but instead may have partners or other adult support networks. Fish (2006) similarly challenges the heterosexism that runs throughout health and social care services.

Age

As we have seen, the dominant concern of the care-giving literature was conventionally the burden faced by those caring for frail elderly relatives, rather than the preferences and needs of older people themselves; older people were 'conceptualised as a passive object to be cared for' (Arber and Ginn 1992b: 87). This reflects the ageism in the caring literature, a literature that largely neglected, ignored and stereotyped the experiences of older people. The reality, as we have seen, is much more complex and contradictory, with older people both providing and receiving care, and older people choosing to remain independent and outside either informal or formal care services for as long as possible.

One of the themes in current sociological research is the involvement of grandparents, reflecting the growth in the number of grandparents who are providing some level of care for their grandchildren. Secondary analysis of the Office of National Statistics Omnibus Survey revealed that there was great diversity in the characteristics of grandparents and their families, and in the amount of caring grandparents did for their grandchildren (see Clarke and Roberts 2004). A follow-up interview study by Mason *et al.* (2007) found that the grandparents in their study were involved in considerable amounts of hands-on care for their grandchildren. But, more interestingly, they discovered that grandparents felt they had to tread a careful line between 'not interfering' and 'being there'. This suggests that grandparenting is as much about moral ideas (doing the 'right thing') as it is about more pragmatic concerns.

Perhaps the most emotive, and indeed contentious, issue within the caring literature is summed up in the term 'young carer'. Since the early 1990s when this first emerged as a matter of public concern, a considerable amount of research and policy attention has gone into considering the experiences of children and young people with a parent or sibling who is ill or has a disability (see, for example, Aldridge and Becker 1993, Banks *et al.* 2002, Becker 2007, Becker *et al.* 2001, Cree 2003, Dearden and Becker 1995, Department of Health 1999, Department of Health 2009, Tucker and Liddiard 1998). Much of this literature highlights that caring for others in the family can have an adverse effect on children's education, play, mental health and lives in general, turning 'normal' expectations of parent/child relationships upside-down, and putting pressure on children and young people at a time in their lives when they should be free to enjoy their childhoods.

There are problems with this characterisation, however, just as we have seen in relation to other kinds of caring. Firstly, there is no absolute definition of a young carer and organisations vary in the definition they adopt. This leads to estimates of total populations of young carers that are hugely at variance with one another; recent estimates indicate that there may be between 19,000 and 51,000 young carers in Britain (Banks *et al.* 2002). The presentation of young carers as 'victims' in much of the literature is also highly offensive to parents who continue to take responsibility for their children in spite of being reliant on them, as well as to children themselves. A 2009 Department of Health strategy document on carers states that 'many young carers value the contribution they are able to make within their families and that caring can be a positive experience – enhancing independence and strengthening family ties'. The report goes on to add that 'Extensive or inappropriate caring roles, however, can harm children's ability to attend and achieve at school and make them more vulnerable to negative experiences such as bullying, as well as making the transition to adulthood more difficult' (2009: 29). This demonstrates, again, that caring is a relative experience, and one which happens in context. And, as we have seen, this context is social, cultural and political as well as familial. This point is developed further by Haugen (2007) in a study of children's care in families after divorce. She demonstrates that care is not unidirectional, and that children are competent actors and yet vulnerable at the same time. This requires a more layered approach to understanding the issues, something she refers to as 'caringscapes'.

Disability

Morris argues that the failure of the feminist researchers on informal care to consider the experiences of disabled and older people betrays the ways in which white, middle-class women have viewed disabled and older people; they have 'colluded with prejudicial social attitudes which are commonly held about older and disabled people' (1995: 71). This is in spite of the fact that disability is strongly differentiated in terms of gender: because of women's greater longevity, twice as many older women as men (14 per cent to 7 per cent) are severely disabled (Arber and Ginn 1992b: 94).

In reviewing the topic of disability and care, Macfarlane asserts that, for most disabled people, care is a difficult word to define. This is because most of the 'care' received by disabled people was, in the past, 'not of their choosing or under their control' (1996: 13). Much care has been oppressive, often custodial in nature and provided in a controlled way. The 'enforced isolation' experienced by many disabled people is made worse by the lack of accessible public transport, by discriminatory employment practices and by inaccessible buildings; disabled people have, at times, felt unable to complain about the care they received because of fear of reprisals or punishment (1996: 13–14). This is not, however, to suggest that disabled people have been prepared to accept this state of affairs without question. Campaigns by the Disabled People's Movement have led to major improvements in service delivery in recent years. Hasler goes so far as to say that the introduction of 'direct payments' schemes 'represented for the first time a shift of power to disabled people' (2004: 219), allowing them to take control of their own lives and make decisions about the kinds of care they wished to receive. Disabled people have fought to reinvent their identities as people who are 'equal but different'. French and Swain describe this well:

> For many disabled people the tragedy view of disability is in itself disabling. It denies their experiences of a disabling society, their enjoyment of life, and even their identity and self-awareness as disabled people. The affirmation of positive identity is both collective and individual. Disabled identity, as non-disabled identity, has meaning in relation to and constructs the identity of others. To be disabled is to be 'not one of those'. The affirmation of positive identity challenges the tyranny of the personal tragedy theory of disability and impairment.
>
> (2004: 39)

Mental illness

For those with mental health problems, as with older people and those with disabilities, 'care' in the past has meant institutionalisation and separation from society. Asylums were, asserts Jones (2002: 11), 'part of the same system as the workhouse and the prison; they were places where those whose behaviour threatened the social order could be gathered together and controlled (Foucault 1967; Scull 1979)'. In more recent years, new methods of controlling mental illness through drugs and psychological therapies have heralded a move towards care 'in the community'. Nevertheless, there are still high levels of fear and stigma attached to those with mental health problems, which make it doubly difficult to ask for help. Mental health carries with it old ideas of 'madness', 'insanity' and 'dangerousness', particularly if, as Fernando and Keating (2008) argue, the diagnosis is schizophrenia. This has an impact, not just on care givers but also on people experiencing mental illness themselves, leading them to put off seeking help and further increasing their isolation.

Research demonstrates, again as previously discussed, the structural issues that are at work here. It is known that women are more likely than men to be in receipt of mental health services

(Chesler 2000). Moreover, there is a high predominance of black and minority ethnic people in compulsory detention in mental health facilities, and it is young men who make up the highest numbers here (Graham 2007). Fenton and Sadiq (2000) point out that there are also special factors for Asian women. Western cultures, they state, give a lot of importance to people as individuals. Asian traditions, in contrast, set store by people's relationship with others, and mostly those with their family and community. This means that a breakdown in family relationships can be seen as a threat to the roles by which individuals define themselves. This can lead to great mental and emotional turmoil. Finally, class and age also play an important part in determining care experiences in relation to mental health: class, because, as we have seen, income and social class affects the resources and opportunities available to care-givers and recipients; and age, because of the ever-present impact of ageism (Bytheway 1995).

Perhaps the biggest challenge currently facing health and social care services in the UK is the increasing number of older people with dementia, predicted to rise from 700,000 people in 2009 to 1 million by 2021 (Alzheimer Society 2007). Again, the language that is used to describe this is most often couched in terms of 'risk' and 'burden'; there is little interest in the emotional impact of dementia on people with dementia and their families. Barnes discusses this in relation to the professional care given to her mother. She argues that there is a tendency for care 'to be reduced to responding to functional needs in the present' (2006: 29), rather than seeing individuals as whole people with a past and a future. Drawing on the insights of Tronto (1993), Barnes argues that we need to get away from the stereotypes of the 'tragic heroine' and the 'needy client' (2006: 176), and realise that we are all care givers and care recipients; that we all need care, for ourselves and for others.

The politics of caring

I cannot leave this chapter on caring without referring to the policy context within which caring takes place. The meaning and organisation of care in the community or 'community care' has changed considerably. After the Second World War, community care meant care provided by the state for those unable to care for themselves (Payne 1995). Since that time, there has been a major shift towards care *by*, not *in*, the community, as explained in a government report published in 1981:

> . . . the primary sources of care are informal and voluntary. These spring from the personal ties of kinship, friendship and neighbourhood. They are irreplaceable. It is the role of public authorities to sustain and, where necessary, develop – but never to displace – such support and care. Care *in* the community must increasingly mean care *by* the community.
>
> (DHSS 1981)

All subsequent legislation has followed on from this starting point, reflecting both the wishes of those who receive care to remain at home as long as possible (as evidenced in the caring research) and also government fiscal pressures. The impetus to remove people from institutional care is a long-standing one. It can be seen in the 1948 Children Act, which sought to replace very large children's homes with more locally based 'family group homes', and in the expansion of fostering and adoption as alternatives to residential care for children. The critique was extended to psychiatric patients and older people by exposés of standards of care in institutions (notably Goffman's 1968 study of asylums and Townsend's 1962 study of residential care), which revealed the dehumanising and coercive nature of institutionalised care.

While it is easy to agree that people requiring care would rather live at home than in large, impersonal institutions, it is important to consider again the context in which the drive towards community care has taken place. Johnson identifies 'an historical shift in priorities from caring for the dependent to providing support to sustain independence, or at least reduce dependence on the state, and to providing protection for the vulnerable. In this sense, it might be argued that care as a policy concept is in decline' (1998: 152). The emergence of new electronic care systems in recent years is, in this context, just another step on this road, as, progressively, care professionals are commissioning 'stand-alone' and networked assistive technological services and home care packages (see Horgan 2009, Hudson 2002, Rafferty and Steyaert 2007).

How are we to understand this shift? Is it part of a positive plan to support individuals better and broaden and extend social welfare, or simply a cynical ploy to cut costs? Or is it, more probably, a bit of both? Similarly, will care in the community lead to more and better standards of care in society, or is it intended to take power and responsibility away from local authorities, and place an increasing burden on family members and unpaid or low-paid workers in our communities? Similar questions are being asked today of the drive towards so-called 'personalised' services in social care (see Hunter and Ritchie 2007). How far will the consumerist culture which is increasingly characterising service delivery reduce or, alternatively, mask inequalities in society? When will care be understood and valued, as Barnes urges, as 'a positive contribution to social justice'? (2006: 178). These questions are fundamental at a theoretical and policy level; they are also faced by social workers working in the field of adult care on a daily basis.

Implications for practice

- The literature suggests that we need to think about care and caring in a more fluid, complex way. Although structural issues inevitably underpin and influence care, experiences are not fixed for all time. Instead, changes do take place across the life course, identities can be resisted and renegotiated as well as accepted, and oppressive systems can, and must, be challenged. Moreover, we are all, in our daily lives, givers and receivers of care.

- We also need to bear in mind that there is always ambivalence in care, whether formal or informal; there are good and bad things about it, for those individuals and agencies who give care and for those who receive care. This is not an 'either/or' situation, but one which is better summed up as 'both/and' (see Hill Collins 1990). Caring is both a moral and a social issue. Social workers must therefore keep an open mind in their assessments, being prepared to listen to and work alongside people in ways that respect their viewpoints and value their differences.

- Finally, it is important to remember that people's need for care is likely to be directly related to services that are, or are not, available. Hence good transport and health systems, which enable access to all members of society, will reduce the need for additional care support. This suggests that care and caring are political as well as individual and structural issues. Because of this, social workers must be prepared to come together with service users and carers to fight for equality of access and outcome in society.

Conclusion

This chapter has argued that care and caring, like all other main topics in this book, is a social construct; it is historically, socially and culturally specific. Care takes place across a range of different contexts, both unpaid and paid, and is affected to a large degree by structural factors such as class, gender, 'race' and ethnicity, age and disability. The sociological literature has shown that caring is a complex phenomenon, highly personal and yet at the same time rooted in social and cultural normative expectations and kinship obligations. It is therefore fundamentally a moral issue. It is also about resources, opportunities and alternatives, and in that respect, it is political. Those of us who work in the 'caring professions' must strive to work alongside those who use our services to ensure that the care that we provide is, as Tronto describes, attentive, responsible, competent and responsive. A sociological understanding of care and caring can help us to do that.

Recommended reading

Balloch, S. and Hill, M. (eds) (2007) *Care, Community and Citizenship*, Bristol: The Policy Press. Includes a large number of short chapters demonstrating a range of contemporary perspectives.

Barnes, M. (2006) *Caring and Social Justice*, Basingstoke: Palgrave Macmillan. Written by one of the most interesting current voices in the field.

Fink, J. (ed.) (2004) *Care: Personal Lives and Social Policy*, Bristol: The Policy Press in association with the Open University. A good introduction to key debates involved in the development of understanding about care and caring.

7 Health and illness

Introduction

Health and illness are 'part of our everyday lives', to such an extent that we often take them for granted (Marsh *et al.* 2009: 513). Yet health and illness have become increasingly a central part of social work's sphere of interest in recent years. This reflects the reality that, thanks to better prevention and treatment of a whole range of physical and mental conditions (including simply growing older), more people are living with, and living longer with, complex illnesses and disabilities, requiring engagement, at some level, with social work and social care. The repositioning of adult care services within Departments of Health in the UK demonstrates this development, as does the preoccupation of successive governments with health promotion (healthy eating, sensible drinking, stopping smoking, etc.).

As long ago as 1946, the World Health Organization (WHO) defined health as 'a state of complete physical, mental and social well-being' (1946: 3). This offers a good beginning to this chapter, which aims to explore the sociology of health and illness, taking in its broad sweep an exploration of health, illness, medicine, disease and disability. We will start, as in previous chapters, with a discussion about meanings.

Definitions

As we will see, there is a lot of overlap in the ways in which people think and write about health, illness and disease, as well as some polarisation between what might be termed 'medical' discourses and those that are described as 'non-medical' or 'lay'. I will try to unpack this further.

In medicine and epidemiology, health is defined as 'the absence of disease' (Mulhall 2001: 47). But this definition in no way captures the image of health held by most people. Nor does it fit with the much broader WHO definition given above. Much of our knowledge about lay conceptions of health in the UK derives from the outcomes of the 'Health and Lifestyles' survey conducted in 1985. The question 'what is health?' was posed to 9,000 individuals. In presenting the findings, Blaxter (1990) concludes that people saw health in different terms, which she characterised as either negative or positive. Those who used negative definitions tended to understand health to mean not being ill: not suffering any symptoms or having any pain, never having to see the doctor, not having a disease or disability. Positive definitions of health tended to describe health in terms of healthy lifestyles, being fit and having lots of energy. For many, health was also associated with psycho-social well-being; health was 'a state of mind', being able to 'live life to the full', 'feeling the joys of spring'. Beyond these generalisations, Blaxter uncovered considerable divergence between the definitions of those who already had an illness and those who did not, and between individuals across the life course. This meant that some of those who had chronic illness or disability (especially older people) still saw themselves as healthy, in spite of, for example, their arthritis or diabetes. Young people, in contrast, were more likely to stress physical strength and fitness as key component of health. Interestingly, women gave much wider and more expansive answers than men. In addition, many more women than men defined health in terms of relationships with other people; the 'healthy person' was someone who was able to get out and about and do things with, and for, others.

What this survey does, in a very simple way, is to remind us that health is a contested area. The same is true for the concept of illness. Senior and Viveash suggest that like health, illness is a 'subjective notion that depends on people's own interpretation of their mental and physical condition and what symptoms they count as illness' (1998: 8). They introduce a number of examples and ask whether they 'count' as being ill: pregnancy, having a hangover, migraine, cancer, having an alcohol problem, a broken ankle, etc. Their conclusion is that there is no simple agreement as to what is defined as an illness. In Western societies, it is doctors who have the power to label illness, but doctors can and do disagree with one another about whether or not a reported illness is 'actual sickness', and we cannot take it for granted that this is an objective process (ibid.)

This leads us, inevitably, to another question: what is disease? For medicine and epidemiology, disease implies an 'abnormality of structure or function, the need for correction, and the idea that abnormalities are undesirable' (Mulhall 2001: 47). This is a clear illustration of what has been called the 'bio-medical model'. This way of thinking is so much a part of our lives we have come to think of it as *the* way of thinking about health, illness and the body (Marsh *et al.* 2009: 515). The main features of the bio-medical model are as follows:

- *Mind/body dualism*: it is assumed that the mind and body can be treated separately (Marsh *et al.* 2009). As Giddens adds, 'the patient represents a *sick body* – a pathology – rather than a whole individual' (2006: 260).

- *Mechanical metaphor*: the body is likened to a machine that, when ill, breaks down. Doctors then take on the role of engineer to repair the machine (Marsh *et al.* 2009: 515). Giddens concurs with this interpretation, indicating that it is assumed that trained medical specialists are the only experts in the treatment of disease. There is, he argues, 'no room for self-taught healers or "non-scientific" medical practices' (2006: 261).

- *The role of technology*: there is an emphasis on technology in defining and treating illness at the expense of the patient's experience (Marsh *et al.* 2009: 516).

- *Biological focus*: there is a search for a specific identifiable cause for disease – for example, a virus (ibid.) – and, I would add, a neglect of social and psychological factors. The assumption behind this, Giddens argues, is the late 1800s' idea 'that there is a specific identifiable agent behind every disease' (2006: 260).

- *Scientific neutrality of medicine*: medicine is presented as being objective and neutral, which in turn enhances its claims to discovering the truth about the body, health and illness (Marsh *et al.* 2009: 516).

This model has dominated medical practice because 'it has been seen to work': it has made a massive contribution to key areas of health through, for example, vaccination; the 'anatomical and neurophysiological structures of the body have been mapped out' and the genetic mapping of the body is already well under way (Bilton *et al.* 2002: 356). The bio-medical model underpins both national and international strategies for healthcare; so, for example, the WHO's long-term health goal is 'eradication of disease' (Bilton *et al.* 2002: 357). But the story is, of course, much less clear than this might seem to suggest. Not everyone with a disease feels ill. Ovarian cancer carries the unfortunate label 'the silent disease', because many women with early-stage cancer of the ovary do not report any symptoms at all. There are also widespread differences in the diseases that are treated by medical practitioners. For example, in the UK, low blood pressure is usually considered to be unimportant, unless caused by blood loss, trauma, severe infection or toxic shock. But in countries such as Germany and France, many people take regular medication for low blood pressure. There are, furthermore, a great many people who suffer from illness without having a recognisable 'disease'; for example, persistent sore throats, migraine or chronic back pain. There may even be conflict as to whether something is indeed a disease. There are said to be 250,000 people in the UK who suffer from chronic fatigue syndrome (CFS), also known as myalgic encephalomyelitis (ME). CFS causes major problems in people's everyday lives and can last for years, yet there is no cure; treatment tends to focus on easing the symptoms (www.nhs.uk/). In his landmark book on risk, Beck (1992) points out that the improvements that we have seen over the last 100 years in diagnosing illnesses have not been matched by 'the presence or even the prospect of any effective measures to treat them' (1992: 204).

On the contrary, just as fewer people die of acute (short-term) illnesses, so many more live with, and die from, chronic (long-term) illnesses. He writes:

> A cure in the original sense of medicine becomes more and more the exception ... Yet this is not the expression solely of a failure. Because of the *successes* medicine also discharges people into illness, which it is able to diagnose with its high technology.
>
> (1992: 205)

Ivan Illich (1975) is even more critical of modern medicine, arguing that it has done more harm than good because of 'iatrogenesis', that is, self-caused disease. Illich identifies three types here: clinical iatrogenesis, where medical treatment makes the patient's condition worse or causes a new health problem; social iatrogenesis, where medicine expands into new areas, creating ever more demand for its services; and finally, cultural iatrogenesis, which is caused by social iatrogenesis, 'where the ability to cope with the challenges of everyday life becomes progressively reduced by medical explanations and alternatives' (Giddens 2006: 262). The solution, for Illich and others, is for the scope of modern medicine to be reduced. Of course thirty years on, we know that there has been no such reduction. On the contrary, the range and breadth of modern medicine has grown exponentially. In part, I believe this is because medicine has been prepared to move beyond the bio-medical model to embrace a more social approach to illness and disease, at the same time as investing increasing amounts of energy into ever more sophisticated bio-technological responses to illness. Lupton (1995) would agree. She identifies a shift away from a strictly bio-medical approach within conventional medicine. She suggests that we can see this in health promotion campaigns' calls for changes in diet and exercise regimes, rather than only offering medical solutions to the problems – of heart disease, for example. Modern medicine has also had to deal with the challenges posed by the major growth in the availability and use of alternative or complementary ways of understanding and treating illness over the last forty years or so. Whilst professional associations sought (and still seek) to limit and regulate this activity, we can also see the increasing incorporation of alternative therapies, including homeopathy, massage and relaxation, yoga, etc., both within general practice and hospital settings. Arguably, the introduction of social workers to healthcare environments over 100 years ago is another illustration of the application of a more social approach within medicine. Although the task of early hospital social workers (almoners) was partly financial (assessing who could and could not pay for treatment), they were always concerned to explore the patient within her or his social context (see Baraclough *et al.* 1996).

The discussion so far suggests that the categorisation of illness and disease is not a neutral, technical matter, but rather, that it depends on social and cultural factors. It is also, importantly, highly political. The reluctance of some medics to treat CFS seriously cannot be seen as unconnected to wider moral questions and public attitudes towards 'malingering' and the so-called 'work-shy'. Another controversial example demonstrates this well. In the late nineteenth century, and throughout most of the twentieth century, it was standard practice in medicine to see homosexuality in terms of pathological models. It was not until 1973 that the American Psychiatric Association declassified homosexuality as a mental disorder (Bayer 1987). Homosexual acts remain criminalised in many countries today (see McBrewster *et al.* 2009).

Implications for practice

- If illness is a social construct as well as a physical condition, then it is evident that practitioners need to be circumspect about both its manifestation and its treatment, not taking either for granted.

- In seeking to adopt a 'professional' mantle, social work has often embraced a medical model, seeing social problems as being akin to diseases and explaining them in terms of individual 'pathology'. This led practitioners to see the causes of problems in an individual's background or personality, rather than in the social, cultural or political environment within which their problems were located. This approach is still common, and can lead to 'blaming' of individuals and oppressive practice.

- Social work practitioners may, at times, feel that 'social work' or lay knowledge is somehow inferior to medical knowledge. The discussion so far reminds us that all knowledge is imperfect, socially and culturally specific, open to challenge, dynamic and subject to change.

Historical accounts

Historical accounts provide ample evidence to support the contention that health and illness are socially and historically specific. We will explore this by examining two accounts of historical development: firstly, of causes of illness and death; and secondly, of medicine.

Patterns of death and disease have changed significantly since the end of the nineteenth century. Fulcher and Scott (2007: 289) identify a 'health transition' – that is, a change in patterns of disease – and as a result, a change in the nature and scale of the main diseases which cause illness and death. They set this down in three stages:

- In stage 1, in pre-modern, agrarian societies, the principle causes of illness and death are acute infectious diseases, which are spread through direct contact, through polluted water or through parasitic carriers (fleas, mosquitoes, etc.) Diseases such as tuberculosis, malaria and plague are endemic, as well as cholera, typhoid, etc. Whilst all pollutions are at risk, only the very wealthy have any immunity.

- In stage 2, the 'industrialising society' brings some improvement to the standard of living, though urban poverty increases. Acute infectious diseases remain at a high level, but are particularly concentrated amongst the new urban poor, whose living conditions make them vulnerable. Improved public health (sanitation, better housing and nutrition) has some effect on the diseases of the poor, and serves to protect the majority of the population from their worst effects.

- In stage 3, the 'industrialised society' has greater control over infectious diseases (thanks largely to better public health, although vaccination has also made a contribution to this). Since the 1940s, there has been a rapid growth in medical and surgical techniques. This has brought reductions in infant mortality and increases in life expectancy. In stage 3, levels of degenerative diseases, such as cancer, heart disease and stroke, are high, and these are the principal causes of chronic illness and death: 'people now live long enough to suffer from different kinds of disease'. These diseases are therefore most common amongst older people. Conversely, road-traffic deaths (which affect all ages) account for almost 40 per cent of all accidental deaths (2007: 289–90).

This account not only demonstrates changes that have taken place over time, but also the impact that industrialisation and urbanisation have had on the process of change. This will be picked up further in the discussion on cross-cultural societies. The history of medicine also provides insight into the issues. Duffin (2000) presents an illuminating and highly entertaining history of medicine. She begins with a discussion of anatomy, which is seen as integral to the study of medicine today, but in previous years has been considered not just irrelevant, but even taboo. In ancient Greece, embalmers were 'adept at situating and extracting organs through tiny holes and slits in the body', yet physicians did not use anatomy, preferring to explain disease in terms of physiology, 'in which breath was the essence of life' (2000: 12). In the Middle Ages, the rise of secular universities and challenges to religious teaching meant that dissections became more frequent, and Renaissance art contributed to anatomy at this time. By the eighteenth century, dissection became more respectable, as part of a new philosophy of knowledge known as sensualism, which valued observation over abstract theorising. At the beginning of the nineteenth century, anatomy and dissection became essential for medical training. The result was a wave of new crimes: grave robbing and murder for the sale of corpses, reported in the US and Canada, in Paris and in the UK, where in a notorious case in Edinburgh in 1823, William Burke and William Hare were found guilty of murdering sixteen people and selling their bodies to the medical school anatomist, Robert Knox (2000: 34). Since that time, dissection gradually came to be seen as more acceptable to the general public, and today, some people are prepared to leave their bodies to science 'for the greater good', as an act of public generosity.

Looking back over this period, Duffin says it is easy to see it as a 'logical series of progressive steps leading to openness and tolerance about the body that is the essence of medical wisdom and practice' (2000: 35). But, she argues, the story is not as straightforward as this. Historical practices are, in reality, strongly connected to the beliefs of the day (religious, cultural and moral), and the same is true today. Duffin points out that the future of anatomy is uncertain. Medical students today rarely do their own dissecting; detailed anatomy is not reinforced by the general practice of medicine (2000: 37). Duffin tells similar tales of the history of healthcare, paediatrics, surgery, etc., and in each, she demonstrates that medics have been successful over time in fighting for, and asserting, their predominance over their craft. She writes: 'The history of medical professionalization is the shift from pluralistic health care [offered by a range of wise-women, quacks, charlatans and the adepts of alternative theories] to a monopoly of a powerful orthodoxy' (2000: 120). Medical professionals have achieved this by forming professional societies at both local and national levels, by founding medical schools and by regulating practitioners. Major discoveries of anaesthesia and antisepsis meant that diseases that had been accepted as fatal or chronic could now be cured; patients from here on 'expected a "technical fix" for every pain, but by acquiescing to medical expertise, they lost individual autonomy over their well-being' (2000: 123).

The advent of healthcare systems in the nineteenth and early twentieth centuries in Europe and Canada demonstrate the new faith in medicine as the panacea or 'cure-all' for individuals and society. Duffin suggests that the purpose of these systems, whether private insurance schemes or publicly funded state schemes, was threefold: first, to remove the onus for payment from the sick and the poor; second, to ensure that those providing care are paid; and third, to prevent disease. The first two goals, she asserts 'are often met; the third, however, is not' (2000: 128). In her *History of Medicine*, Duffin presents example after example of mistakes being made, of unintended consequences, of advances in one area leading to greater awareness of what is not known, as well, of course, of improvements and advances along the way. Perhaps most tellingly for social work, she states that while information might be increasing, knowledge is not. She writes:

> How can any doctor profess to 'know' the tens of thousands of medical periodicals filled with so-called new knowledge? Ideas that are true at the beginning of a medical education are sometimes false by the end. Faced with a labyrinth of conflicting information, how do doctors learn when to reject what they have been taught in favour of something new ? . . . Is it better knowledge? And has it come with no cost?
>
> (2000: 125–6)

Cross-cultural studies

We have already noted that industrialisation and urbanisation have an impact, both positive and negative, on health and illness. We have also noted that the dominant view of health and illness in the developed world is strongly influenced by the bio-medical model. Cross-cultural analysis demonstrates that understandings of health, illness and the body are extremely variable across different cultures and societies, and across different groups within a specific society.

Burch (2001) introduces two helpful examples of this. She cites research by Morgan (1996) into the meaning attached to high blood pressure (hypertension) by white and African Caribbean patients in an area of London. Morgan found that the African Caribbean patients in her study were less likely to take their prescribed medication than the white patients, and preferred instead to use herbal remedies that they were already familiar with. They were also less worried about the condition, because of its high prevalence in the community; it was seen as 'normal'. A further important difference was highlighted between the two groups. African Caribbean patients were more likely to see strokes as a possible outcome of hypertension, whereas white patients identified heart conditions. This led to very different interpretations of what the future held, and different approaches to taking treatment. In other words, African Caribbean patients were more fatalistic than their white neighbours. Another very different example is Adelson's 1998 study of the Cree of Whapmagoostui in Northern Quebec. Adelson explains that the Cree have no equivalent word for 'health', and instead see this in terms of 'being alive well', a concept which, she argues, 'is inseparable from community, history, identity, and ultimately resistance' (Adelson 1998 quoted in Burch 2001: 152). 'Being alive well' is about more than simple physiology. Instead, it 'relates more to a way of life associated with practices', including physical activity, keeping warm and eating traditional Cree foods (2001: 152). The Cree believe that their capacity to 'be alive well' is threatened by the customs and conditions introduced by the 'whiteman'.

Hahn's 1999 anthropological investigation of public health introduces many equally pertinent illustrations of cultural differences in perceptions of health. For example, Green writes in this volume about the importance of engaging the participation and support of traditional healers in the prevention of HIV and other sexually transmitted infections in sub-Saharan Africa, where it is estimated that 80 per cent of the population relies on healers for the treatment of all conditions, though many also visit hospitals. In countries scarred by war, this percentage may be even higher (1999: 64). He argues that health promotion must build on methods that are 'culturally appropriate': finding out how health knowledge is passed on in families; how concepts such as sickness, contagion, pollution, etc. are understood; and then exploring what common ground might exist before beginning a dialogue with healers about the possible alternative treatments they might use. This approach is likely to be much more successful, he asserts, than using 'trained workers' from bio-medical back-grounds (1999: 74). Graham would agree wholeheartedly with this. She sets out the principles and values that underpin what she calls the 'African-centred worldview' (2002: 69):

- the interconnectedness of all things;
- the spiritual nature of human beings;
- collective/individual identity and the collective/inclusive nature of family structure;
- oneness of mind, body and spirit;
- the value of interpersonal relationships.

Finally, it is important to remember that the body itself is viewed very differently in different cultural settings. This is demonstrated by considering different perceptions of what an 'attractive' body should look like (for example, fat or slim?) and how the body should be covered (for example, with Western clothes, the hijab, a traditional Muslim head covering, or the burqa?). Burch argues that the body is constructed within Western science and philosophy as separate from the mind. It is also gendered (male or female, with male as the norm), as well as being a 'site for consumption' (2001: 143). It must be disciplined (Foucault 1975), and goods and services must be purchased for it. In other words, it has become a 'project' (Giddens 1991), as demonstrated by the abundance of health and fitness clubs, slimming aids, sportswear, and increasingly, I would add, cosmetic surgery aimed at controlling and improving the body.

Implications for practice

- The discussion shows that we must be careful, as always, not to judge others on the basis of our own ways of thinking about health and illness, because these ways of thinking are always partial, and sometimes may turn out to be wrong.

- Practitioners need to remember that 'treatment' may bring its own risks, through, for example, side effects of drugs and unanticipated consequences of surgery. Even a stay in hospital is hazardous; for example, a patient might catch a hospital-acquired infection such as methicillin-resistant Staphylococcus aureus (MRSA).

- Because medics are trained in Western bio-medical views of the world, they may know little about the health beliefs, practices and illnesses of other groups. This may, in part, explain some individuals' non-compliance with treatment regimes and reluctance to use services, behaviour just as likely to be seen in people from minority ethnic communities in the UK as in those in the developing world.

Traditional sociological approaches

In introducing a reader on health and illness, Bury and Gabe (2004) note that medical sociology, although successful in research and teaching in medical settings, made very little impact on mainstream sociology until relatively recently. This has changed radically, as we will see, and today health and illness is central to sociology's concerns.

Functionalist perspectives

As discussed in previous chapters, functionalism sees society as an organic whole; all the different elements within society (family, education, political systems, the economy, etc.) work together ('function') for the good of society and its members. From this perspective, a well-managed, cohesive society creates happy, healthy individuals; a poorly run society where norms and values are not shared generates unhappy, unwell individuals. The 'founding father' of functionalism, Emile Durkheim, set out to demonstrate this in his study *Suicide* (1952 [1897]), where he examined suicide rates across countries. Finding suicide rates to be relatively consistent year on year, Durkheim offered explanations for the individual act of suicide based on the relationship between the individual and society. What he argued essentially was that suicide rates depended on the group's level of social integration: groups

Chapter 1

with high levels of social integration had low suicide rates; societies with low levels of integration had high suicide rates. Durkheim's notion of 'anomic' suicide is of particular relevance to the sociology of health and illness (Berkman *et al.* 2000). Anomic suicide is conceptualised as being caused by major societal crises, both economic and political, which occur during periods of rapid social change. For Berkman *et al.*, this presents a useful way of thinking about crises in Russia and Eastern Europe in the late twentieth century. It may also, I would add, have useful lessons relevant for the early twenty-first-century worldwide economic recession.

The person who is most often associated with the sociology of health and illness is Talcott Parsons. Mirroring Durkheim's approach to suicide, Parsons set out to demonstrate that illness was a social phenomenon, rather than simply a physical one relating to individuals. He argued that ill health needed to be understood in terms of the functioning of society as a whole. As he wrote in *The Social System*, 'too low a general level of health, too high an incidence of illness, is dysfunctional: this is in the first instance because illness incapacitates the effective performance of social roles' (1964 [1951]: 430). Parsons's analysis is underpinned by a number of key assumptions: firstly, that the patient–doctor relationship is best understood as a social system, governed by norms about appropriate behaviour; secondly, that health is a basic requirement of being able to fulfil one's place in the social order (as breadwinner, spouse, parent, etc.); thirdly, that illness is, in contrast, a kind of deviance which is potentially disruptive to the social order. The function of the medical system, according to this way of thinking, is to manage the disruption caused by illness by creating the 'sick role'; that is, a socially sanctioned way of being ill that functions to constrain the potentially dysfunctional properties of illness. Parsons saw the sick role as a temporary, medically sanctioned form of deviant behaviour. He argued that, from the patient's perspective, the sick role is structured by two rights and two obligations:

Rights of sick people:

1. The sick person is exempt from 'normal social roles'; that is, he or she is allowed to give up normal activities, such as work or school, although they may require some legitimation of this; for example, in the form of a sick note from a GP.

2. The sick person is not responsible for his or her condition, so cannot be blamed for the incapacity.

Obligations on sick people:

1. The sick person should try to get well as quickly as possible (thereby relinquishing the sick role as soon as possible).

2. The sick person should seek technically competent help and co-operate with the medical professional.

These rights and obligations are echoed in the 'physician role', though Annandale suggests that this is 'less well defined by Parsons' (1998: 10). This, she argues, involves winning the patient's trust and access to their body, and, in turn, the obligation to apply the highest levels of competence in caring for the patient and to be guided by the patient's best interests, not personal gain.

Roger Jeffery (1979) makes use of the idea of the sick role in his study of three hospital casualty departments in England. Here he found that hospital staff divided patients into two distinct groups: 'good' patients (those with head injuries, cardiac arrests, road traffic accidents) and 'normal rubbish' (attempted suicides, alcoholics, etc). He unpicks this further, identifying that staff 'liked' the 'good' patients either because they were able to practice the skills necessary for passing their examinations (because they could use their chosen specialities); or because they 'tested the general competence and maturity of the staff' (1979: 93). The 'normal rubbish', by way of contrast, offered no such challenges. They were either 'trivia' (they arrived at the hospital with a condition which was neither due to trauma nor urgent); 'drunks' (often abusive and threatening); 'overdoses' (viewed as 'self-injury' rather than attempted suicide); 'tramps' (who came in to try to get a warm bed for the night); or, less frequently, 'nutcases' (psychiatric patients and drug users), and 'smelly', 'dirty' or 'obese' patients (1979: 97). Jeffery goes on to suggest that patients were considered 'rubbish' because they had broken one or more of four unwritten rules; rules which he argues are consistent with Parsons's notion of the sick role:

1. 'Normal rubbish' – for example, 'drunks', 'tramps', 'overdoses' – *were* seen as responsible for their illnesses, and because of this staff felt no moral obligation to treat them although the legal obligation remained. They were also 'not really ill' (1979: 100).

2. Some patients had *not* been restricted from carrying out their normal activities, for example, 'trivia' who had delayed coming to the department or patients who were otherwise deviant, such as 'hippy types' (1979: 101).

3. Some patients did *not* see illness as an undesirable state; for example, 'overdoses' or 'tramps'.

4. Some patients did *not* 'cooperate with the competent agencies in trying to get well' (ibid.); for example, 'drunks' and 'overdoses'. Some refused to co-operate, others were unable to do so. It was felt that some would go on to do the same thing again, so staff felt that they were wasting their time.

Jeffery describes the ways in which patients try to manage the sick role by stressing the accidental nature of their injury, or saying that they are keen to get back to work soon. For those who are considered 'rubbish', various punishments (like being kept waiting or treated rudely) ensue. He concludes that although his own study was of hospital staff, he believed that what he found was 'probably a general feature of medical encounters' (1979: 106). This is a sobering thought, not least because many of social work's service users are likely to fit the criteria of 'normal rubbish'.

Critics of Parsons's presentation of the sick role argue that it makes more sense of short-term, acute illnesses than it does of long-term or incurable conditions. It may also make more sense in relation to physical illness than to mental illness where, as Fulcher and Scott indicate, there may be some ambiguity about whether a person is ill or not. Those who experience mental disorder may be unwilling to admit their symptoms. Moreover, the public understanding of some conditions may be low, so that people who are depressed may be told to 'pull themselves together' (2007: 300). It is also argued that Parsons failed to see that some people *are* blamed for their incapacity. HIV is probably the most obvious case-example here. Whenever someone is found to be HIV positive, the question, 'how did it happen?' is never far from the surface. For those who are 'innocent victims' of a defective blood transfusion, sympathy and support are absolute; for men who have sex with men or those who use intravenous drugs, there may be little in the way of concern for their condition. On the contrary, they may even be told that this is their 'just deserts' or God's punishment for their behaviour. Susan Sontag explores this in her polemic essay, 'AIDS and its Metaphors' (2001) (see also Green and Sobo 2000).

One of the foremost critiques of Parsons's theorising comes from Eliot Freidson (1970). Drawing on interactionist ideas, Freidson asserts that the encounter between the doctor and patient is not governed by consensus, legitimate authority and trust; instead, it is characterised by 'medical dominance' and 'suppressed conflict', as patients struggle to be treated as individuals and medics struggle to 'adjust or fit any single case to the convenience of practice (and other patients)' (quoted in Annandale 2004: 184). Annandale takes this further. She points out that functionalist approaches ignore the impact of structural issues on illness. She asserts that seriousness, legitimacy and cultural expectations based on class, 'race', gender and age all have an impact on how we behave (and are allowed to behave) when we are ill. In reviewing Parsons's contribution to the understanding of health and illness, she accepts that he brought to the surface a 'nascent social model'. But he also, she believes, 'solidified medicine's power base' and, arguably, 'its ability to set research agendas' (1998: 11). Nettleton takes a different view. She maintains that the concept of the sick role is an ideal type, which does not necessarily respond to empirical reality. Its principal merit, she suggests, is that 'it provides us with a heuristic device against which actual illness behaviours and experiences can be assessed' (2006: 75). She goes on to illustrate this by pointing out that most people, most of the time, do not go to the doctor when they feel unwell. They delay accessing the sick role, demonstrating that there is a moral dimension to seeking help: people do not want to be, or appear to be, 'timewasters', and instead are keen to 'use services responsibly' (ibid.). Moreover, the decision to ask for a doctor's appointment is likely to be due to a range of factors other than the severity of symptoms. Nettleton describes seeking help as 'an ongoing social process, rather than a straightforward response to physical symptoms' (2006: 77). From this, she concludes that accessing the sick role is a complex process. Over and above this, the interpretation of symptoms is itself context dependent; influenced by social and cultural factors, not just physical ones.

Critical perspectives

Annandale identifies the 1970s as a time when medical sociology struggled to rid itself of the 'political straitjacket' of the bio-medical model (1998: 11). It did so by looking in three very different directions: towards Marxist ideas, towards feminism, and, as will be discussed in the next section, towards interpretive perspectives.

Marxist approaches

The earliest example of a Marxist approach to health and illness is seen in Engels's study, *The Condition of the Working Class in England in 1844*, in which he argued that the typhoid, tuberculosis, scrofula and rickets that he encountered in Manchester were in reality diseases of poverty and class; medical intervention alone would not be able to eradicate them, not least because medicine operated on the basis of profit and was part of the capitalist system (1892). So from a Marxist perspective, industrialisation creates health-related risks to workers and to the general population. But more than this, it is believed that capital creates the very problems that medicine then seeks to contain, if not cure (that is, unemployment, pollution, stress, etc.). Annandale argues that there is, from this viewpoint, 'an inevitable contradiction between safety and the pursuit of profit' (1998: 13). The creation of the National Health Service (NHS) is itself an example of this contradiction. It may be presented either as a ploy to ensure that workers are healthy enough to continue to make profits for their capitalist employers or as a working-class victory, or perhaps as a bit of both (see Senior and Vieash 1998).

Annandale explores this further by considering the continued use of silicone breast implants long after their risks for women became known. Her overall assessment is that although new technologies will always carry risks, the pursuit of profit makes these risks far higher than they need to be. In short, 'capitalism despoils both health and health care' (1998: 15). Annandale also examines the way in which 'late capitalism' fosters an ideology of health that, she argues, underplays social and cultural factors and instead stresses individual responsibility. Drawing on the work of Beck (1992), she explores the ways in which in recent times, new markets have been created for products which aim to counter risks to health; risks which have, on closer inspection, been created by capitalism. For example, vitamin complexes have been introduced and sold to consumers in ever-greater numbers to enhance nutrition in an era of 'fast food'.

Feminist approaches

Feminist sociologists have also sought to challenge conventional acceptance of the bio-medical paradigm. Feminist sociologists have highlighted the gender imbalance in the medical profession as a whole, as well as the take-over by men and medicalisation of traditional aspects of women's healthcare, including childbirth and obstetrics (see Abbott and Wallace 1990, Oakley 1980, 1984 and 1993). Feminists have also pointed out that women's health problems (depression, for example) have not been treated seriously by the male-dominated medical profession (see Barnes and Maple 1992, Showalter 1987). Nettleton asserts that the attempts of women to reclaim control of their bodies is demonstrated in the success of *Our Bodies, Ourselves*, a book that was first published by the Boston Women's Health Book Collective in 1970, and republished in successive years (2006: 106).

Interpretive perspectives

Interactionist sociology turns our attention away from large-scale structures to small-scale, intimate encounters. As outlined in previous chapters, interactionist or interpretive accounts rose to prominence in the 1960s and 1970s, emphasising the ways in which selves are produced in relation to others; the self develops through role-taking, and in this way, everyday life becomes 'a process of negotiation, impression management and meaning creation' (Annandale 1998: 21). A large number of sociological studies demonstrate this approach, almost all written from the perspective of the patient's experience. Three examples stand out as especially useful for social work: studies of the meaning of illness; analysis of illness and disability as stigma; and labelling theories applied to the medical setting.

The meaning of illness

The eminent medical sociologist Robert Dingwall acknowledged in 1976 that there is no such thing as 'essential illness'; instead, illness is construed through the meanings and interpretations that are given to certain experiences. Moreover, 'there is', he argues, 'no necessary relationship to any biological happening' (1976: 26). He goes on to differentiate between 'illness behaviour' (the way people behave when they have certain symptoms) and 'illness action' (the sick person's continuing efforts, with others, to make sense of what is happening to them). Dingwall urges that sociologists should attempt to understand illness action, not simply observe illness behaviour.

Studies of chronic illness often make use of a narrative perspective. The individual's narrative is especially important here, because conventional medicine may not provide answers or cures for chronic conditions, and, as a result, people have to find ways of telling the story of their lives with illness as a constant or recurring feature. For example, Williams (1984) identifies two key features in the narratives of people suffering from rheumatoid arthritis: narrative reconstruction, through which people attempt to rebuild the story of their lives – or as Williams writes, to 'reconstruct and repair ruptures between body, self and world' (quoted in Bury and Gabe 2004: 254); and genesis, where people seek the origins or causes of their illness. Williams indicates that narratives are always 'co-authored'; doctors, family members and friends all play a part in building the story. Interestingly, some people may not see themselves as the authors of their lives at all, putting their life experiences down to 'God' or some other higher being. Williams suggests that it is important for medical sociologists and for medics themselves to be cautious of jumping to conclusions about people's narratives based on only part of the story. This point is developed further by Kleinman (1988) who urges practitioners to listen to, and take heed of, the patient's story. Likewise, Frank (1995) identifies three types of illness narratives:

1. *The 'restitution' narrative*: like Parsons's sick role, the person is ill, finds out what is wrong, uses medication and gets well again.

2. *The 'quest' narrative*: this is 'defined by the person's belief that something is to be gained through the experience' (1995: 115), possibly self-awareness, or the ability to help others. We can see many illustrations of this in writing by 'survivors' of cancer. Some people will even go as far as to say that being ill has been a positive experience for them, allowing them to 'take stock' or 'change direction' in their lives.

3. *The 'chaos' narrative*: this has no clear beginning and no end; no purpose and no meaning. Frank notes that this is hardest for practitioners (as well as patients) to deal with because it is accompanied by a sense of failure and uncertainty. People who suffer from symptoms that are medically unexplained fit this representation (Nettleton 2006: 84).

Stigma

Probably the most influential sociologist writing from this perspective is Erving Goffman. Goffman's classic 1963 study of stigma suggests that stigma is essentially about 'differentness' (we stigmatise those we perceive to be different from ourselves) and he makes an important distinction between 'the discredited' (where the 'differentness' is known about immediately, or has been disclosed) and 'the discreditable' (whose 'differentness' is not immediately noticeable, or is not disclosed). He describes the lengths people go to in order to mask their 'differentness' and 'pass' as 'normals' (1963: 100). Those who are prepared to admit their 'differentness' may nevertheless play down the effects of this, in a process Goffman calls 'covering' (1963: 125). 'Passing' and 'covering' behaviour applies equally to those who have a discrediting condition and their associates, who experience 'courtesy stigma' by virtue of their connection with the stigmatised person (1963: 44). Significantly, Goffman indicates that distaste for the stigmatised does not come only from 'normals'; people incorporate society's ideas about perfection and come to discredit themselves. Self-hatred and shame thus 'spoils' their social identity and their interactions with others, so that they come to see themselves only in terms of their 'spoiled identity'.

Subsequent studies have demonstrated the pervasive effects of stigma on a range of chronic illnesses; a significant body of this work explores the relationship between HIV, AIDS and stigma. This research indicates that HIV and AIDS are especially stigmatising, in part because they demonstrate the three types of stigma referred to by Goffman:

1. *'Abominations of the body'*: AIDS brings with it disfiguring and painful physical transformations and eventual death. Significantly, it is also a transmissible and deadly disease which carries with it ideas of 'contagion'.

2. *'Blemishes of character'*: because HIV has been identified as a disease affecting 'high-risk groups', those who get HIV infection are commonly viewed as 'bad' or 'sinful' (IV drug users, gay men, prostitutes, promiscuous men and women) or 'incompetent' (people who are too foolish to protect themselves from infection).

3. *'Tribal stigma of race, nation and religion'*: there is a strong racist undercurrent in much of the antagonism towards those with HIV and AIDS (Cree *et al.* 2004).

Bor and Elford (1998) argue that it is the stigmatised nature of HIV that separates it from other chronic illnesses. Green and Sobo (2000) take this further, asserting that AIDS has become the threat to encourage people away from what are perceived to be 'dangerous identities'. It is not surprising given this characterisation that many people with HIV choose not to disclose their diagnosis to others; they try to 'pass' as 'normals' and hide their discrediting condition from others, including their children (Green and Sobo 2000). Children who are affected by parental HIV also hide their parents' illness for fear of retribution; Goffman calls this 'courtesy stigma'. One fourteen-year-old in a study of affected children in Scotland describes what stigma meant to her:

> It's just like they treat you differently than – not like a normal person. They just treat you different, they either feel sorry for you and treat you like, sympathetic, they don't treat you like the way they would have if they didn't know. Or they'd be really horrible to you and like, don't want anything to do wi' you.
>
> (quoted in Cree *et al.* 2004)

Labelling theory

Chapter 8

We have already noted that it is doctors to whom we look in order to label or define symptoms as 'illness'. Interpretive studies demonstrate that this is by no means as simple as it might seem. Patients may accept or reject a given diagnosis, just as doctors may see something as 'not a proper illness'. In this way a negotiation takes place; one in which doctors are very much 'in charge'. Medics use a range of 'props' to convince others of their authority in the medical situation: white coats, medical equipment, medical notes, medical language (see Senior and Viveash 1998). This does not suggest, however, that patients are always passive. Senior and Viveash cite research which indicates that patients use a number of strategies to influence the encounter: they may ask questions, request further information, suggest a 'lay' diagnosis, doubt or disagree with the doctor's diagnosis. For example, Boulton *et al.* (1986) found that middle-class patients were much more likely to seek further information of their GPs. Interestingly, however, both middle-class and working-class patients were equally likely to dismiss or disbelieve their doctors' views and advice. Boutlon *et al.* conclude that it is important to examine the process of doctor–patient interactions, not just the outcomes.

New directions

All the approaches discussed so far continue to have a major influence on sociological theory and research on health and illness. What is new in recent years is a growing understanding of the impact of social structure on health and illness: it is acknowledged that factors such as social class, gender, ethnicity and age all influence how we experience health and illness, together and separately. Moreover, post-modern writing about the body has changed sociological and common-sense ideas about both health and illness.

The impact of social structure on health and illness

This subject has received extensive research attention over the last forty years or so, much of it preoccupied with the notion of health inequalities. We have already noted that Engels first drew attention to health inequality in 1844, pointing out that 57 per cent of working-class children died before their fifth birthday, compared with only 20 per cent of those of the higher classes. Subsequent end-of-century social surveys reiterated the connections between inadequate housing, poverty and ill health. For example, Charles Booth's seventeen-volume *The Life and Labour of the People in London*, which appeared between 1889 and 1903, showed that one-third of the population lived at or below the 'poverty line', a concept invented by Booth. At the same time, Seebohm Rowntree's survey of York, *Poverty: A Study of Town Life* (1901), found 28 per cent of the population living in poverty. The creation of the National Health Service (NHS) in 1948, following on from the Beveridge Report's (1942) commitment to combat the 'five giants of Want, Disease, Ignorance, Squalor and Idleness', should be understood as an attempt to eradicate health inequalities once and for all, by making healthcare free to all citizens at the point of delivery.

In the 1970s a series of government publications drew attention to the uncomfortable realisation that, despite the NHS having existed for thirty years, inequalities in health remained. The government commissioned a report to look into this, under the chair of Sir Douglas Black (*Inequalities in Health*, DHSS 1980). The Black Report stated that mortality rates for both sexes had declined over the last 100 years. But, more worryingly, inequalities still existed and they were getting wider. Men and women born into Social Classes IV and V had twice the risk of dying before retirement age than those born into Social Class I. The differences were apparent at all stages in the life cycle (including infant mortality), and also in reports of chronic illness. The report further notes that the risk of early death for men in all classes was almost twice that of women, leading women to experience greater isolation and health needs in later life. Mortality rates were found to vary considerably across the UK, with southern Britain experiencing the best health. Ethnicity was also felt to be an important factor, with New Commonwealth immigrants experiencing similar mortality rates to indigenous working classes, but lack of adequate data on 'race' and health, for either first- or second-generation immigrants, made it difficult to assess this further. The report highlights the considerable body of research evidence that middle-class people made more use of GP services and received better care from them, in spite of the fact that their actual needs were less than those of working-class people. The report also states that inequalities appeared to be greatest in the case of the 'preventive services'; that is, antenatal care, cancer screening, immunisation, etc.

Four possible explanations for health inequalities are offered in the Black Report:

1. *'The artefact explanation'*: the idea that we are not comparing like with like, because the rise in 'white collar' occupations as compared with unskilled and semi-skilled manual jobs means that there has been, and will continue to be, a drop in the numbers of those poorest classes. The report suggests that this is not a sufficient explanation; that indicators of poor health affect a much wider group than simply the poorest class (quoted in Townsend and Davidson 1982: 113).

2.   *'Natural and social selection'*: the idea that the healthier you are, the more upwardly mobile you are likely to be and vice versa; 'people *drift* to the bottom rung of the Registrar General's occupational scale' (ibid.).

3.   *'Materialist or structuralist explanations'*: these prioritise economic and socio-structural factors; poverty and exploitation are believed to cause disease and premature death (what the report calls 'the radical Marxian critique' (1982: 114)). Reflecting on this, the report notes that 'the killer diseases of modern society – accidents, cancer and heart disease – seem less obviously linked to poverty' (ibid.). However, it goes on to argue that poverty is a relative concept: those who are unable to play a full part in society 'can properly be regarded as poor. They may also be relatively disadvantaged in relation to the risks of illness or accident or the factors positively promoting health' (1982: 115). The report goes on to explain that by the time the health of those in the lowest socio-economic groups has 'caught up' with contemporary levels, the health of those in higher groups will have 'forged ahead'. The result is that inequalities do not simply persist, they increase (1982: 116–17).

4.   *'Cultural/behavioural explanations'*: the idea that there is something in the culture of working-class people that is unhealthy; 'people harm themselves or their children' through their use of tobacco and alcohol, poor diet, lack of exercise, low take-up of immunisation, antenatal services, contraception, etc. (1982: 118). The report notes, however, that there is unequal access to knowledge and education about healthy living, and good food and sports facilities may be prohibitively expensive. There may also be some cultural differences between groups, but the report's authors remain unconvinced that working-class culture can be held responsible here.

In reviewing the evidence overall, the report concludes that the 'best answer' lies in some form of the 'materialist' approach, although it suggests that different types of explanation apply more strongly, or more appropriately, to different stages of the life cycle (1982: 122–3). This is spelt out as follows:

*   The greatest risk in childbirth was among mothers who were older and had had several children, but class differences were also significant here.

*   Children aged between one and four years were most at risk from accidents, with working-class children at highest risk.

*   Health differences between adults of different classes had remained and widened.

*   Health became literally 'a matter of life and death' for the over-sixty-fives, with men more likely to die than women, and working-class people more likely to die across the board; in other words, 'inequalities in health perpetuated from the cradle to the grave' (1982: 132–3).

The report ends by calling for more research, for strategic planning, for better care for children, disabled people and older people, and for more health education.

Since the Black Report was published, a considerable amount of social policy, health and sociological research has attempted to tease out further the association between social inequalities and ill health (for example, Davey Smith *et al.* 1990, Whitehead 1992, Wilkinson 1984 and 1996). Much of this research has confirmed that although the conditions of the 'well off' may have been improving, those of the poor have changed very little and 'may even have deteriorated by some indicators' (Annandale 1998: 89). In 1997, the government commissioned Sir Donald Acheson to 'review and summarise inequalities in health in England and to identify priority areas for the development of policies to reduce them' (Acheson 1998: v). The Acheson Report adopts what it calls a 'socio-economic' model of health and its inequalities, 'in line with the weight of scientific evidence' (1998: 5). It introduces Dahlgren and Whitehead's (1991) social ecological model, which suggests that determinants of health can be seen as layered, one over another. It begins with the individual's unique genes at the centre, surrounded by personal factors (for example, smoking habits, physical activity, etc.), then social and community influences, followed by structural factors (housing, working conditions, access to services, etc.) and finally the outer layer (conditions in society as a whole).

The Acheson Report argues that the health gap between socio-economic groups must be considered in both relative and absolute terms, because both have an adverse impact on individuals and society. Moreover, it asserts that 'the economic and social benefits of greater equality seem to go hand in hand' (1998: 8). The report concludes that policies aimed at improving average health may have the undesired effect of increasing health inequalities overall, because the most 'well off' may benefit most from this (for example, cervical screening campaigns which have a higher take-up amongst the middle classes). Conversely, the report argues that strategies aimed at reducing inequality in general will benefit the health as well as the economic and social situation of the less 'well off'. This, the report suggests, could provide 'a new direction for public policy' (1998: 30).

The question of what should and can be done to reduce health inequalities remains very much a 'live' issue, for social researchers and politicians alike. Some have focused on the inadequacies of earlier explanations and models. For example, there has been some debate about just what has been measured in the research to date, most crucially, what is social class, and does it remain 'a useful marker for people's life chances' (Annandale 1998: 89)? What is the difference (if any) between the terms 'social class', 'social status' and 'socio-economic status', when many researchers use them interchangeably? Bartley asserts that: 'The measures used tend to be mainly . . . based on convenience or on rather casually developed ideas about what might be important for health inequality' (2004: 22). This is a damning indictment. Moreover, lack of conceptual clarity means that it is difficult to be sure how health inequality might be addressed. One of the most common areas of confusion emerges in the concepts of absolute and relative difference. 'Absolute difference' means the difference between two groups in real numbers; 'relative difference' refers to the percentage difference between two groups. It is possible for an absolute difference to be small, but a relative difference large, if the overall numbers are small. The reverse is also true: a large absolute difference can lead to a small relative difference if total numbers are large. Because of this, a government may decide to take action to reduce what is a relatively small relative difference, if there are large absolute numbers of cases of, say, heart disease (see Bartley 2004: 40).

Bartley (2004) identifies a range of 'aetiological pathways' (that is, causes of ill health). Firstly, she introduces 'behavioural and cultural explanations', as already illustrated in the Black Report and in Blaxter's (1990) *Health and Lifestyles*, which stressed the importance of health education to promote healthier lifestyles, as well as in Mackenbach *et al.*'s 2002 European study, which found differences between countries that could not simply be explained in terms of socio-economic inequalities. Secondly, the psycho-social model is discussed, which emphasises the psychological effects of stressful conditions at work or at home, or of having low social status. This model acknowledges that explanations based on health behaviours (as in the first option) or on narrowly materialist concerns (as in a Marxist approach) do not provide sufficient reason for continued health inequalities. Instead, concepts such as social support, stress and job strain emerge, as in the work of the prominent epidemiologist Richard Wilkinson (1984, 1996), who argues that relative poverty is as damaging as absolute poverty because of the psycho-social stress (and hence ill health) that it brings. Wilkinson describes Britain as a 'cash and keys' society in which 'cash equips us to take part in transactions in the market', and keys to our homes (if we are fortunate enough to have one) 'protect our private gains from each other's envy and greed' (1996: 226). As individualism and the market economy grow, so civic morality declines and public health is compromised; people drink too much, eat unhealthy 'comfort' foods and become

depressed. (This sounds very like Durkheim's notion of 'anomie', discussed in Chapter 2.) In his more recent books, Wilkinson (2005) and Wilkinson and Pickett (2009) argue that the problem of relative poverty will not be solved by everyone becoming richer. On the contrary, Wilkinson asserts that societies with more equal distribution of incomes also have better health outcomes; this should then be the target for intervention (thus mirroring the Acheson Report's findings).

Bartley's third aetiological pathway is the 'materialist model', which was the one accepted by the authors of the Black Report and the Acheson Report, as well as by many researchers including Davey Smith *et al.* 1990. Bartley draws attention, however, to the diverse nature of what is encompassed by 'materialist' explanations, including income, class, housing and work. She finds that these factors do not always tie up with one another, so that, for example, the link between income and employment is not the same as the link between income and housing, since one is about production and the other consumption. She argues that we need to adopt a more complex definition of 'materialist' (2004: 96). One of the issues facing this model, she continues, is that there are widespread differences within groups according to age, gender, ethnicity, etc., not just between groups. This has led to the introduction of a 'neo-materialist' explanation, which pays less attention to the individual, and is more interested in societies as a whole (see for example, Wilkinson and Pickett 2009). Bartley's final presentation is based on the 'life-course' approach, which emerged in the 1980s. Researchers from this perspective suggest that illness or deprivation in early childhood have a later impact on health chances. Some have investigated whether there might be particular 'critical periods' which have a later adverse effect on individuals; others have explored the ways in which social advantages and disadvantages might 'add together' in a cumulative way over time. For example, Hilary Graham (1998) found that although only 22 per cent of women were smokers, this rose to 46 per cent of those with no educational qualification, 50 per cent of those with no qualifications and a low-skilled job, 67 per cent of those who also lived in social housing and 73 per cent of women who also claimed social assistance benefits.

Reflecting on the models and explanations overall, Bartley argues that these are not necessarily mutually exclusive; on the contrary, they may be seen as working together to affect someone's chances of health or illness (2004). Graham (2007) agrees, proposing that social and health researchers need to work together more; that bridges need to be built between social epidemiologists and sociologists. More than this, she argues that there are whole fields of interest that have barely been touched on by researchers to date, including the very different patterns of women's health and illness and the ways in which socio-economic and gender inequalities are 'mediated by ethnicity' (2007: xvii). This very much reflects the message of Annandale's earlier book, where she argues that 'there may be important similarities as well as differences between men and women' (1998: 159). Furthermore, she asserts that there is little real understanding of the ways that racism on the one hand, and ethnic diversity on the other, interact with each other and with other structural factors in relation to health and illness.

Post-modernism and the sociology of the body

Post-modern thinking has had a major influence on the sociology of health and illness; Michel Foucault's writing is central to these developments. We have already acknowledged that illness is a social construction as well as a physical condition. A Foucauldian perspective drives social constructionism much further than this, according to Annandale, who argues that what we know as diseases are themselves 'fabrications of powerful discourses, rather than discoveries of "truths" about the body and its interaction with the social word' (1998: 35).

In *The Birth of the Clinic*, Foucault (1975) documents the construction of a new way of thinking about the body and health in the period since the Enlightenment. He identifies a shift between the eighteenth and nineteenth centuries in the way that the body was seen; new disciplines emerged within medical science (physiology, embryology, immunology) to sit alongside anatomy in 'speaking about' and analysing the body. Foucault extends this analysis in an article in which he argues that demographic changes at this time led not only to the identification of population as a problem, but to its emergence 'as an object of surveillance, intervention, modification, etc.' (1980: 171). More recently, Fox argues, psychology and sociology have also had an impact on medical discourse, as a 'biopsychosocial model of medicine transforms the early biomedical body' (1998: 11). Post-modern and post-structuralist writers have sought to make visible the issues of power which are at the heart of medical discourse, highlighting the ways in which both health and illness are defined and treated by the medical profession, while other 'regimes of truth' (lay accounts, complementary therapies, etc.) are presented as illegitimate or dangerous. But Foucault's thesis is much deeper than this might suggest. There is no simple 'top-down' notion of power here; instead, power is viewed as a relationship which is 'localised, dispersed, diffused and typically disguised through the social system, operating at a micro, local and covert level through sets of specific practices' (Turner 1997: xi–xii). Moreover, modern civilisation is itself a 'project' which relentlessly writes the body, transforming it into a cultural object. Fox explains further:

> There is no escape: even 'liberating' movements contribute to this writing. For example, twentieth century sexual 'liberation' from 'repression' is not liberation at all, but the domination and subjection of the body in a normalising discourse on sexuality and desire. Any theory of resistance is merely a further discourse of power and knowledge, creating a new subjectivity.
>
> (1998: 13)

In reflecting on Foucault's work overall, Turner suggests that his main contribution to medical sociology lies in his emphasis on the importance of regulation and administration as key features of 'modern society'. Turner is less sure, however, about what Foucault has to say about the 'risk' society in which we now live. Turner argues that welfare and health systems today demonstrate a mixture of 'risk culture' (where risks are macro and externalised) and 'McDonaldisation of services' (that is, the application of Fordist production methods and rational managerialism to the fast-food industry, now extended to all sectors of society). He suggests that followers of Foucault need to 'address the new environment of risk cultures, political contingencies and deregulated welfare systems' (1997: xix). He lists the following as challenges to Foucault's ideas: the fact that it is private medicine and 'a doctrine of obligation' which is increasingly meeting the needs of the ageing populations in Western societies; that the notion of citizens' rights is being replaced by ideas of 'individual obligation'; that the problem of mental health is increasingly being resolved not by more surveillance, but by de-institutionalisation; and that rising healthcare costs have led to increased privatisation, internal markets and de-institutionalisation (ibid.)

For myself, I do not see any necessary contradiction between a Foucauldian perspective and current systems of health and welfare. On the contrary, his analysis of power and regulation makes a lot of sense of the current emphasis on individualisation (what Foucault calls the 'technology of the self'; that is, self-discipline and bodily management), which is a prominent feature of health and welfare practice today (see Foucault 1988). Lupton argues that Foucault's notion of the practices of the self can be brought into play to analyse the ways in which people respond to the medical encounter (1997: 105). They may struggle to subvert medical and disciplinary techniques which they see as restricting their autonomy, or they may strive to present themselves as 'good patients'. Of course, they may not always be aware of what they are doing; the self is often fragmented and contradictory, pulling between conscious and unconscious states. As Lupton writes, 'subjectivity may be understood as dynamic and contextual rather than static, and as often fraught with ambivalence, irrationality and conflict' (1997: 106). This, she argues, offers new insight, as people are often as complicit in the reproduction of medical power as they are in challenging it.

The emergence of the sociology of the body in recent years bears witness to a continuing interest in Foucault's ideas. Nettleton and Watson outline the main developments which have taken place, paraphrased below (1998: 4):

- *Body politics*: recognition that the physical body has a social and political status, such that having a different body (whether that is female as opposed to male, or a body with a disability) helps to determine an individual's life chances. Feminism and the Disabled People's Movement have been central to raising awareness here.

- *Demographic changes*: an ageing population, and the consequences of living with an ageing body.

- *The prevalence of chronic illness*: infectious diseases have been replaced by chronic conditions; this has led to questions of identity and living with pain and discomfort.

- *Consumerism*: increased emphasis on the appearance and health of the body; looking and feeling 'good', where good means slim, active and youthful.

- *Technological changes*: physical limitations can be overcome, appearance changed, organs and limbs repaired. It becomes increasingly difficult to distinguish between the 'natural' and the 'technological' body.

- *The body as an expression of our identity*: diet, exercise and lifestyles can be portrayed as 'moral', 'immoral' or 'irresponsible'.

Annandale is also interested in this area, arguing that the rise of cosmetic surgery, a 'boom industry' in the developed world, demonstrates the 'emergence of the self as a reflexive project' (Annandale 1998: 18). For Annandale, the body is 'not passive'; instead, it needs to be monitored and controlled, as individuals literally re-create themselves 'under conditions of considerable uncertainty' (ibid.). This theme is taken further by Shilling, who sees the body as 'a project' which is always 'unfinished' (2003: 5). Drawing on Giddens (1991), she suggests that in a society which is dominated by risk and uncertainty, the body has come to form a secure site over which individuals are able to exert control: 'If one feels unable to exert control over an increasingly complex society, at least one can have some effect on the size, shape and appearance of one's body' (2003: 6). From this perspective, death represents the end of that control; it becomes a failure of control. Shilling also identifies class differences, as well as gendered differences, in the way that we seek to control our bodies, so that working-class people have a more functional view of the body, treating it as 'a means to an end', whereas the middle classes are more likely to treat it 'as an end in itself'; for example, participating in sport for its intrinsic value, rather than to get fit. This, of course, raises another set of questions about what 'intrinsic' value means, and who decides? New reproductive technologies create similar kinds of issues for women, as these treatments have brought opportunities to women for empowerment, choice and control of their fertility, while simultaneously increasing medical intervention in their bodies and lives. As Nettleton concludes, 'Bodies form a key site of political struggle, and their presence forms a key dimension of the interactions between health carers and those who are being cared for' (2006: 135).

Implications for practice

Chapter 1

- It has been stated that social work's origins lie in functionalist and modernist ways of thinking. It is therefore not unexpected that social work in health settings has often played the part of bolstering the bio-medical model, while accepting unquestioningly the authority of medics.

- In recent times, however, we can see social work playing a more contradictory role in healthcare, valuing people's narratives and supporting those who are ill and those with disabilities to challenge the medical orthodoxy, at the same time as continuing to act in an ancillary capacity in traditional, doctor-led hospital and clinic settings. There have also been significant moves within social work to highlight and confront structural inequalities in health.

Conclusion

This chapter has demonstrated that health and illness has, in recent years, taken centre-stage in sociological literature, just as it has moved to the heart of the social work enterprise. Neither health nor illness can be taken for granted. Both are socially constructed, and both are equally affected by structural inequalities and by power. At the heart of health and illness is the body, and sociological writing on the body has shown that individuals can, and do, resist the claims that others make of them, and can and do struggle to assert their personhood in the face of an existence characterised by risk and uncertainty. As ever, it has been argued that social work has the capacity to be a force for good; to make a difference in people's lives. An uncritical, non-reflective practice may exacerbate people's experience of inequality and disadvantage. McLeod and Bywaters (2000: 8) argue that social work can play a significant role in producing more equal chances of physical health and greater equality when ill. They see the following as elements of such practice:

- A direct contribution to increasing the material, environmental, personal and social resources required: e.g. maximising income; securing safe, appropriate accommodation; strengthening interpersonal and social support, and improving access to information.

- Collaboration in building up the infrastructure of interest groups, locality-based activism or self-help organisations in the interests of redressing discrimination.

- Advocacy and brokerage with the professionals concerned to ensure greater equity in accessing available professional care and treatment and in the quality of care received.

(2000: 9)

Recommended reading

Bury, M. and Gabe, J. (2004) *The Sociology of Health and Illness: A Reader*, London: Routledge. A useful collection of highly relevant papers.

Bywaters, P., McLeod, E. and Napier, L. (eds) (2009) *Social Work and Global Health Inequalities: Practice and Policy Developments*, Bristol: The Policy Press. Presents an international social work perspective.

McLeod, E. and Bywaters, P. (2000) *Social Work, Health and Equality*, London: Routledge. This offers encouragement to social work practitioners.

Wilkinson, R. and Pickett, K. (2009) *The Spirit Level: Why More Equal Societies Almost Always Do Better*, London: Allen Lane. A polemic and important book.

8 Crime and deviance

Introduction

This chapter examines from a sociological perspective a subject which looms large in the public imagination and in rhetoric from both the Left and the Right of the political divide. When New Labour came to power in 1997, its manifesto promised that it would be the 'Law and Order' party, 'tough on crime and tough on the causes of crime'. Since that time, statistics indicate that overall crime, including violent crime, has fallen by almost 40 per cent (www.crimestatistics.gov.uk/). But at the same time, the prison population in England and Wales rose from about 66,000 in 2001 to more than 80,000 in 2009, while the prison population in Scotland stood at a record 7,835 in 2009, up from less than 6,000 in 2000. The Labour government is not alone in wanting to lock up more people. The Conservative Party website stated in December 2009 that if successful at the next general election it planned to increase prison capacity by 5,000 places above Labour's plans.

This chapter begins by considering definitions of crime and deviance, arguing that the definitions we use have fundamental implications for our understandings of crime, criminal behaviour and the management and control of crime. As in previous chapters, there is a discussion of historical and cross-cultural accounts of crime. The main thrust of the chapter is on the many and varied sociological explanations of crime and deviance. The chapter does not set out to review the whole field of criminology, which is an eclectic discipline drawing on perspectives as diverse as psychology, psychiatry, political economy, history, anthropology, ecology, law and, of course, sociology.

Definitions

The question 'what is crime?' may seem straightforward enough. After all, there can be no doubt about what is, and is not, a crime, since a criminal act is defined as such by law, and criminals are those who break the law. But what about acts that are not defined as criminal by law, but that we may believe are criminal nonetheless? Until 1991, rape within marriage was not a crime in law, although it was widely recognised as unacceptable, 'criminal' behaviour. Hester and Eglin (1992: 27) argue that virtually every form of human action has in some time or place been deemed warranted, if not desirable, including slavery, non-consensual intercourse within marriage and all forms of execution. And what about acts which are defined as criminal by law, but which we may not see as criminal? It was not until 1967 that the UK government decriminalised homosexuality, and, as we will see, it remains an offence in many countries around the world.

Taken together, these questions suggest that crime is a relative rather than an absolute concept; it is defined by society and it changes over time. But there is another complicating factor. Emsley suggests that crime is 'an action defined by the law which, if detected, will lead to some kind of sanction being employed against the perpetrator' (2007: 123). Two additional elements have been introduced here. Firstly, an act must be 'detected' in order to be considered criminal, and secondly, a 'sanction' or punishment of some kind must be the end result for the perpetrator. As we will discuss, criminologists and sociologists have demonstrated over many years that figures for detected crime and 'invisible' or 'hidden' crime are at great variance, with figures for detected crime representing only a fraction of total criminal activity (Maguire *et al.* 2007). In addition, the nature and range of sanctions or punishments for wrong-doing are highly variable and change over time. For example, we know that in the past the crimes of heresy, sacrilege and blasphemy were punishable by hanging. At the same time, the murder of one commoner by another was seen as less serious, meriting only a cash fine to the relatives of the deceased (Giddens 1989: 121). This suggests that a given society will, at a particular moment in time, decide not just what a criminal act is, but also how far it is prepared to go to police that act, and what sanctions it will impose on those who are found guilty of the criminal act.

But this approach to crime may be criticised on the grounds of cultural relativism. Is there no such thing as a crime which is *always* a crime; perhaps, for example, murder or rape or a racist assault? This gets us into further difficult areas, however. All criminal acts are open to diverse interpretations and located in specific circumstances. This means that the abused woman who finally 'cracks' and stabs to death her violent husband of twenty years may be seen as less guilty than the jealous husband who suffocates his wife in a violent rage. The same act (murder) may be viewed quite differently, and questions such as intentionality and self-defence come to the fore. Intentionality is also an issue in rape trials. When men are accused of rape, juries have to decide whether to believe the man who says he thought that the woman agreed to sexual intercourse, even if she said 'no'. As a consequence, courts find it notoriously hard to secure a conviction, especially when the victim knows the accused and has chosen to be with him in the first place (Brown *et al.* 1993). Racist attacks have also been difficult to prove, not least because of all the complex issues around institutional and personal racism in the police force, the courts and society as a whole (Brake and Hale 1992). (See also Sir William McPherson's (1999) Report into the Stephen Lawrence Enquiry.)

If crime is difficult to define, then what about deviance? Giddens states that deviance may be defined as 'non-conformity to a given set of norms that are accepted by a significant number of people in a community or society' (2006: 794). Again, this simple definition leads us into the murky waters of ambiguity. Who decides what 'non-conformity' is? Which norms, and whose norms, are being transgressed? How many is a 'significant number'? Most of us have broken social rules at some point in our lives; for example, by driving too fast, parking illegally, not paying for something in a shop, smoking marijuana, etc. Evidence suggests that legislation introduced in the UK in December 2003 to prevent the use of hand-held mobile phones while driving has not yet significantly changed behaviour, though the decision by insurance companies to increase premiums for motorists found guilty may have an impact on drivers' behaviour in the longer term. This suggests that it is not the criminalisation of the act which changes behaviour, but the likelihood of getting caught and of receiving some kind of penalty, financial or otherwise. Additionally, not all behaviours that are viewed as deviant are also criminal. The term 'deviance' is much broader than 'crime': it is possible to deviate from a number of cultural norms, including health norms, sexual norms and religious norms (Macionis and Plummer 2008: 542). So, for example, New Age travellers or rave culture may be studied as forms of deviance, as might Hare Krishnas or, as Giddens controversially suggests, the permanently homeless.

The argument so far is that a crime is an action defined by law as criminal and punishable if detected; deviance is non-conformity and may or may not be deemed criminal. Social work, probation services and social workers all play a part in defining on a daily basis the limits and boundaries of criminal and deviant behaviour, as do law-makers and law-enforcers, criminals and victims of crime, politicians, judges, sheriffs and magistrates, the media, police officers, members of the public and pressure groups, and, of course, sociologists and criminologists.

Implications for practice

- Definitions of crime and deviance determine our views about sentencing, punishment, treatment or deterrence. This suggests that we need to constantly ask questions of ourselves, of others and of society, about what we think the problem is and why.

- Practitioners also need to be cautious about some of the terms that are commonly used to describe those we work with. The terms 'offender' and 'perpetrator' are often used in a shorthand, uncritical way, as if this was unproblematic and as if this somehow summed up the whole person. This is discriminatory and is also likely to lead to incomplete assessments being made.

Historical accounts

Two key questions dominate any discussion of crime, historically and in the present day. How much crime is there? Is it increasing or decreasing? To answer these questions, we need to know something about how crime statistics are collected, now and in the past.

Emsley (2007) highlights the difficulties in making judgements about the nature and extent of crime over time. He points out that official statistics for crime in England were not collected until 1805; before this time, although certain court records were kept, there was no attempt by government to keep annual countrywide records. When national crime records began in 1805, statistics only registered committals for trial. The system for collection was refined in 1834 and again in 1856, by which time statistics were gathered on indictable offences, committals for trial and persons convicted and imprisoned. The changes in record-keeping have led to serious disagreement amongst historians about the value of statistics. Some maintain that the figures are meaningless for serious analysis; others argue that whilst they cannot give any exact picture of the extent of crime, they do nevertheless give an indication of the pattern of crime. Emsley (2007) suggests that the late eighteenth century witnessed a steady increase in crime, particularly property crime, becoming sharper from the first decade of the nineteenth century until about 1850, when the pattern levels out; except, most notice-ably, for the offence of burglary. After the First World War, there was another steady increase which halted briefly during and after the Second World War, then began to rise sharply once again in the 1950s. Emsley relates this pattern to what is known about society more generally; it makes sense in terms of shifts in population and the economy in the eighteenth century and the concerns about the urban poor and the threat of revolution in the nineteenth century. But the picture is far from straightforward, and it remains impossible to know whether social conditions actually caused an increase in crime, or whether people were more sensitive to offences and so reported them (and indeed prosecuted them) more frequently. For example, the increase in burglary may reflect an increase in prosperity, because people had more possessions in their homes. Similarly, the decrease in crime during both world wars may suggest that the police forces were too busy to attend to ordinary criminal activities; or it may reflect the fact that many young men were either out of the country or under stricter control at home. Neither example tells us anything absolute about either the nature or the extent of crime.

Emsley (2007) presents another set of complicating factors that interferes with any notion of reliability in historical analyses of crime figures: that is, changes in the organisation and management of policing. Although the Metropolitan Police Force was established in London in 1829, and larger towns in England and Wales were required in 1835 to institute local watch committees to set up police forces, there was no national system of policing until the 1850s. Before this time, a range of different policing measures was in operation. In 1856, an Act of Parliament set up for the first time a system of county-based police forces for England and Wales, with only the larger towns maintaining their independent police, under 'watch' committees. Similar legislation was passed a year later in Scotland. Emsley is doubtful about whether the new police force actually achieved its stated objective of preventing crime. What is apparent, however, is that the police demonstrated their efficiency by arresting anyone whose behaviour was seen as offensive, including drunks, prostitutes and street sellers.

There is one final development that makes the comparison of crime figures across time questionable. Emsley records that throughout the eighteenth and into the nineteenth centuries, it was the victim or the victim's relatives who made the decision to prosecute an offender in England and Wales (not so in Scotland, where this was already the procurator fiscal's decision by the beginning of the eighteenth century). Emsley (2007) indicates that there were major problems with the system in England and Wales. Victims were reluctant to proceed with a prosecution because of the expense of paying for legal documents and fees, and because of fear of reprisal, or fear of having to take time away from paid work. During the nineteenth century, the new police forces increasingly took on the role of prosecutor, so that by the end of the century, most prosecutors were police officers, leading to an inevitable rise in the number of prosecutions and, hence, the number of convictions.

It is worth thinking a bit more about why there was a shift towards official record-keeping, a paid police force and professional prosecution at this time. The answer lies, as in previous chapters, in the upheaval which was the industrial revolution:

> It was not until the early nineteenth century that crime became an object of scientific enquiry in its own right. In important respects, a concept of 'crime' only came to replace a concept of 'sin' when a burgeoning legal apparatus, designed to protect property and the interests of the nation-state, evolved out of the social, economic and cultural transformations of the industrial revolution. As concern over the 'problem of crime' intensified, so crime became the object of more systematic observation and measurement.
>
> (McLaughlin *et al.* 2003: 1)

Before this time, crime was regarded for the most part as the deliberately chosen behaviour of rational, free-willed actors. It was believed that those who broke the law weighed up the calculations of pain and pleasure and then acted purposefully and selfishly. According to this so-called classical tradition, the objective of the law was to identify the right measure of punishment to fit the crime. Punishment was designed principally as a deterrence, to stop the individual's criminal behaviour, and to deter others from committing similar offences. There was no particular interest in trying to understand the causes or the meaning of crime. The circumstances behind the criminal act, either individual or social, were largely irrelevant to the wider project of delivering justice. The nineteenth century witnessed widespread concerns about rising crime rates, poverty and disorder in rapidly growing towns and cities throughout Europe and the United States, as illustrated in the social surveys of the living and working conditions of the poor, conducted by Andrew Mearns, Henry Mayhew, Edwin Chadwick and others, which highlighted the links between poverty, disease, vice and crime.

As concern about crime intensified, so the second-half of the nineteenth century saw the emergence of a specialist 'science of the criminal': a deliberately scientific approach to crime which was 'concerned to develop a "positive" factual knowledge of offenders, based on observation, measurement and inductive reasoning' (Garland 1997: 31). The new 'science of the criminal' developed in diverse ways. Some scholars such as Cesare Lombroso, working from an anthropological tradition, focused on the physical nature of human beings, seeking to uncover inherited characteristics and assumed abnormalities that might separate out the criminal from the citizen. For example, Lombroso identified a number of physical characteristics that he attributed to habitual delinquents, including thinning hair, lack of strength and weight, prominent foreheads, thick curly hair, large ears, etc. He believed that these were all indications of regression to a less developed human form; a return to being 'savages'. Others, using Freudian psychoanalytic theory, attributed criminal conduct to serious mental pathology or at least to some unresolved emotional conflicts. Offenders were said to break the law because of a need to act out emotional conflicts (that is, to 'ventilate'); from a desire to be punished (masochism); or because of an inability to control sexual impulses that derived from traumatic periods in their psychological development. A third area of investigation pioneered sociological approaches to crime, exploring social conditions and social factors (for instance, incomplete socialisation) that might explain crime and criminality. These will be explored more fully later in the chapter.

Cross-cultural studies

Macionis and Plummer assert that all societies have crime and deviance; there is no such thing as a 'crime-free society' (2008: 543). Studies suggest that crime rates across Europe and the United States increased throughout the twentieth century, before beginning to fall at the beginning of the twenty-first century. Macionis and Plummer urge caution in making inter-country comparisons, however. For example, victim studies suggest that the Netherlands is the most criminal environment, but it transpires that this is because of the high incidence of people reporting the theft of bicycles! (2008: 544).

Two particular case-study examples demonstrate that there is widespread variation between countries in their approaches to crime, deviance and crime control: these feature homosexuality and capital punishment. For example, it is perfectly legal to be homosexual in the UK today, supported by legislation in 2004 which gave civil partnerships similar rights to those of heterosexual marriage (see Chapter 2). But homosexual acts are viewed in a very different light in some other countries. On 18 March 2009, the United States, under President Obama's leadership, finally endorsed a United Nations (UN) statement calling for the worldwide decriminalisation of homosexuality, a statement that the former president, George W. Bush, had refused to sign. When the UN statement was voted on in December 2008, 66 of the UN's 192 member countries signed the non-binding declaration, which was endorsed by all 27 European Union members as well as Japan, Australia and Mexico. But importantly, 70 UN member countries still outlaw homosexuality, and in several, homosexual acts can be punished by execution. More than 50 nations, including members of the Organisation of the Islamic Conference, opposed the declaration, which was also opposed by the Vatican (*Guardian*, 18 March 2009, www.guardian.co.uk/).

Different approaches to crime are also demonstrated in the use of capital punishment. This issue was very publicly aired in late December 2009, when a British man, Akmal Shaikh, was executed for attempting to smuggle drugs into China. This was in spite of pleas for leniency by his family and the British government on grounds of his mental health problems. Shaikh was the first European to be executed by China for twenty-five years. Between 1,700 and 10,000 people are executed there each year; the exact number is unknown, but it is claimed that even by the most conservative estimates, China accounts for seven out of every ten executions in the world (*Guardian*, 29 December 2009, www.guardian.co.uk/). Amnesty International indicates that a wide range of offences carry the death penalty in China, including bribery, embezzlement and stealing gasoline (Marsh *et al.* 2009: 585). The former head of China's State Food and Drug Administration, Zheng Xiaoyu, was executed in 2007 for having accepted bribes to authorise sub-standard and counterfeit medicine (*Guardian*, 13 July 2007, www.guardian.co.uk/). Capital punishment is also legal in the United States. Since the Supreme Court overturned the ban on the death penalty in 1976, thirty-eight of the fifty US states provide for the death penalty by law (Marsh *et al.* 2009: 586).

Implications for practice

- The discussion demonstrates that crime and deviance are historically, socially and culturally relative; crime and deviance are both social constructions.

- Social workers and probation officers must analyse critically their own values and attitudes to discern where they stand in relation to the discussion so far. They must also seek to interrogate their own institutional settings, so that they can fully appreciate the nature of the job they are being asked to do on behalf of society.

Traditional sociological approaches

Although we tend to think of deviance in terms of free choice or individual failings, all behaviour, deviant and conforming, 'is shaped by society' (Macionis and Plummer 2008: 561). Some sociological approaches illustrate functionalist, consensus underpinnings: they assume that society's norms and values are shared by all. Other approaches have grown out of a conflict tradition, locating crime and disorder firmly in class inequality and the workings of capitalism.

Functionalist theories

Writing in 1895, the French sociologist Emile Durkheim argues that crime is a 'social fact': normal and universal in all societies and at all times, and therefore endemic to social organisation:

> In the first place crime is normal because a society exempt from it is utterly impossible. Crime . . . consists of an act that offends certain very strong collective sentiments. In a society in which criminal acts are no longer committed, the sentiments they offend would have to be found without exception in all individual consciousnesses, and they must be found to exist with the same degree as sentiments contrary to them. Assuming that this condition could actually be realised, crime would not thereby disappear; it would only change its form, for the very cause which would thus dry up the sources of criminality would immediately open up new ones.
>
> (Reprinted in McLaughlin *et al.* 2003: 66).

According to Durkheim, not only is crime normal and universal, but deviance is 'necessary' because it performs four functions that are essential to society (Macionis and Plummer 2008: 562):

1. Deviance affirms cultural values and norms. It does so by confirming good and evil, crime and justice; it is 'indispensable to the process of generating and sustaining morality'.

2. Responding to deviance clarifies moral boundaries; a line is drawn between right and wrong.

3. Responding to deviance promotes social unity; people unite to react against serious deviance, reaffirming 'the moral ties that bind them'. (Critics have argued that Durkheim is wrong here, that fear of crime can force people to withdraw from public life, not come together to fight it.)

4. Deviance encourages social change, because deviant people 'push a society's moral boundaries, suggesting alternatives to the status quo and encouraging change'. Moreover, today's deviance 'sometimes becomes tomorrow's morality'.

Durkheim concludes that criminals are not 'totally unsociable beings' or parasites introduced into the midst of society. Instead, they play a 'definite role in social life'.

Anomie and strain theories

Although Durkheim sees crime as a normal and potentially positive feature, this does not imply that he was unconcerned about rising crime in his own society. On the contrary, much of his scholarly work was devoted to seeking to understand what he saw as a breakdown in social organisation and an increase in crime and deviance. In his first major work, of 1893, Durkheim examines the transition taking place in France from a rural, agrarian society to an industrial urban one. *The Division of Labour in Society* presents two very different social arrangements. Pre-industrial society typifies for Durkheim 'mechanical solidarity'; that is, a high degree of social solidarity based on similar lifestyles and strong relationships and inter-connectedness between people. There would be little chance of crime becoming widespread in this kind of society, Durkheim asserts, because the 'collective conscience' would be robust and effective. Modern industrial society, in contrast, is said to epitomise a state of 'organic solidarity', characterised by a complex division of labour which sets people apart from each other. This encourages a state of 'egoism', which was contrary to the maintenance of social solidarity and to conformity to law (Heathcote 1981: 347). Durkheim argues that in this kind of society, social order and collectivity cannot be taken for granted. Instead, institutions and structures have to be created to build and maintain a consensus in society (Rock 2007).

Durkheim's distinction between pre-industrial and industrial societies has been criticised as being over-simplified and inaccurate in terms of its understanding (Rock 2007). Nevertheless, key aspects of his conceptualisation of the impact of social change have been highly influential. In *The Division of Labour in Society*, Durkheim asserts that in times of rapid social change, 'anomie' occurs. Anomie refers here to an absence of clear-cut moral rules and a lack of certainty as to how to behave in the changed social circumstances: a kind of individually perceived 'normlessness' (Heathcote 1981: 347). Durkheim expresses this vividly: 'man's nature [is to be] eternally dissatisfied, constantly to advance, without relief or rest, towards an indefinite goal' (Durkheim 1984 [1893]: 256). Durkheim also uses the concept of

anomie in his later study of *Suicide*, published in 1897. Here anomie refers not to a break-down in social organisation at a societal level, but to an individual response to societal pressures. Durkheim suggests that in periods of sudden prosperity or severe economic depression, there is no longer any effective regulation of people's ambitions. Competitive individualism (what Durkheim calls 'egoism') and unlimited aspirations lead to a state of anomie, where people become disoriented and anxious, and a number of them commit suicide. Durkheim's analysis of suicide figures confirms his proposition: those who commit suicide are more likely to lack effective familial and social affiliations (for example, divorced or single people) than those who have high levels of these attachments. He writes: 'The more weakened the groups to which the individual belongs, the less he depends on them, the more he consequently depends only on himself and recognises no other rules of conduct than what are founded on his private interests' (1952 [1897]: 209).

Durkheim's conceptualisation of anomie has been developed by subsequent sociologists and criminologists, who have each brought their own slant to the discussion. The idea of anomie remains popular today, and has been applied in places as diverse as housing estates in the UK and Paris, poor areas of Los Angeles, parts of Africa and the state of Chechnya (Rock 2007).

Durkheim's ideas about social disorganisation were put into practice between the 1910s and the 1930s at the University of Chicago's School of Sociology, as part of the development of an ecological approach to crime. The so-called 'Chicago School', led by Park, Burgess, McKenzie and Wirth, took forward ideas from the late nineteenth-century social surveys that had identified the notion of 'criminal areas', where poverty, overcrowding and crime were high. They set out, through a combination of survey technique and participant observation, to chart the ways in which various areas of Chicago had become

specialised around activities and occupied by the many different groups who had come to live in the city from the 1860s onwards. They argued that, like plants in the natural environment, different social groups competed for space and colonised areas of the urban environment. Their objective was not just to investigate communities, but to bring about social change. To this end, the academics also worked as probation officers, community workers and consultants on housing and anti-poverty agencies. (See also Chapter 5.)

It was Robert Merton who gave Durkheim's notion of anomie a distinctly American flavour (Rock 2007). Merton argued that American society in the 1930s produced anomie, or 'strain', by giving people the idea of equality of opportunity and access to success in society, but then put structural obstacles in their way that prevented them from achieving their aspirations. For Merton, the 'American dream' was a myth, since class, 'race' and other social differences systematically restricted opportunities. Unable to meet their unrealistic aspirations through legitimate means, individuals turned to illegitimate careers instead, hence generating crime and deviance. Merton encapsulates this as follows: 'the culture makes incompatible demands . . . In this setting, a cardinal American virtue – "ambition" – promotes a cardinal American vice – "deviant behavior"' (1957: 145). Merton suggests that anomie gives rise to a series of possible adaptations, each reflecting the range of choices that are open to the individual. Apart from conformity, Merton identifies four 'deviant' adaptations (Muncie and Fitzgerald 1981: 407):

1. *Innovation*: this is the adaptation most frequently associated with crime. It is depicted as a typically working-class adaptation, leading poor people with no legitimate access to financial success to get involved in burglary, robbery and other property crimes.

2. *Ritualism*: this is an adaptation of the lower-middle-class bureaucrat, who chooses to 'play it safe', keeping his or her head down and zealously conforming to rules. It is lack of ambition that singles out this person as deviant.

3. *Retreatism*: instead of coping with the structural strains in society, retreatists opt out altogether and seek their own rewards through drug addiction, vagrancy, alcoholism and psychosis.

4. *Rebellion*: this is the adaptation adopted by those who not only reject society's norms and goals but also challenge their legitimacy. Their aim is to change the social system which has created the goals in the first place.

Subcultural explanations

Although Merton's analysis was both historically and culturally specific, his ideas were taken up and adapted in Britain and in the United States. For example, Albert Cohen (1955) in his study, *Delinquent Boys*, points out that it was lower-class young men who were most likely to experience strain and become delinquent: young men formed gangs out of 'status frustration', to gain the status and achievement that was denied to them by the dominant culture. Through a process of 'reaction formation' they rejected the dominant values that they could not achieve and turned them upside-down: 'the practical and utilitarian in middle-class life was transformed into non-utilitarian delinquency; respectability became malicious negativism, the deferment of gratification became short-run hedonism' (Rock 2007:10). Delinquency was characterised, therefore, by short-term pleasures, toughness, excitement and thrills; typical offences were vandalism, joyriding and fighting (Smith

1995). It was also, significantly, portrayed as a masculine activity. Cohen (1955) asserts that if strain had any meaning in the context of girls, this could only be explained in terms of frustrations in their sexual relationships. The girls who became involved in delinquent acts are portrayed as doing so because of 'thwarted affections', not 'status frustration' (Naffine 1987: 13).

Cloward and Ohlin (1961) extend Merton's and Cohen's analysis. They accept Merton's concept of a connection between aspirations and opportunities, but argue that the critical factor here is not simply the blocking of legitimate opportunities. Instead, deviance and delinquency are based on the *availability* of legitimate and illegitimate opportunities. Cloward and Ohlin argue that lower-class neighbourhoods possess both legitimate and illegitimate opportunities for success: young men who cannot achieve success through legitimate means may turn to illegitimate means to fulfil their aspirations. Whether they do so or not will depend on their access to these opportunities: on the circles (or subcultures) in which they are moving, and on learning and opportunity within these subcultures. Cloward and Ohlin refer to this process of learning criminal behaviour as 'differential opportunity'. They identify three different subcultures that lower-class young men might be connected with (Cloward and Ohlin 1961, Macionis and Plummer 2007):

1. *The criminal subculture*: which is closely connected with adult crime, and is characterised by property crime, including robbery, burglary and theft.

2. *The conflict subculture*: which has strong parallels with Albert Cohen's notion of a negativistic, violent subculture.

3. *The retreatist or escapist subculture*: offences involving possession or supply of drugs feature strongly here.

Subsequent researchers have sought to test the reliability of these ideas in practice. For example, Matza and Sykes (1961) take issue with the essentialism in strain theory, arguing that a commitment to delinquent norms is only ever likely to be partial; those seen as delinquent share many values with the middle-class citizen, and as a result delinquency is an occasional activity rather than a defining characteristic of their lives. Matza and Sykes conclude that what separates young working-class men from the rest of society is the high value they place on leisure; it is through leisure that they try to recover some of the autonomy which is unavailable to them in school and work. The first study to attempt to apply American subcultural theory in the British context was conducted by David Downes (1966) in East London. Downes discovered that the working-class boys in his study did not experience status frustration or strain. 'They neither hankered after the middle-class world nor repudiated it' (Rock 2007: 10). Instead, they were well located in their shared working-class identity. Neither school nor work held any special meaning for them except as a source of income, and instead they turned their energies and aspirations to leisure-time pursuits, engaging in delinquent activities only when access was limited to 'the necessary symbols of subcultural leisure' (for example, clothing and entertainment) or when 'the expectation of action is met with "nothing going on"' (Muncie and Fitzgerald 1981: 410).

Reviewing strain theory overall, Macionis and Plummer suggest that Merton's ideas may explain some types of crime, notably property crimes, better than other kinds of crime, such as crimes of passion or mental illness. They also express reservations about the tacit assumption in anomie and strain theory that everyone shares the same cultural values, and that the only deviants to merit scrutiny are those who are poor and working class. Importantly, they argue that if crime 'is defined to include stock fraud as well as street theft, offenders are more likely to include affluent individuals' (2008: 564). Smith (1995) offers another, equally valid objection. Strain theories, he argues, do not do well in explaining why most young men who commit delinquent acts as youths do not go on to become adult criminals. After all, he asserts, 'the strain of frustrated ambition' is likely to continue and probably even to get worse over time. Yet we know that in reality, 'very few people follow this pattern' (1995: 35). But Smith does find these ideas useful nonetheless. As he summarises: 'In policy terms, strain theories suggest a progressive, redistributive agenda which deserves to be defended against more repressive alternatives' (1995: 36). Strain theories also serve as a counterbalance to individualistic approaches to crime and deviance, reminding us that poverty and inequality have real effects on the lives of some people.

There is, however, one further issue that seriously undermines this approach. Strain theory and the subcultural studies are predicated on an assumption that the core subject is male and that the position of young women is quite different (and inferior) to that of young men. It is young men who are said to endure strain in relation to their career and employment prospects; it is young men who experience a disjuncture between their aspirations and their opportunities. Young women, in contrast, are seen as only interested in success in their relationships with men; their offending behaviour is trivial and insignificant. This, for Naffine and other feminist criminologists, is 'flawed theory' (1987: 23).

Control theories

Control theories have a very different starting point from other theories of crime. Instead of asking 'why do people commit crime?', the question becomes 'why *don't* people commit crime?' Control theories have a long history in criminology, and explanations as diverse as psychoanalytic theories on the one hand, and Durkheim's ideas of anomie on the other, demonstrate a concern for the notion of insufficient control mechanisms in the individual or in society.

It was Travis Hirschi who took up and developed control theory in the 1960s. Hirschi (1969) argues that as human beings, we have the capacity for both moral and immoral, criminal and non-criminal behaviour. What prevents us from indulging in criminal activities is neither our inherent goodness, nor subcultural grouping, nor social class. Rather, it is what he calls the 'social bond'; that is, the connection between the individual and society. The social bond is said to have four interrelated components: attachment, commitment, involvement and belief. Delinquent acts result 'when the individual's bond to society is weak or broken' (1969: 16), so that there is nothing to prevent that person from engaging in a criminal act. The components of the social bond may be outlined as follows:

- *Attachment*: that is, the connection an individual has to conventional people and those in authority, particularly parents and schoolteachers. The stronger the attachment (and thus the greater the sensitivity to the opinions of others), the stronger the control.

- *Commitment*: that is, the investment an individual is prepared to make in terms of time, effort, money and status, versus the costs associated with the choice not to conform. The greater the commitment, the more an individual has to lose.

- *Involvement*: that is, participation in legitimate activity, including employment, clubs and organisations, sport. Again, the greater the commitment to this kind of activity, the less time will be available for non-conforming activity.

- *Belief*: that is, acceptance of the conventional value system. Lack of acceptance of the rule of law, for example, makes lawbreaking more likely.

The empirical evidence for control theories is inconclusive, although there does seem to be a correlation between strong attachment to school and family and low rates of delinquency in young people (Smith 1995). A study by Harriet Wilson cited by Rock (2007: 14–15) found that what separated delinquent from non-delinquent children in 'socially deprived' families in Birmingham was the extent of parental supervision. Parents who acted as 'chaperones' effectively prevented their children from offending, by keeping them indoors and under close supervision. Smith points out a more profound complaint with control theories. Because they provide no motivation for offending beyond the absence of controls, it is implied that any of us might commit crimes. Yet, Smith reasons, most of us would never think of committing armed robbery or murder, let alone weigh up the costs and benefits of doing so. Control theories may therefore explain better some acts of youthful misbehaviour than persistent and serious crime. In addition, control theories fail to give attention to the ways that opportunities for different crimes become available and are sustained over time, or to the reality that crime rates are higher in certain neighbourhoods (1995: 39–40).

Naffine highlights the early control theories' lack of interest in women and girls, in common with all sociological theories so far examined. When Hirschi tested his theory in 1964, his subjects were 1,300 American schoolboys. Naffine finds this surprising: given that Hirschi was explicitly interested in why people do *not* offend (that is, he was interested in conformity, not deviance), why then did he not study girls, since females are known to be more law-abiding and conforming than males? Naffine finds an explanation for this in the strong convention in criminology of investigating the male; of valuing the male while devaluing the female, even when they are exhibiting exactly the same behaviours. Consequently, she is scathing of studies that went on to verify Hirschi's ideas, presenting conforming males as responsible, hardworking, energetic, intelligent breadwinners, whereas women who conformed were portrayed as passive, dependent, and 'generally lacking any of these critical faculties' (1987: 67). Feminist research subsequently took up the challenge of investigating 'the new and intriguing riddle of the conforming woman' (Rock 2007: 15). Some of this research confirms that women's greater conformity is best explained by the greater control and supervision of women's behaviour, in the family and in public arenas. Carlen (1988) suggests that it is when domestic family controls are removed altogether – for example, when young women leave home or are taken into care – that they are more likely to be exposed to controls (and freedoms) traditionally associated with young men.

Control theories re-emerged in the UK and the United States in the late 1970s as part of a new 'law-and-order' approach to crime in both countries. What has been called 'Right Realism' portrays deviance as 'an individual pathology: a set of destructive, lawless behaviours actively chosen and perpetrated by individual selfishness, a lack of self-control and morality' (Giddens 2006: 806). The solution is therefore not greater social equality or the redistribution of wealth in society, but greater control and prevention of crime through harsher punishment (deterring some offenders and locking others away for longer periods) and better prevention and detection measures. Conservative governments in the UK and the US, influenced by the Right Realist perspective, began to intensify law enforcement activities, extending police powers, expanding the criminal justice system and calling for longer prison sentences as the most effective deterrent against crime (ibid.). The New Labour government elected in 1997 carried on in this vein, while at the same time also drawing on ideas that, as we will see, owe much to 'Left Realism'.

Interpretive approaches

Interpretive or 'interactionist' approaches present a very different perspective on the social world in general and crime and deviance in particular. Instead of conceptualising the basic values of society as a unitary system, and the actions of individuals as determined by external, structural forces, society is viewed as a plurality of different possibilities – individuals can and do make choices about their actions, including their criminal and deviant actions. The object of research becomes an investigation of why individuals choose to behave in a certain way (and equally why they do not).

Differential association theory

One of the most influential theories to draw on an interpretive framework is that of 'differential association' (also known as cultural deviance theory). Edwin H. Sutherland originally proposed this theory in 1939 in *Principles of Criminology*, and then revised his ideas in subsequent editions of this book. The 1978 edition sets out the nine propositions that he maintains are generally applicable to all crime in modern society (spelling as original):

1. Criminal behavior is learned.

2. Criminal behavior is learned in interaction with other persons in a process of communication.

3. The principal part of the learning of criminal behavior occurs within intimate personal groups.

4. When criminal behaviour is learned, the learning includes (a) techniques of committing the crime, which are sometimes very complicated, sometimes very simple, and (b) the specific direction of motives, drives, rationalizations and attitudes.

5. The specific direction of motives and drives is learned from definitions of the legal codes as favorable or unfavorable.

6. A person becomes delinquent because of an excess of definitions favorable to violation of law over definitions unfavorable to violation of law.

7. Differential associations may vary in frequency, duration, priority, and intensity.

8. The process of learning criminal behavior by association with criminal and anti-criminal patterns involves all of the mechanisms that are involved in any other learning.

9. While criminal behaviour is an expression of general needs and values, it is not explained by those general needs and values, since non-criminal behavior is an expression of the same needs and values.

(Sutherland and Cressey 1978: 80–3)

From this conceptualisation, it is apparent that crime is caused not by social disorganisation or individual pathology, but by a process of learning, interaction and communication within subcultures. Modern society is no longer seen as a homogeneous whole. Instead, different and separate social worlds are envisaged, each transmitting their own goals, and people grow up with different and conflicting definitions of, and attitudes towards, legal codes. They are socialised into criminal behaviour in exactly the same way that people are socialised into non-criminal behaviour. The effectiveness of that process of socialisation and learning depends on the frequency, duration, priority and intensity of this 'differential association' (Sutherland 1939, Sutherland and Cressey 1978).

Sutherland's work has been criticised for being too generalised and for not sufficiently recognising human purpose and meaning. It is also criticised for not offering a good enough explanation for all crime and deviance (Muncie and Fitzgerald 1981). Nevertheless, his ideas do offer an extremely plausible explanatory framework for some kinds of delinquent and criminal activity; for example, heroin use. Most people, claims Smith (1995), have little idea how to obtain heroin, let alone how to use it. 'Even if the actual use of the drug is a solitary activity (which often it is not), it is made possible by learning what to do, necessarily with one another, often in a group' (Smith 1995: 43). Sutherland has also been criticised for his presentation of women (Naffine 1987). Although he states at the outset that his propositions are gender and class neutral, he later admits that women do not fit the general pattern; that because girls and women are traditionally conditioned and supervised more closely than boys and men, anti-criminal norms are not available to them in the same way. Feminist researchers have subsequently explored this idea more fully, suggesting that differential association theory (along with control theory) may explain both women's conformity and their offending behaviour: women commit less crime because of their restricted access to illegitimate or criminal opportunities.

The crimes women do commit (for example, shoplifting) are available to them in the course of their normal daily lives; specialist tasks such as safe-breaking or the use of weapons and tools are not (Smart 1976: 15).

Labelling theory

Labelling theory asks an entirely different kind of question from the theories discussed so far. Instead of asking 'why do they do it?' – or even 'why don't they do it?' – it asks 'what processes have led to this act being labelled as deviant and treated as such?' The focus therefore shifts away from the individual and her or his motivations, family background, subcultural grouping, relationships to the labelling agencies themselves, the police, courts, media, social work agencies, and the state in general. Labelling theory assumes that we all commit crimes, although we are not all caught. Once caught, we are not all labelled as criminal; behaviour may be ignored, excused or the police may respond by issuing a caution. The distinction between 'criminals' and 'non-criminals' is, Bilton *et al.* assert, 'fortuitous and highly problematic' (2002: 389). Macionis and Plummer argue that, in its narrowest sense, 'labelling theory asks what happens to criminals after they have been labelled, and suggests that crime may be heightened by criminal sanctions'. In its broadest sense, labelling theory suggests that criminology has given too much attention to criminals as types of people and not enough 'to the panoply of social control responses – from the law and the police to media and public reactions – which help to give crime its shape (2008: 565).

Smith states that the basic idea behind labelling theory was not new: 'if you give the dog a bad name, things are likely to go badly for the dog' (1995: 76). But it was in 1938 that Tannenbaum first used this idea in a criminological context, recognising that: 'The person becomes the thing he is described as being ... The harder they [agents of control] work to reform the evil, the greater the evil grows under their hands ...' (quoted in Smith 1995: 76). These ideas were then developed more fully by Lemert in the 1950s and Becker in the 1960s, although Smith (1995) suggests that it was not until the 1980s that labelling theory began to have a major impact on policy and practice. Lemert made an important distinction in 1951 between 'primary' deviance and 'secondary' deviance. Primary deviance was presented as an isolated act of wrong-doing, which may have little significance to the person concerned (for example, a childish prank in the classroom). Secondary deviance occurs in response to social reaction to the primary deviance (for example, the child chooses to play the 'bad boy' and sets out to annoy or upset the teacher by further rule breaking). The onset of secondary deviance is viewed by Goffman (1963) as marking the beginning of a 'deviant career': 'As individuals develop a strong commitment to deviant behaviour, they typically acquire a stigma, a powerfully negative social label that radically changes a person's self-concept and social identity' (Macionis and Plummer 2008: 566).

Stigma overpowers other dimensions of identity so that the individual is diminished in others' eyes and becomes socially isolated (see also Chapter 7). Garfinkel (1956) points out that a criminal prosecution is one example of public labelling in this way, much like a university graduation ceremony.

Chapter 7

Lemert refines the policy implications of his 'societal reaction' theory in his later study of juvenile delinquency (1971). Here he equates the large increase in cases of delinquency dealt with by juvenile courts in the United States between 1957 and 1971 with the rise of the 'rehabilitative ideal' among agencies of juvenile social control. The 'rehabilitative ideal' which had encouraged maximum intervention in the lives of young people had led to a much broader range of activities and behaviours coming under the spotlight of the social control agencies. Juvenile delinquency had, in effect, expanded to include behaviour that was not outside the criminal law. Lemert concludes that social control is a cause, not an effect, of deviance. Labelling theory is also demonstrated in Becker's famous (1963) participant observation study of jazz musicians' use of marijuana. Here he describes the set of stages undertaken by the musicians as they learn to use the drug, hide its use from others who might disapprove, and then take on a marijuana-smoker's identity when their behaviour is labelled as deviant. From this, Becker argues that 'deviant behaviour is behaviour that people so label'. He writes:

> Social groups create deviance by making the rules whose infraction constitutes deviance, and by applying those rules to particular people and labeling them as outsiders. From this point of view, deviance is not a quality of the act the person commits, but rather a consequence of the application by others of rules and sanctions to an 'offender'. The deviant is one to whom that label has successfully been applied; deviant behaviour is behaviour that people so label.
>
> (1963: 8–9)

Labelling theory is extended further in the work of Leslie Wilkins (1964), who coined the term 'deviancy amplification theory' to refer to 'the unintended consequences that can result when by labelling a behaviour as deviant, an agency of control actually provokes more of that same deviant behaviour' (Giddens 2006: 802). He argued that if the person who is labelled takes on the identity of a deviant person, this is likely to provoke further responses from agencies of social control. In this way, undesirable behaviour is repeated, and the person labelled as deviant becomes even more resistant to change. The effects of deviance amplification were illustrated by Stanley Cohen in his classic study, *Folk Devils and Moral Panics* (1972), already examined in Chapter 4. Here he argues that the labelling of young 'mods' and 'rockers' as troublemakers backfired, creating even more problems for law enforcement. Sensationalist press reporting led to a 'moral panic'; what Giddens defines as 'a media-inspired over-reaction towards a certain group or type of behaviour' (2006: 802). Moral panics in more recent years in the UK have been fuelled by teenage pregnancy, youth crime, 'bogus' asylum seekers, and, arguably, the threat from Islamic extremists.

In evaluating labelling theory overall, Muncie and Fitzgerald are critical of the approach's inadequate analysis of power: there is no way of understanding the processes by which labels are attached to specific behaviours (1981: 419). Becker's own words indicate something different. In answer to the question 'whose rules?', he writes:

> Differences in the ability to make rules and apply them to other people are essentially power differentials (either legal or extralegal). Those groups whose social position gives them weapons

and power are best able to enforce their rules. Distinctions of age, sex, ethnicity, and class are all related to differences in power, which accounts for differences in the degree to which groups so distinguished can make rules for others.

(1963: 18)

In practice, several studies, both qualitative and quantitative, suggest that official labels do have an impact on delinquent identities and behaviour. Most especially, official labels may have a strong impact on those who are less committed to antisocial behaviour at the time the label is applied, particularly young people. There are, nevertheless, questions that cannot be ignored in relation to labelling theory. Why are some acts and not others labelled as deviant? Does an act have to be noticed and so labelled in order to be deviant? What about behaviour, for example rape or murder, which is regarded as unacceptable almost everywhere? Smith points out that in choosing marijuana smoking for his analysis of deviance Becker chose a relatively safe topic: there is clearly room for doubt about whether this should be considered a criminal offence, whereas more serious crimes fit much less readily into a labelling perspective (1995: 78). Naffine (1987), meanwhile, denounces the sexism in much research which adopts a labelling perspective, including Becker's study. She points out that Becker portrayed the jazz musicians in his study as men; women were typecast as 'squares' who held back their men from the creativity and glamour of their lives. More recent feminist research on delinquent girls presents a much more colourful picture of young women.

Conflict theories

The third broad area of sociological explanations for crime and deviance encompasses what are known as 'conflict theories'. Conflict theories, emerging in the changing social and economic climate of the 1960s and 1970s, demonstrate a new set of understandings about the nature of crime and social order. Like traditional functionalist approaches, conflict theories are concerned with the wider structures of society. But here the similarity ends. While functionalist approaches conceptualise crime and social disorder in terms of a decline in the moral consensus in society, conflict theories explain crime in terms of capitalism, patriarchy and structured systems of inequality in society; the law is perceived as an instrument which supports and perpetuates inequality. Conflict approaches have developed considerably since the 1960s, learning from each other and at the same time taking on insights from the interpretive paradigm. The emergence of a new 'Left Realism' in the mid-1980s has been particularly influential for social policy and practice.

Marxist perspectives

A classical Marxist approach presupposes that all social phenomena can be explained in terms of the society's means of production or economic relations (Muncie 1999: 125). Because capitalism is structured by inequality, there is no consensus in society about norms and values. Instead, society is characterised by class conflict. The law is itself an instrument of the ruling class, designed to protect the interests of the bourgeoisie and at the same time to sustain the exploitation of the working class or proletariat. Although Marx wrote little about crime itself, Muncie identifies five key propositions derived from Marx's general analysis:

- Crime is not caused by moral or biological defects, but by fundamental conflicts in the social order.

- Crime is an inevitable feature of existing capitalist societies because it is an expression of basic social inequalities.

- Working-class crime results from the demoralization caused by labour exploitation, material misery and the appalling conditions at home and in the factories.

- In certain respects, such crimes as theft, arson and sabotage may be considered a form of primitive rebellion – a protest or rebellion against bourgeois forms of property ownership and control.

- The extent and forms of crime can only be understood in the context of specific class relations and the nature of the state and law associated with particular modes of production.

(Muncie 1999: 125.)

Marxist criminologists in the 1970s set out to challenge the taken-for-granted assumptions in criminology, turning attention away from individual offending to the economic structures of society (for example, Taylor *et al*. 1975). From the perspective of this 'new criminology', high levels of crime in capitalist societies are 'unsurprising, because capitalism is a crime-creating system, by virtue of the motivations and aspirations it encourages in people and the class relations and inequalities that characterise it' (Bilton *et al*. 2002: 392). Property crime is 'normal' behaviour, as people resort to illegal means to achieve their material aims and desires. Taylor *et al*. express this forcefully:

Property crime is better understood as a normal and conscious attempt to amass property than as the product of faulty socialisation or inaccurate and spurious labelling. Both working class and upper class crime . . . are real features of a society involved in a struggle for property, wealth and self-aggrandisement . . . A society which is predicated on unequal right to the accumulation of property gives rise to the legal and illegal desire to accumulate property as rapidly as possible.

(1975: 34)

The analysis goes further, however. It is argued that any notion of 'objectivity' and 'neutrality' in criminology is a myth: that criminology has focused too much on working-class crime at the expense of crimes carried out by powerful individuals and corporations, including 'white collar' crimes, fraud, tax evasion, industrial pollution, etc. The result is that the 'crime problem' has come to be associated almost exclusively with working-class 'street' crime, and not upper-class 'suite' crime, both officially and in the minds of working-class people themselves (Bilton *et al*. 2002: 394). The solution for Marxist criminologists is to get rid of capitalism; piecemeal tinkering with the system simply allows capitalism to continue.

The period from the mid-1970s onwards has been characterised by a series of debates and disagreements about the nature of crime and crime control by writers from within the conflict tradition. These debates have been focused on a number of key issues, which it is argued cannot be resolved by an analysis from within a pure (sometimes called a 'crude' or 'idealist') Marxist perspective:

- If crime is caused by material deprivation and poverty, why is it that not all poor people commit crime? And, equally importantly, why do rich and professional people commit crime?

- If crime is related only to structural factors, how can this account for individual choice, opportunity and meaning?

- If crime is a form of 'primitive rebellion', why is so much crime intra-class, and directed against the poorest and most vulnerable in society?

- If crime is related only to class oppression, how can this explain crimes such as racist assault and sexual violence?

- If crime is a feature of capitalism and class inequality, how can this explain the reality that most offenders are men? The Marxist approach has shown little interest in the female offender (Naffine 1987).

- If the law is an instrument of the ruling classes, why does it work at times in favour of poor people and against the interests of the powerful?

New studies have reworked and amalgamated versions of anomie, subcultural and interactionist theories alongside ideas of power and social control (for example, the groundbreaking 1978 study of mugging by Hall and colleagues). The key subject in this becomes a critical understanding of the social order and of the power to criminalise and control. The aim, Muncie asserts, is 'to transform criminology from a science of social control into a fully politicised struggle for social justice' (Muncie *et al.* 1996: xix). Scraton and Chadwick outline what they see as the central argument in 'critical criminology':

> Critical criminology recognizes the reciprocity inherent in the relationship between structure and agency but also that structural relations embody the primary determining contexts of production, reproduction and neocolonialism. In order to understand the dynamics of life in advanced capitalist societies and the institutionalization of ideological relations within the state and other key agencies it is important to take account of the historical, political and economic contexts of classicism, sexism, heterosexism and racism . . . The criminal justice process and the rule of law assist in the management of structural contradictions and the process of criminalization is central to such management. While maintaining the face of consent, via negotiation, the tacit understanding is that coercion remains the legitimate and sole prerogative of the liberal democratic state.
>
> (1991: 85)

Left Realism

A new agenda emerged within the conflict tradition in the mid-1980s, in large part as a reaction to the appearance of neo-liberal, neo-classical ideas of law and order ('Right Realism') which were gaining ascendancy in the UK and the United States (see, for example, Van Den Haag 1975, Wilson 1975). The sociologists Jock Young, John Lea and Roger Matthews came together to try to reinforce the relevance of social explanations for crime and deviance, while at the same time distancing themselves from what they saw as the naïvety of a crude Marxist approach (they called this 'Left Idealism') which, they claimed, underestimated how much of a problem crime really was. The self-styled 'Left Realists' stressed the seriousness of crime, arguing that it has real, damaging consequences for the most disadvantaged in society. According to Young, the central tenet of Left Realism is

> to reflect the reality of crime, that is in its origins, its nature and its impact. This involves a rejection of tendencies to romanticize crime or to pathologize it, to analyse solely from the point of view of the administration of crime or the criminal actor, to underestimate crime or to exaggerate it.

> (1986: 11)

Left Realists argue that crime tends to be committed *by* working-class people *on* working-class people; in other words, it is intra-class, not inter-class. This means that instead of being a problem of the capitalist system, crime is largely a problem for inner cities and for working-class housing estates. Drawing on delinquent subcultural ideas, Left Realists assert that the most probable cause of most criminality is relative deprivation and marginalisation; people who are on the edge of society feel that society is unjust and that they have been treated unfairly (for example, young black African Caribbean men in the UK). Young (1986) asserts that at a societal level feelings of disenchantment and alienation may lead to rioting. At an individual level, theft and burglary may seem an appropriate means to redress the balance. Crime is therefore not conceptualised as some kind of revolutionary challenge to the ruling class. Instead, it is seen as reactionary behaviour which demonstrates the absence of real political solutions to the experience of degradation and exploitation suffered by the working class. Individual crime therefore has no political agenda. Left Realists argue that a full understanding of crime will only come through a consideration of the 'square of crime': the state, the public, offenders and victims.

Young argues that criminology must have a practical imperative; it must address the climate of 'impossibilism' and set out to reduce crime (1986: 29). Bilton sets out the three different levels of action required:

- At the 'macro' level, the pursuit of social justice is essential, requiring the government to improve material rewards, employment opportunities and housing and community facilities by fundamental shifts in government economic and educational policies. (Young reaffirms the need for society-level change in his later book (1999) which demonstrates the damaging effects of social exclusion for society as a whole.)

- At the 'intermediate' level, it requires more enlightened penal policies which reduce the prison population and replace sentences of imprisonment, where appropriate, with non-custodial alternatives. It also requires more democratically controlled and accountable police forces sensitive to the communities in which they work, and hence a shift in police attitudes to, for example, black youths.

- At the 'immediate' level, it requires 'target-hardening' strategies based on environmental and design changes that will inhibit the ability to commit crime, such as better security measures, better street lighting, vandal-proof phone boxes, etc.

(2002: 398)

In reviewing the contribution of Left Realism to the criminological debate, critics accuse Left Realists of stigmatising individuals and groups. It is said that by concentrating largely on working-class street crime, they perpetuate the idea of the 'dangerousness' of working-class and minority ethnic people. In addition, not enough attention is given to questions of social justice, because they are so caught up in questions of control and deterrence (Muncie 1999: 139). Nevertheless, all of the measures outlined above have been visible in the New Labour government's agenda since it came to power in 1997, accompanied by a large dose of 'Right Realist' ideas leading to the increased stigmatisation of some groups (for example, working-class young people becoming known as 'hoodies') and the incarceration of more people than ever before across the countries of the UK.

New directions

Returning to the sociological literature, a number of challenges to conventional explanations of crime and deviance emerged from the 1970s onwards, all of which have had a major impact on sociological thinking today, as well as on social policy solutions.

Gender and crime

There is a strong link between gender and crime. All the data indicate that crime is an activity carried out mainly by men; about 80 per cent of those convicted of serious offences in England and Wales are males (Office of National Statistics 2007, reported in Marsh *et al.* 2009: 572). Feminist theory has presented a powerful challenge to conventional criminology from the 1970s onwards, asking new questions about the ways in which society is structured and the nature of power relations. The feminist critique emerged in 1976 with the publication of Carol Smart's *Women, Crime and Criminology*.

Since then, feminists have highlighted the neglect and distortion of women in criminology at the same time as raising a new set of critical questions about gender and crime (Heidensohn and Gelsthorpe 2007). Conventional criminological theories, as already indicated in this chapter, assume the male as the norm. When the female appears, she is on the edges of male behaviour, most frequently stereotyped as a sex object for men's use, or as a conforming, home-loving, colourless creature (Naffine 1987). Feminist criminologists have sought to redress the balance; to bring women back into criminology. For some feminists, this has meant re-examining traditional sociological theories, such as anomie, strain theory, labelling perspectives, etc., from the viewpoint of women in general and women offenders in particular. Others have turned their attention to new subjects and areas of investigation, including the gendered nature of crimes such as domestic violence (for example, Dobash and Dobash 1979) and women's experience of the criminal justice system (for example, Walklate 1989). The underlying philosophy throughout draws on a conflict analysis: explanations for crime again lie in unequal power structures in society. But within this, it is possible to identify a range of feminist perspectives.

Radical feminists such as Susan Brownmiller (1975) and Andrea Dworkin (1981, 1988) conceptualise crimes such as rape and sexual violence in terms of structures of male power and privilege in patriarchy. From this perspective, crimes against women are only extreme forms of behaviours that are viewed as 'normal' for men in patriarchal societies. For example, in her well-known and highly controversial book, Brownmiller asserts that rape 'is nothing more or less than a conscious process of intimidation by which *all men* keep *all women* in a state of fear' (1975: 15). Liberal feminists are also interested in societal expectations of men and women, but their focus of attention is on gender role socialisation, not patriarchy. Oakley points to the male aspect of almost all crime, observing that the 'dividing line between what is masculine and what is criminal may at times be a thin one' (1972: 72). Socialist feminists such as Rowbotham (1973) take a very different approach, arguing that criminality is 'the product of the unequal distribution of power in both the market and the home' (Muncie 1999: 131).

Just as Marxist criminology has been criticised for presenting too one-dimensional an approach, so feminist criminologies have been challenged by those sympathetic to, and critical of, the feminist project more generally. The radical feminist approach has been criticised by feminists and others for its essentialism and its reductionism; it is claimed that there are more ways of being a man (and indeed a woman) than this analysis would seem to suggest. Liberal feminist perspectives are seen to lack a structural analysis of power: there is no adequate explanation of how gender roles are assigned and why some women (including those who commit crime) manage to break free from the ties of their socialisation. Socialist feminist criminology has been accused of falling into the same trap as Marxist criminology, failing to recognise the structuring context of 'race' and ignoring human action and choice (Muncie 1999: 132). More recently, feminist criminologists (both women and men) have sought to deconstruct the language and concepts of criminology in a new, post-modern approach, examining the gendered nature of both crime and the law, and the impact of ideas of 'masculinity' and 'femininity' on constructions of crime and deviance (for example, Campbell 1993, Connell 1995, Hudson 1989, Jefferson 1992, Phillips 1993, Segal 1990).

Some researchers have continued to focus on the behaviour of women and girls as perpetrators and victims of crime. Wilczynski (1995), in a study of parents who kill their children, discovers that women who kill their children are dealt with very differently than men: 'When a woman kills her own child, she offends not only against the criminal law, but against the sanctity of stereotypical femininity: it is therefore assumed that she must have been "mad"' (1995: 178). This observation has resonance with accounts of the treatment of 'troublesome' girls; that is, girls who find themselves in juvenile court for criminal offences. Hudson asserts that such young women are subject to a 'double penalty': they are 'punished both for the offence itself and for the social crime of contravening normative expectations of "appropriate" female conduct via "promiscuity", "wayward" behaviour, "unfeminine" dress and so on' (1989: 206–7). Not only this, the most common cause of anxiety at the point of referral is likely to be that the girls are 'beyond control' and/or at risk morally. The gendered nature of crime has also been explored in studies that have investigated women and children as victims of crime. Studies of rape, domestic abuse and child sexual abuse have examined not just the experience of crime itself, but also the ways in which courts, police officers and the media have dealt with these issues (for example Carlen and Worrall 1987, Dobash and Dobash 1979). More recent studies have widened out the discussion of victimisation to consider the reality that both women and men may be victims of crime. Newburn and Stanko (1994) point out that although men in general continue to occupy an advantaged position in relation to women, this does not mean that they are not capable of suffering criminal victimisation. They assert that we must give up 'our essentialist models of gender which undifferentiatedly present women as victims and men as oppressors, and confront the social reality in which men not only routinely victimise women, but also victimise each other' (1994: 165). We must also, some feminists argue, face up to the gaps and silences within feminist analysis, for example, examining women's violence (see Badinter 2006, Pullar 2009).

Ethnicity and crime

Just as crime has been shown to be gendered, so black and Asian people's experience of crime and the criminal justice system is markedly different to that of white people, as demonstrated in official statistics in both the UK and the United States. So, for example, although the percentage of black and Asian people living in the UK is very low overall, black people were 6.4 times more likely to be stopped and searched than white people, and Asian people twice as likely; similarly, black people were over three times more likely to be arrested than white people (2003–4 England and Wales figures, reported in Marsh *et al.* 2009: 575). Black and Asian people are also more likely to be victims of crime than white people (Macionis and Plummer 2008: 572). Black people are, in the United States, more likely to be executed. Although only 12 per cent of the US population is black, 42 per cent of the nation's condemned prisoners are black and 35 per cent of those executed since 1977 have been black (Marsh *et al.* 2009: 576). Sociologists have been concerned to ask key questions arising from this. Firstly, why is the crime rate higher amongst black people than amongst white people? And secondly, why is the crime rate higher amongst black people of African Caribbean (UK) and African American (US) origin than amongst other black people? Marsh *et al.* (2009) and Smith (1995, 1997) explore a number of different kinds of explanations, all of which demonstrate familiar themes from sociological literature (see also Gabbidon and Greene 2005). Smith begins with a warning that research carried out in London indicates that there is only ever a suspect in 16 per cent of offences. This suggests that we need to be wary of drawing wider conclusions on such a limited sample (1995: 136). Furthermore, it should be acknowledged that the official crime index in the UK excludes arrests for offences as wide-ranging as drink-driving and so-called 'white collar' violations such as insider trading, embezzlement and tax evasion. This omission, Macionis and Plummer assert, distorts the crime picture overall and 'clearly contributes to the view of the typical criminal as a person of colour' (2008: 572).

Sociological explanations for the difference in crime rates between white and black people may be characterised as follows:

- Demographic and social and economic factors: there is a higher proportion of young people among minority ethnic populations, and black people are more likely to live in poor, inner-city areas; hence there is more black crime (Marsh *et al.* 2009: 576). Critics have pointed out that this cannot offer sufficient explanation for why certain individuals and groups living in the same situation are more or less likely to get involved in crime.

- Black crime is a form of political resistance, a legacy of colonialism and slavery. Marsh *et al.* are cautious about accepting this kind of explanation, suggesting that young black people are as conformist as other young people to the values of wider society (2009: 577).

- Racial prejudice amongst police officers and institutional racism in the criminal justice system leads to young black people being criminalised. 'Stop and search' policy in the UK has been shown to have been used disproportionately in relation to black people (Macionis and Plummer 2008: 573). Meanwhile, Smith points out that African Caribbean people in England and Wales are more likely than whites or Asians to be stopped by the police on suspicion of having committed an offence, and are more likely (other things being equal) to be arrested rather than receive a caution. They are also more likely to be charged after arrest with offences which carry a high risk of a prison sentence, especially street robberies and drug offences, and they are more likely to be remanded in custody. A higher proportion of black people are sentenced in the Crown Court, and they are also more likely to be given custodial sentences, rather than probation or community service (1995: 136, 141–3).

- Cultural explanations suggest that some behaviours, such as the use and sale of illegal drugs, are culturally 'normal' in some minority ethnic communities, yet prohibited by society. This affects crime rates for black African Caribbean people (Smith 1995). In contrast, Moore (1988) explains the low levels of crime amongst Asian groups in the UK as being due in part to their stronger family and community ties and more cohesive culture, as well as to their greater economic success.

- As well as appearing in offenders' statistics in disproportionately high numbers, black people are at greater risk of victimisation. This is partly, argues Smith, because many are young and live in high-crime areas (1995: 145). But it is also because they experience high levels of racist attacks and racially motivated crime, as the British Crime Survey regularly demonstrates.

Post-modern and post-structural perspectives

It is clear from the discussion in this chapter that criminology and sociological perspectives of crime and deviance are rooted in the 'modernist' project: their aim throughout has been to find explanations and causes of crime so that intervention strategies can be identified. Post-modern perspectives see this as an unattainable goal: it is argued that we cannot make sense of 'crime' (or the family, or youth, etc.) in any complete sense, because the social world is characterised by complexity and contradiction, relativity and difference. Post-modernists therefore reject grand terms and totalities such as 'the state', 'patriarchy' or 'capitalism' as providing adequate explanations for people's experience. They also reject the idea that criminology can have any necessary theoretical coherence or unity. As Smart writes, 'The core enterprise of criminology is profoundly problematic' (1990: 77).

Moving away from 'grand theories', Foucault (1977) urges the introduction of a more historically specific analysis which examines the minute mechanisms of control, rather than concentrating on power in terms of ideology or structure. In his seminal book, *Discipline and Punish*, he contrasts earlier brutal and sometimes chaotic punishment of the body with more recent forms of surveillance and imprisonment. He criticises the conventional identification of power with repression, and argues instead that power is broader than the state, and should be considered in its productive aspects as well as its negative ones. From a Foucauldian perspective, therefore, there is no distinction to be made between 'hard' and 'soft' measures of social control. They are both part of the process of 'policing' (of managing populations and individuals) and they have the capacity for drawing on different techniques, inspectorial and regulatory, to achieve this end. Social work and probation services are both part of this social control system, and they themselves draw on 'hard' measures such as offence-focused work and 'soft' measures such as counselling and relationship-building.

Macionis and Plummer (2008) indicate that systems of control have been greatly extended and strengthened in recent years. There has been a dramatic increase in the use of closed circuit television (CCTV) in shops, motorways and all kinds of public places. There are also ever more sophisticated records kept on individuals by an increasing number of public and private agencies. Informal systems of control have increased too, evidenced by the major growth in Neighbourhood Watch Schemes in the UK. Likewise, systems of electronic tagging have been introduced in a number of countries in Europe and in the US, so that offenders can now be confined at home, their behaviour monitored and modified. Macionis and Plummer identify a recent development in the introduction of the Anti-Social Behaviour Order (the ASBO), which serves a restriction on someone (usually a young person) and relates to various activities including truancy, public drunkenness and graffiti. They conclude that there has been a major expansion in social control and surveillance in modern societies: 'Boundaries of control are being blurred and many new deviants are being "created" through this system' (2008: 556).

Implications for practice

- The sociological literature on crime and deviance suggests a number of key lessons for practice; most fundamentally, that in trying to understand these phenomena we need to look to social, economic, cultural and political factors, not simply to individual and psychological ones.

- The very different kinds of explanations also indicate that no one 'grand theory' can explain all crime and deviance. On the contrary, different types of explanation are more helpful in explaining particular kinds of criminal behaviour. This suggests that different kinds of solutions will also be needed.

- The literature reminds us that social work and probation are both social control agencies. As such, they need to be aware of the dangers of 'net widening' (Whyte 1998), because early intervention and preventive strategies may risk unnecessarily drawing people into the social control system.

Conclusion

It has been argued that crime is historically and socially constructed: it changes over time, and it exists because we give it a name and choose to take action to control it. In this respect, it is always political. And crime is reflective of wider structural issues of class, 'race' and ethnicity, age and gender: inequalities affect what is seen as crime and targeted as worthy of social control. Crime is also about individual and social circumstances: about individual choices and meanings, and about individual family backgrounds and social and cultural circumstances. There can be no one satisfactory, all-embracing explanation for crime and deviance, and no one solution. This should not lead us to despair. As André Gorz writes: 'The beginning of wisdom is in the discovery that there exist contradictions of permanent tension with which it is necessary to live and that it is above all not necessary to seek to resolve' (1982: 118).

Recommended reading

Maguire, M., Morgan, R. and Reiner, R. (eds) (2007) *The Oxford Handbook of Criminology*, 4th edn, Oxford: Oxford University Press. An extremely large volume, demonstrating the breadth and depth of current perspectives in criminology.

McLaughlin, E., Muncie, J. and Hughes, G. (eds) (2003) *Criminological Perspectives: Essential Readings*, 2nd edn, London: Sage and Open University. Includes classic texts from within the sociology of crime and deviance and criminology.

Muncie, J. (2009) *Youth and Crime*, 3rd edn, London: Sage. A useful account of the sociological literature as it affects young people.

9 Towards sociological practice

In reviewing the book as a whole, a number of important themes arise that provide a way forward for a critical and reflexive sociological practice for social workers and probation officers.

Interrogate the commonplace

Be prepared to ask questions and refuse to accept 'as read' the concepts, ideas and perspectives that are part of everyday knowledge and practice wisdom. The family, crime, community, etc. are not the same for all time and in all places. Meanings change, and are created by the very discourses that name and classify the notions they describe (Foucault 1972). Moreover, the 'knowledge' on which concepts are based is itself open to question, as we have discovered in our examination of official statistics about crime. Until we have begun to deconstruct the concepts we are using, we will not understand the complexities and contradictions that are likely to affect our practice. We will also fail to appreciate the vested interests that seek to forefront specific kinds of meanings, definitions and evidence.

Think historically

Social work is frequently accused of failing to learn from the lessons of the past – of repeating its mistakes, and swinging backwards and forwards from one solution to another and then back again.

Social work's ambivalence about residential care and adoption provide two pertinent illustrations of this. A critical or post-modern outlook on history helps us to see that there is no 'continuous smooth text that runs beneath the multiplicity of contradictions' (Foucault 1972: 155). History is not a story of continual progress or gradual improvement towards a better society, or even the story of inevitable decline and impending disaster. As a consequence, the solutions we put forward today may not (as we might wish them) be qualitatively better than those of the past. Instead, continuities and change are inevitable features of social work. I explored this in an earlier book:

> The history of social work is not the story of ever-increasing knowledge, expertise or human enlightenment. Neither is it the story of an ever-expanding state machine designed to find ever-more sophisticated means of controlling the working class or women. On the contrary, every new intervention in social work has been accompanied by both gains and losses along the way, and consequences which are not always expected and predictable.
>
> (Cree 1995: 10)

A historical, sociological approach encourages us to examine those 'gains and losses', so that we might make informed decisions about how practice might be organised in the future. This approach also invites a degree of humility, however, because of an awareness that our 'answers' may be no less problematic than those of our forebears.

Beware of ethnocentrism

I have made the point throughout this book that it is easy to fall into the trap of being culturally and ethnically blinkered, judging other people and other societies from our own perspective without seeing that our way of thinking and being is simply that – it is our way; not the best way, and certainly not the only way.

Locate issues in their wider social, political and economic context

I have argued throughout the book that individual experience is structured by class, 'race' and ethnicity, gender, age, disability and sexuality. Inequality and oppression exist at both individual and structural levels; they occur between people, and are expressed through organisational policy and practice and through society's institutions (Braye and Preston-Shoot 1995: 3). While post-modern perspectives usefully remind us that there are no 'essential' categories by which to define people's experiences, this should not delude us into underestimating either the power or the durability of structured inequalities. The daily lives of black and Asian people, working-class people, women and disabled people continue to be constituted by exclusion and oppression. Social workers and probation officers work predominantly with people who are discriminated against, marginalised and otherwise on the edges of social life. Individual and psychological approaches to practice cannot adequately address the broader issues of their lives and experience.

Place value on individual experience and meaning

Draw on the wealth of experience that you have already, from your life, reading, films, family and friends, and use this positively to create a provisional framework in which to assess both theory and practice. At the same time, seek to discover and respect the experiences and perspectives of service users. This means not 'first-guessing' what people feel like and believe, but instead treating them as experts in their own lives, able to bring meaning and understanding to the the matters in hand, if we are prepared to listen (Thompson 1981).

Do not expect to find simple answers

Sociology does not provide simple answers to the complex issues of life. The classical sociologist Weber himself argued that sociology 'could not tell the members of society what values to hold, but it could demonstrate the possibilities and constraints facing them within their social structure' (1970, in Bilton *et al.* 2002). Sociology offers a range of perspectives, commentaries and interpretations of social life and experience, which may help us to make informed decisions about our lives and work. This

Chapter 1

is a more optimistic message for social work than that presented by Davies (1991) and discussed in Chapter 1. Sociology may not be able to provide social work practitioners with answers, but the questions themselves lead to the potential development of sensitive, anti-oppressive practice. This leads to my final point.

Act with integrity

Chapter 1

'Integrity' may seem like an old-fashioned word, but it is, I believe, a useful one. It reminds us of a point made early in Chapter 1, that all theories, ideas and practices are based on a particular set of political and moral principles. We therefore have choices to make about which theories we believe are most useful, and what actions will be most helpful (or perhaps least damaging) for those with whom we are working. Social work is fundamentally about values and about value-judgements. Sociological knowledge can provide us with a framework for anti-discriminatory, anti-oppressive practice, by giving us the analytical tools with which to begin to explore the relationship between individuals and society, between 'personal troubles' and 'public issues' (Mills 1959).

Bibliography

Abbott, P. and Wallace, C. (1990) *An Introduction to Sociology: Feminist Perspectives*, London: Routledge.

Abbott, P., Wallace, C. and Tyler, M. (2005) *An Introduction to Sociology: Feminist Perspectives*, 3rd edn, London: Routledge.

Abrams, L. (1998) *Orphan Country: Children of Scotland's Broken Homes from 1845 to the Present Day*, Edinburgh: John Donald.

Abrams, P. (1978) *Neighbourhood Care and Social Policy*, Berkhamsted: The Volunteer Centre.

—— (1982) *Historical Sociology*, London: Open Books Publishing.

Abrams, P., Abrams, S., Humphrey, R. and Smith, R. (1989 [1978]) *Neighbourhood Care and Social Policy*, London: HMSO.

Acheson, D. (1998) *Independent Inquiry into Inequalities in Health Report* (Acheson Report), London: The Stationery Office.

Adams, R. (1996) *The Personal Social Services: Clients, Consumers or Citizens*, London: Longman.

Ahmed, S. (2000) 'Boundaries and connections', in Ahmed, S., Kilby, J., Lury, C., McNeil, M., Skeggs, B. (eds) *Transformations, Thinking through Feminism*, London: Routledge.

Ahmed, S., Kilby, J., Lury, C., McNeil, M., Skeggs, B. (2000) 'Introduction: thinking through feminism', in Ahmed, S., Kilby, J., Lury, C., McNeil, M., Skeggs, B. (eds) *Transformations, Thinking through Feminism*, London: Routledge.

Alanen, L. (1994) 'Gender and generation: feminism and the "child question"', in Qvortrup, J., Bardy, M., Sgritta, G. and Wintersberger, H. (eds) *Childhood Matters: Social Theory, Practice and Politics*, Aldershot: Avebury.

Aldridge, J. and Becker, S. (1993) *Children who Care: Inside the World of Young Carers*, Loughborough: Department of Social Science, Loughborough University.

Alibhai-Brown, Y. (2001) *Mixed Feelings: The Complex Lives of Mixed-Race Britons*, London: The Women's Press.

Allan, G. (1991) 'Social work, community work and informal networks', in Davies, M. (ed.) *The Sociology of Social Work*, London: Routledge.

—— (1996) *Kinship and Friendship in Modern Britain*, Oxford: Oxford University Press.

Allan, G. and Crow, G. (2001) *Families, Households and Society*, Basingstoke: Palgrave Macmillan.

Alzheimer Society (2007) *Dementia UK. The Full Report*, London: Alzheimer Society. Available at: www.alzheimers.org.uk/

Amit, V. (2002) 'Reconceptualising community', in Amit, V. (ed.) *Realizing Community: Concepts, Social Relationships and Sentiments*, London: Routledge.

Anderson, B. (1991) *Imagined Communities*, 2nd edn, London: Verso.

Anderson, M. (1980) *Approaches to the History of the Western Family 1500–1914*, London: Macmillan.

—— (1983) 'What is new about the modern family?', *The Family* 31: 2–16.

Annandale, E. (1998) *The Sociology of Health and Medicine: A Critical Introduction*, Cambridge: Polity Press.

—— (2004) 'Working on the front-line: risk culture and nursing in the new NHS', in Bury, M. and Gabe, J. (eds) *The Sociology of Health and Illness: A Reader*, London: Routledge.

Apter, A. (1990) *Altered Loves: Mothers and Daughters during Adolescence*, Herts: Harvester Wheatsheaf.

Arber, S. and Gilbert, N. (1989) 'Men: the forgotten carers', *Sociology* 23 (1): 111–18.

Arber, S. and Ginn, J. (1991) *Gender and Later Life: A Sociological Analysis of Resources and Constraints*, London: Sage.

—— (1992a) 'Class and caring: a forgotten dimension', *Sociology* 26: 619–34.

—— (1992b) '"In sickness and in health": care-giving, gender and the independence of elderly people', in Marsh, C. and Arber, S. (eds) *Families and Households: Divisions and Change*, Basingstoke: Macmillan.

Archard, D. (2004) *Children: Rights and Childhood*, 2nd edn, London: Routledge.

Ariès, P. (1962) *Centuries of Childhood*, London: Jonathan Cape.

Badinter, E. (2006) *Dead End Feminism*, translated by Julia Borossa, Cambridge: Polity Press.

Bailey, R. and Brake, M. (1975) *Radical Social Work*, London: Edward Arnold.

Baldwin, D., Coles, B. and Mitchell, W. (1997) 'The formation of an underclass or disparate processes of social exclusion? Evidence from two groupings of "vulnerable youth"', in MacDonald, R. (ed.) *Youth, the 'Underclass' and Social Exclusion*, London: Routledge.

Ballantyne, J.H. and Roberts, K.A. (2009) *Our Social World: Introduction to Sociology*, 2nd edn, Thousand Oaks, CA: Sage.

Balloch, S. and Hill, M. (eds) (2007) *Care, Community and Citizenship*, Bristol: The Policy Press.

Banks, M., Bates, I., Breakwell, G., Brynner, J., Emler, N., Jamieson, L. and Roberts, K. (1992) *Careers and Identities*, Buckingham: Open University Press.

Banks, P., Gallacher, E., Hill, M. and Riddell, S. (2002) *Young Carers: Assessment and Services Literature Review*, Edinburgh: Scottish Executive Central Research Unit.

Banks, S. (2007) 'Becoming critical: developing the community practitioner', in Butcher, H., Banks, S., Henderson, P. and Robertson, R. (eds) *Critical Community Practice*, Bristol: The Policy Press.

Banton, M. (1965) *Roles: An Introduction to the Study of Social Relations*, London: Tavistock.

Baraclough, J., Dedman, G., Osborn, H. and Willmott, P. (1996) *100 Years of Health Related Social Work 1895–1995: Then-Now-Onwards*, Birmingham: BASW.

Barclay Committee (1982) *Social Workers: Their Roles and Tasks*, London: Bedford Square Press.

Barnes, M. (2006) *Caring and Social Justice*, Basingstoke: Palgrave Macmillan.

Barnes, M. and Maple, N. (1992) *Women and Mental Health: Challenging the Stereotypes*, Birmingham: Venture Press.

Barrett, M. and McIntosh, M. (1982) *The Anti-Social Family*, London: Verso.

Barry, M. (2005) 'Youth transitions', in Barry, M. (ed.) (2005) *Youth Policy and Social Inclusion: Critical Debates with Young People*, London: Routledge.

—— (ed.) (2005) *Youth Policy and Social Inclusion: Critical Debates with Young People*, London: Routledge.

Bartley, M. (2004) *Health Inequality: An Introduction to Theories, Concepts and Methods*, Cambridge: Polity Press.

Bauman, Z. (1990) *Thinking Sociologically*, Oxford: Basil Blackwell.

—— (1993) *Postmodern Ethics*, Oxford: Blackwell.

—— (1997) *Postmodernity and Its Discontents*, Cambridge: Polity Press.

—— (2001) *Community: Seeking Safety in an Insecure World*, Cambridge: Polity Press.

—— (2003) *Liquid Love: On the Frailty of Human Bonds*, Cambridge: Polity Press.

—— (2006) *Liquid Times: Living in an Age of Uncertainty*, Cambridge: Polity Press.

—— (2008) *The Art of Life*, Cambridge: Polity Press.

Bauman, Z. and May, T. (2001) *Thinking Sociologically*, 2nd edn, Oxford: Basil Blackwell.

Bayer, R. (1987) *Homosexuality and American Psychiatry: The Politics of Diagnosis*, Princeton: Princeton University Press.

Becher, H. (2008) *Family Practices in South Asian Muslim Families: Parenting in a Multi-Faith Britain*, Basingstoke: Palgrave Macmillan.

Beck, U. (1992) *Risk Society: Towards a New Modernity*, London, Sage.

—— (1999) *World Risk Society*, Cambridge: Polity Press.

Beck, U. and Beck-Gernsheim, E. (1995) *The Normal Chaos of Love*, Cambridge: Polity Press.

Becker, H. (1963) *Outsiders*, New York: Free Press.

Becker, S. (1997) *Responding to Poverty: The Politics of Cash and Care*, London: Longman.

—— (2007) 'Global perspectives on children's unpaid caregiving in the family', *Global Social Policy* 7 (1): 23–50.

Becker, S., Dearden, C. and Aldridge, J. (2001) 'Children's labour of love? Young carers and care work', in Mizen, P., Pole, C. and Bolton, A. (eds) *Hidden Hands: International Perspectives on Children's Work and Labour*, London: Routledge.

Berkman, L.F., Glass, T., Brisette, I. and Seeman, T.E. (2000) 'From social integration to health: Durkheim in the new millennium', *Social Science and Medicine* 51: 843–57, reprinted in Bury, M. and Gabe, J. (eds) (2004) *The Sociology of Health and Illness: A Reader*, London: Routledge.

Beechey, V. (1986) 'Familial ideology', in Beechey, V. and Donald, J. (eds) *Subjectivity and Social Relations*, Milton Keynes: Open University Press.

—— (1987) *Unequal Work*, London: Verso.

Beechey, V. and Perkins, T. (1987) *A Matter of Hours: Women, Part-time Work and the Labour Market*, Cambridge: Polity Press.

Bell, C. (1968) *Middle Class Families*, London: Routledge & Kegan Paul.

Bell, C. and Newby, H. (1971) *Community Studies*, London: Allen & Unwin.

—— (1976) 'Community, communion, class and community action: the social sources of the new urban politics', in Herbert, D.J. and Johnson, R.J. (eds) *Social Areas in Cities*, London: Wiley.

Berger, P.L. (1967) *Invitation to Sociology: A Humanist Perspective*, Harmondsworth: Penguin.

Berger, P.L. and Kellner, H. (1971) 'Marriage and the construction of reality', in Cosin, B.R. (ed.) *School and Society*, London: Routledge & Kegan Paul.

Berger, P.L. and Luckman, T. (1966) *The Social Construction of Reality*, Harmondsworth: Allen Lane.

Bernard, J. (1972) *The Future of Marriage*, New York: Bantam.

Bernardes, J. (1997) *Family Studies: An Introduction*, London: Routledge.

Beveridge, W. (1942) *Social Insurance and Allied Services*, London: HMSO.

Bhavnani, K. (ed.) (2000) *Feminism and Race (Oxford Readings in Feminism)*, Oxford: Oxford University Press.

Bhavnani, K. and Coulson, M. (1986) 'Transforming socialist-feminism: the challenge of racism', *Feminist Review* 23: 81–92.

Bilton, T., Bonnett, K., Jones, P., Lawson, T., Skinner, D., Stanworth, M. and Webster, A. (2002) *Introducing Sociology*, 4th edn, Basingstoke: Palgrave Macmillan.

Blaxter, M. (1990) *Health and Lifestyles*, London: Tavistock-Routledge, reprinted in Davey, B., Gray, A. and Seale, C. (eds) (2001) *Health and Disease: A Reader*, 3rd edn, Buckingham: Open University Press.

Black, D. and Cottrell, D. (1993) *Seminars in Child and Adolescent Psychiatry*, London: Gaskell.

Blau, P.M. (1964) *Exchange and Power in Social Life*, New York: Wiley.

Bor, R. and Elford, J. (1998) *The Family and HIV Today: Recent Research and Practice*, London: Cassell.

Bornat, J., Johnson, J., Pereira, C., Pilgrim, D. and Williams, F. (1997) *Community Care: A Reader*, 2nd edn, Basingstoke: Macmillan and Open University.

Boulton, M., Tuckett, D., Olson, A. and Williams, A. (1986) 'Social class and the general practice consultation', *Sociology of Health and Illness* 8 (4): 325–50.

Boushel, M. (2000) 'Childrearing across cultures', in Boushel, M., Fawcett, M. and Selwyn, J. (eds) *Focus on Early Childhood: Principles and Realities*, Oxford: Blackwell.

Boyden, J. (1997) 'Childhood and the policy makers: a comparative perspective on the globalization of childhood', in James, A. and Prout, A. (eds) *Constructing and Reconstructing Childhood: Contemporary Issues in the Sociological Study of Childhood*, 2nd edn, London: Routledge.

Brake, M. and Hale, C. (1992) *Public Order and Private Lives: The Politics of Law and Order*, London: Routledge.

Braye, S. and Preston-Shoot, M. (1995) *Empowering Practice in Social Care*, Buckingham: Open University Press.

Brechin, A., Walmsley, J., Katz, J. and Peace, S. (1998) *Care Matters: Concepts, Practice and Research in Health and Social Care*, London: Sage.

Brittan, A. and Maynard, M. (1984) *Sexism, Racism and Oppression*, Oxford: Basil Blackwell.

Brody, E.M. (1981) 'Women in the middle and family help to older people', *The Gerontologist* 21: 471–80.

Brook, E. and Davis, A. (eds) (1985) *Women, the Family and Social Work*, London: Tavistock.

Brow, J. (1990) 'Notes on community and hegemony and the uses of the past', *Anthropological Quarterly* 63 (1): 12–35.

Brown, B., Burman, M. and Jamieson, L. (1993) *Sex Crimes on Trial*, Edinburgh: Edinburgh University Press.

Brown, B.B. and Larson, R.W. (2002) 'The kaleidoscope of adolescence', in Brown, B.B., Larson, R.W. and Saraswathi, T.S. (eds) *The World's Youth: Adolescence in Eight Regions of the Globe*, Cambridge: Cambridge University Press.

Brown, B.B., Larson, R.W. and Saraswathi, T.S. (eds) (2002) *The World's Youth: Adolescence in Eight Regions of the Globe*, Cambridge: Cambridge University Press.

Brown, M.A. and Powell-Cope, G.M. (1992) *Caring for a Loved-One with AIDS*, Seattle, WA: University of Washington.

Brown, S. (2005) *Understanding Youth and Crime: Listening to Youth?* Maidenhead: Open University Press.

Browne, D. (2000) 'The black experience of mental health law', in Heller, T., Reynolds, J., Gomm, R., Muston, R. and Pattison, S. (eds) *Mental Health Matters: A Reader*, Basingstoke: Palgrave Macmillan.

Browne, J. (1995) 'Can social work empower?', in Hugman, R. and Smith, D. (eds) *Ethical Issues in Social Work*, London: Routledge.

Brownmiller, S. (1975) *Against Our Will: Men, Women and Rape*, Harmondsworth: Penguin.

Bryan, A. (1992) 'Working with black single mothers: myths and reality', in Langan, M. and Day, L. (eds) *Women, Oppression and Social Work*, London: Routledge.

Bulmer, M. (1987) *The Social Basis of Community Care*, London: Allen & Unwin.

Burch, S. (2001) 'Cultural studies', in Naidoo, J. and Wills, J. (eds) *Health Studies: An Introduction*, Basingstoke: Palgrave.

Burr, R. and Montgomery, H. (2003) 'Children and rights', in Woodhead, M. and Montgomery, H. (eds) *Understanding Childhood: An Interdisciplinary Approach*, Milton Keynes: Open University and John Wiley & Sons Ltd.

Bury, M. (1997) *Health and Illness in a Changing Society*, London: Routledge.

Bury, M. and Gabe, J. (2004) 'General introduction', in Bury, M. and Gabe, J. (eds) (2004) *The Sociology of Health and Illness: A Reader*, London: Routledge.

Butcher, H., Banks, S., Henderson, P. and Robertson, R. (eds) (2007) *Critical Community Practice*, Bristol: The Policy Press.

Butler, J. (1992) 'Contingent foundations: feminism and the question of "postmodernism"', in Butler, J. and Scott, J.W. (eds) *Feminists Theorize the Political*, New York: Routledge.

Bytheway, B. (1987) *Informal Care Systems: an Exploratory Study within the Families of Older Steel Workers in South Wales*, York: Joseph Rowntree Memorial Trust.

—— (1995) *Ageing*, Buckingham: Open University Press.

Bywaters, P., McLeod, E. and Napier, L. (eds) *Social Work and Global Health Inequalities: Practice and Policy Developments*, Bristol: The Policy Press.

Cain, M. (1989) *Growing up Good: Policing the Behaviour of Girls in Europe*, London: Sage.

Calvino, I. (1997 [1972]) *Invisible Cities*, London: Vintage.

Campbell, B. (1993) *Goliath: Britain's Dangerous Places*, London: Methuen.

Canaan, C. (1992) *Changing Families: Changing Welfare*, Hemel Hempstead: Harvester Wheatsheaf.

Carlen, P. (1988) *Women, Crime and Poverty*, Milton Keynes: Open University Press.

—— (1992) 'Criminal women and criminal justice: the limits to, and potential of, feminist and left realist perspectives', in Matthews, R. and Young, J. (eds) *Issues in Realist Criminology*, London: Sage.

Carlen, P. and Worrall, A. (1987) *Gender, Crime and Justice*, Milton Keynes: Open University Press.

Carsten, J. (2004) *After Kinship*, Cambridge: Cambridge University Press.

Castells, M. (1983) *The City and the Grassroots*, London: Edward Arnold.

—— (1997) *The Power of Identity*, Oxford: Blackwell.

Cavanagh, K. and Cree, V.E. (eds) (1996) *Working with Men: Feminism and Social Work*, London: Routledge.

Cavanagh, K., Dobash, R.E., Dobash, R.P. and Lewis, R. (2001) '"Remedial work": men's strategic responses to their violence against intimate female partners', *Sociology* 35 (3): 695–714.

Chadwick, E. (1842) *Report on the Sanitary Condition of the Labouring Population of Great Britain*, Edinburgh: Edinburgh University Press.

Chahal, K. (2000) *Foundations: Ethnic Diversity, Neighbourhoods and Housing*, York: Joseph Rowntree Foundation. Available at www.jrf.org.uk/

Cheal, D. (1991) *Family and the State of Theory*, Hemel Hempstead: Harvester Wheatsheaf.

—— (2002) *Sociology of Family Life*, Basingstoke: Palgrave Macmillan.

Chesler, P. (2000) 'Women and madness: the mental asylum', in Heller, T., Reynolds, J., Gomm, R., Muston, R. and Pattison, S. (eds) *Mental Health Matters: A Reader*, Basingstoke: Palgrave Macmillan.

Chester, R. (1985) 'The rise of the neo-conventional family', *New Society* (9 May): 185–8.

Chisholm, L., Brown, P., Buchner, P. and Kruger, H. (1990) 'Childhood and youth studies in the United Kingdom and West Germany: an introduction', in Chisholm, L., Buchner, P., Kruger, H. and Brown, P. (eds) *Childhood, Youth and Social Change: A Comparative Perspective*, London: Falmer Press.

Chodorow, N.J. (1978) *The Reproduction of Mothering*, Berkeley: University of California Press.

—— (1989) *Feminism and Psychoanalytic Theory*, London: Yale University Press.

Christensen, P., Hockey, J. and James, A. (1998) '"You just get on with it": questioning models of welfare dependency in a rural community', in Edgar, I.R and Russell, A. (eds) *The Anthropology of Welfare*, London: Routledge.

Christie, A. (ed.) (2001) *Men and Social Work: Theories and Practices*, Basingstoke: Palgrave.

Clarke, J., Hall, S., Jefferson, T. and Roberts, B. (1976) 'Subcultures, cultures and class', in Hall, S. and Jefferson, T. (eds) *Resistance through Rituals: Youth Subcultures in Post-War Britain*, London: Hutchinson and CCCS, University of Birmingham.

Clarke, L. (1995) 'Family care and changing family structure: bad news for the elderly?', in Allen, I. and Perkins, E. (eds) *The Future of Family Care for Older People*, London: HMSO.

Clarke, L. and Roberts, C. (2004) 'The meaning of grandparenthood and its contribution to the quality of life of older people', in Walker, A. and Hagan Hennessy, C. (eds) *Growing Older: Quality of Life in Old Age*, Milton Keynes: Open University Press.

Clifton, J. and Hodgson, D. (1997) 'Rethinking practice through a children's rights perspective', in Cannan, C. and

Warren, C. (eds) *Social Action with Children and Families: A Community Development Approach to Child and Family Welfare*, London: Routledge.

Cloward, R. and Ohlin, L. (1961) *Delinquency and Opportunity: A Theory of Delinquent Gangs*, London: Routledge & Kegan Paul.

Cohen, A. (1955) *Delinquent Boys: The Culture of the Gang*, Chicago: Free Press.

Cohen, A.P. (1985) *The Symbolic Construction of Community*, London: Routledge.

Cohen, S. (1972) *Folk Devils and Moral Panics: The Creation of Mods and Rockers*, Oxford: Martin Robertson.

—— (1985) *Visions of Social Control: Crime, Punishment and Classification*, Cambridge: Polity Press.

Coleman, J.C. (1979) *The School Years*, London: Methuen.

—— (1990) *The Nature of Adolescence*, 2nd edn, London: Routledge.

—— (1992) 'The nature of adolescence', in Coleman, J.C. and Warren-Adamson, C. (eds) *Youth Policy in the 1990s: The Way Forward*, London: Routledge.

Coleman, J.C. and Hendry, L.B. (1999) *The Nature of Adolescence*, 3rd edn, London: Routledge.

Colton, M., Drury, C. and Williams, M. (1995) *Children in Need: Family Support under the Children Act 1989*, Aldershot: Avebury.

Connell, R.W. (1983) *Which Way is Up?* London: Allen & Unwin.

—— (1995) *Masculinities*, Cambridge: Polity Press.

Cooper, D. (1971) *The Death of the Family*, London: Allen Lane.

Cornwell, J. (1984) *Hard-Earned Lives: Accounts of Health and Illness from East London*, London: Tavistock.

Corsaro, W. (2004) *The Sociology of Childhood*, 2nd edn, Thousand Oaks, CA: Pine Forge Press.

Cotterell, J. (2007) *Social Networks in Youth and Adolescence*, 2nd edn, London: Routledge.

Cree, V.E. (1995) *From Public Streets to Private Lives: The Changing Task of Social Work*, Aldershot: Avebury.

—— (1996) 'Why do men care?' in Cavanagh, K. and Cree, V.E. (eds) *Working with Men: Feminism and Social Work*, London: Routledge.

—— (2000) *Sociology for Social Workers and Probation Officers*, London: Routledge.

—— (2003) 'Worries and problems of young carers: issues for mental health', *Child and Family Social Work* 8 (4): 301–9.

—— (2008) 'Social work and society', in Davies, M. (ed.) *Blackwell Companion to Social Work*, 3rd edn, Oxford: Blackwell.

—— (2009) 'The changing nature of social work', in Adams, R., Dominelli, L. and Payne, M. (eds) *Practising Social Work in a Complex World*, 2nd edn, Basingstoke: Palgrave Macmillan.

Cree, V.E. and Cavanagh, K. (1996) 'Men, masculinism and social work' in Cavanagh, K. and Cree, V.E. (eds) *Working with Men: Feminism and Social Work*, London: Routledge.

Cree, V.E. and Davis, A. (2007) *Social Work: Voices from the Inside*, London: Routledge.

Cree, V.E., Hounsell, J., Christie, H., McCune, V. and Tett, L. (2009) 'From further education to higher education: social work students' experiences of transition to an ancient, research-led university', *Social Work Education* 28 (8): 887–901.

Cree, V.E., Kay, H., Tisdall, K. and Wallace, J. (2004) 'Stigma and parental HIV', *Qualitative Social Work* 3 (1): 7–25.

Cree, V.E. and Myers, S. (2008) *Social Work: Making a Difference*, Bristol: The Policy Press/BASW.

Cree, V.E. and Wallace, S.J. (2009) 'Risk and protection', in Adams, R., Payne, M. and Dominelli, L. (eds) *Practising Social Work in a Complex World*, 2nd edn, Basingstoke: Palgrave Macmillan.

Cross, W.E. (1991) *Shades of Black: Diversity in African-American Identity*, Philadelphia: Temple University Press.

Cullingford, C. and Din, I. (2008) *Ethnicity and Englishness: Personal Identities in a Minority Community*, Newcastle upon Tyne: Cambridge Scholars Publishing.

Cunningham, J. and Cunningham, S. (2008) *Sociology and Social Work*, Exeter: Learning Matters.

Dahrendorf, R. (1957) *Class and Class Conflict in Industrial Society*, London: Routledge & Kegan Paul.

Dahlgren, G. and Whitehead, M. (1991) *Policies and Strategies to Reduce Social Inequality in Health*, Stockholm: Institute of Futures Studies.

Dalley, G. (1988) *Ideologies of Caring*, Basingstoke: Macmillan.

Daniel, B. and Taylor, J. (2001) *Engaging with Fathers: Practice Issues for Health and Social Care*, London: Jessica Kingsley.

Davey Smith, G., Bartley, M. and Blane, D. (1990) 'The Black Report on socio-economic inequalities in health 10 years on', *British Medical Journal* 301: 373–7.

David, M.E. (2003) *Personal and Political: Feminisms, Sociology and Family Lives*, Stoke on Trent: Trentham Books.

Davies, J. (1993) 'Introduction', in Davies, J., Berger, B. and Carlson, A. (eds) *The Family: Is It Just Another Lifestyle Choice?* London: Institute of Economic Affairs, Health and Welfare Unit.

Davies, M. (ed.) (1991) *The Sociology of Social Work*, London: Routledge.

Davis, H. and Bourhill, M. (1997) '"Crisis": the demonization of children and young people', in Scraton, P. (ed.) *'Childhood' in 'Crisis'?* London: UCL Press.

Davis, J. (1990) *Youth and the Condition of Britain*, London: The Athlone Press Ltd.

Davis, K. (1996) 'Disability and legislation: rights and equality', in Hales, G. (ed.) *Beyond Disability: Towards an Enabling Environment*, London: Sage in association with the Open University.

Davis, L. (ed.) (1997) *Disability Studies: A Reader*, London: Routledge.

Dawson, A. (2002) 'The mining community and the ageing body: towards a phenomenology of community?' in Amit, V. (ed.) *Realizing Community: Concepts, Social Relationships and Sentiments*, London: Routledge.

Day, G. (2006) *Community and Everyday Life*, London: Routledge.

Day, P.R. (1987) *Sociology in Social Work Practice*, Basingstoke: Macmillan.

Daykin, N. (2001) 'Sociology' in Naidoo, J. and Wills, J. (eds) *Health Studies: An Introduction*, Basingstoke: Palgrave.

Dearden, C. and Becker, S. (1995) *Young Carers: the Facts*, Sutton: Reed Business Publishing.

Delamont, S. (2003) *Feminist Sociology*, London: Sage.

Delphy, C. (1984) *Close to Home: A Materialist Analysis of Women's Oppression*, London: Hutchinson.

Delphy, C. and Leonard, D. (1992) *Familiar Exploitation: A New Analysis of Marriage in Contemporary Western Societies*, Cambridge: Polity Press.

Dench, G., Gavron, K. and Young, M. (2006) *The New East End: Kinship, Race and Conflict*, London: Profile Books.

Dennis, N. and Erdos, G. (2000) *Families without Fatherhood*, 3rd edn, London: Civitas/Institute for the Study of Civil Society.

Dennis, R. and Daniels, S. (1996) '"Community" and the social geography of Victorian cities', in Drake, M. (ed.) *Time, Family and Community: Perspectives on Family and Community History*, Oxford: Blackwell.

Denzin, N.K. (1987) 'Post modern children', *Society* 24 (3): 32–5.

Department of Education and Skills (2006) *Widening Participation in Higher Education*, London: Department of Education and Skills. Available at: www.dius.gov.uk/higher_education/~/media/publications/E/EW Participation/

Department of Health (1995) *Child Protection: Messages from Research*, London: HMSO.

—— (1999) *Caring about Carers: A National Strategy for Carers*, London: Stationery Office.

—— (2009) *Report of the Standing Commission on Carers 2007 to 2009*, London: HMSO. Available at: www.dh.gov.uk/en/Publicationsandstatistics/Publications/PublicationsPolicyAndGuidance/DH_107305/

Department of Health and Social Security (DHSS) (1980*) Inequalities in Health, Report of a Research Working Group* (Black Report), London: DHSS.

—— (1981) *Growing Older*, Cmnd. 8173, London: HMSO: 3.

Dingwall, R. (1976) *Aspects of Illness*, Oxford: Martin Robertson.

Dingwall, R., Eekelaar, J. and Murray, T. (1995 [1983]) *The Protection of Children: State Intervention and Family Life*, 2nd edn, Aldershot: Avebury.

Dobash, R.E. and Dobash, R.P. (1979) *Violence against Wives: a Case Against Patriarchy*, New York: Free Press.

—— (eds) (1992) *Women, Violence and Social Change*, London: Routledge.

Dobash, R.P. and Dobash, R.E. (2004) 'Women's violence to men in intimate relationships: working on a puzzle', *British Journal of Criminology* 44: 324–49.

Doel, M. and Best, L. (2008) *Experiencing Social Work: Learning from Service Users*, London: Sage.

Dominelli, L. (1997) *Sociology for Social Work*, Basingstoke: Macmillan.

—— (2002) *Feminist Social Work Theory and Practice*, Basingstoke: Palgrave Macmillan.

Dominelli, L. and McLeod, E. (1989) *Feminist Social Work*, Basingstoke: Macmillan.

Donzelot, J. (1980) *The Policing of Families*, London: Hutchinson.

Downes, D. (1966) *The Delinquent Solution*, London: Routledge & Kegan Paul.

Drakeford, M. and Butler, I. (2006) *Scandal, Social Policy and Social Welfare*, revised 2nd edn, Bristol: The Policy Press.

Duffin, J. (2000) *History of Medicine: A Scandalously Short Introduction*, Basingstoke: Macmillan.

Durkheim, E. (1952 [1897]) *Suicide: A Study in Sociology*, London: Routledge & Kegan Paul.

—— (1964 [1895]) *The Rules of Sociological Method*, New York: The Free Press.

—— (1984 [1893]) *The Division of Labour in Society*, Basingstoke: Macmillan.

Dworkin, A. (1981) *Pornography: Men Possessing Women*, London: Women's Press.

—— (1988) *Letters from A War Zone: Writings 1976–1987*, London: Secker and Warburg.

Eisenstadt, S.N. (1956) *From Generation to Generation*, New York: The Free Press.

Elliot, F.R. (1996) *Gender, Family and Society*, Basingstoke: Macmillan.

Emsley, C. (2007) 'Historical perspectives on crime', in Maguire, M., Morgan, R. and Reiner, R. (eds) *The Oxford Handbook of Criminology*, 4th edn, Oxford: Oxford University Press.

Engels, F. (1892) *The Condition of the Working Class in England in 1844*, London: Swan Sonnenschein & Co.

—— (1902 [1884]) *The Origin of the Family, Private Property and the State*, Chicago: Charles H. Kerr & Company.

Ennew, J. (1986) *The Sexual Exploitation of Children*, Oxford: Basil Blackwell.

—— (ed.) (1994) *Children's Childhoods: Observed and Experienced*, London: Routledge.

Epstein, J.S. (1998) *Youth Culture: Identity in a Postmodern World*, Oxford: Blackwell.

Equal Opportunities Commission (1980) *The Experience of Caring for Elderly and Handicapped Dependants: Survey Report*, Manchester: EOC.

—— (1982) *Caring for the Elderly and Handicapped: Community Care Policies and Women's Lives*, Manchester: EOC.

Erikson, E. (1968) *Identity: Youth and Crisis*, London: Faber.

Etzioni, A. (1995) *The Spirit of Community: Rights, Responsibilities and the Communitarian Agenda*, London: HarperCollins.

Evandrou, M. (1990) *Challenging the Invisibility of Carers: Mapping Informal Care Nationally*, WSP/49, London: STICERD.

Evans, K. and Fraser, P. (1996) 'Difference in the city: locating marginal use of public space', in Samson, C. and South, N. (eds) *The Social Construction of Social Policy: Methodologies, Racism, Citizenship and the Environment*, Basingstoke: Macmillan.

Fawcett, B., Featherstone, B., Hearn, J. and Toft, C. (eds) (1996) *Violence and Gender Relations: Theories and Interventions*, London: Sage.

Featherstone, B. (2009) *Contemporary Fathering: Theory, Policy and Practice*, Bristol: The Policy Press.

Featherstone, B. and Fawcett, B. (1995) 'Oh no! not more isms: feminism, post-modernism, post-structuralism and social work education', *Social Work Education* 14 (3): 25–43.

Fenton, S. and Sadiq, A. (2000) 'Asian women speak out', in Heller, T., Reynolds, J., Gomm, R., Muston, R. and Pattison, S. (eds) *Mental Health Matters: A Reader*, Basingstoke: Palgrave Macmillan.

Ferguson, I. and Woodward, R. (2009) *Radical Social Work in Practice: Making a Difference*, Bristol: The Policy Press.

Fernando, S. and Keating, F. (eds) (2008) *Mental Health in a Multi-Ethnic Society: A Multi-disciplinary Handbook*, London: Routledge.

Ferri, E. and Smith, K. (1996) *Parenting in the 1990s*, London: Family Policy Studies Centre and Joseph Rowntree Foundation.

Finch, J. (1984) 'Community care: developing non-sexist alternatives', *Critical Social Policy* 9 (Spring): 6–18.

—— (1989) *Family Obligations and Social Change*, London: Polity Press.

—— (1995) 'Responsibilities, obligations and commitments', in Allen, I. and Perkins, E. (eds) *The Future of Family Care for Older People*, London: HMSO.

—— (2007) 'Displaying families', *Sociology* 41 (1): 65–81.

Finch, J. and Groves, D. (1980) 'Community care and the family: a case for equal opportunities', *Journal of Social Policy* 9 (4): 487–511.

Finch, J. and Mason, J. (1993) *Negotiating Family Responsibilities*, London: Routledge.

Fink, J. (2004) 'Questions of care', in Fink, J. (ed.) *Care: Personal Lives and Social Policy*, Bristol: The Policy Press in association with the Open University.

Fischer, J. (1978) *Effective Casework Practice*, New York: McGraw-Hill.

Fish, J. (2006) *Heterosexism in Health and Social Care*, Basingstoke: Palgrave Macmillan.

Fisher, M. (1994) 'Man-made care: community care and older male carers', *British Journal of Social Work* 24: 659–80.

—— (1997) 'Older male carers and community care', in Bornat, J., Johnson, J., Pereira, C., Pilgrim, D. and Williams, F. (eds) *Community Care: A Reader*, 2nd edn, Basingstoke: Macmillan and Open University.

Fletcher, R. (1973) *The Family and Marriage in Britain*, Harmondsworth: Penguin.

Fook, J. (2002) *Social Work: Critical Theory and Practice*, London: Sage.

Foster, J. (1996) '"Island homes for island people": competition, conflict and racism in the battle over public housing on the Isle of Dogs', in Samson, C. and South, N. (eds) *The Social Construction of Social Policy: Methodologies, Racism, Citizenship and the Environment*, Basingstoke: Macmillan.

Foucault, M. (1972) *The Archaeology of Knowledge*, London: Tavistock.

—— (1975) *The Birth of the Clinic: An Archaeology of Medical Perception*, New York: Vintage Books.

—— (1977) *Discipline and Punish*, London: Allen Lane.

—— (1980) 'The politics of health in the eighteenth century', in Gordon, C. (ed.) *Power/Knowledge: Selected Interviews and Other Writings, 1972–1977*, Brighton: The Harvester Press.

—— (1988) 'The political technology of individuals', in Martin, L.H., Gutman, H. and Hutton, P.H. (eds) *Technologies of the Self: A Seminar with Michel Foucault*, London: Tavistock.

Fox, N.J. (1998) 'Postmodernism and "health"', in Peterson, A. and Waddell, C. (eds) *Health Matters: A Sociology of Illness, Prevention and Care*, Buckingham: Open University Press.

Frank, A. (1995) *The Wounded Storyteller: Body, Illness and Ethics*, Chicago: University of Chicago Press.

Fraser, D. (2003) *The Evolution of the British Welfare State: A History of Social Policy since the Industrial Revolution*, 3rd edn, Basingstoke: Palgrave Macmillan.

Fraser, H. (2005) 'Four different approaches to community participation', *Community Development Journal* 40 (3): 286–300.

Freeman, D. (1983) *Margaret Mead and Samoa: The Making and Unmaking of an Anthropological Myth*, Boston, MA: Harvard University Press.

Freidson, E. (1970) 'The social organization of illness', in Bury, M. and Gabe, J. (eds) *The Sociology of Health and Illness: A Reader*, London: Routledge.

Freire, P. (1970) *Pedagogy of the Oppressed*, New York: Continuum.

French, S. and Swain, J. (2004) 'Whose tragedy? Towards a personal non-tragedy view of disability', in Swain, J., French, S., Barnes, C. and Thomas, C. (eds) *Disabling Barriers – Enabling Environments*, 2nd edn, London: Sage.

Freud, A. (1937) *The Ego and the Mechanisms of Defence*, London: Hogarth Press.

—— (1958) 'Adolescence', *Psychoanalytical Study of the Child* 13: 255–78.

Frith, S. (2005) 'Youth', in Bennett, T., Grossberg, L. and Morris, M. (eds) *New Keywords: A Revised Vocabulary of Culture and Society*, Oxford: Blackwell.

Frønes, I. (1994) 'Dimensions of childhood', in Qvortrup, J., Bardy, M., Sgritta, G. and Wintersberger, H. (eds) *Childhood Matters: Social Theory, Practice and Politics*, Aldershot: Avebury.

Frost, N. and Stein, M. (1989) *The Politics of Child Welfare: Inequality, Power and Change*, Hemel Hempstead: Harvester Wheatsheaf.

Fulcher, J. and Scott, J. (2007) *Sociology*, 3rd edn, Oxford: Oxford University Press.

Furedi, F. (2009) *Wasted: Why Education Isn't Educating*, London: Continuum Press.

Furlong, A. and Cartmel, F. (2007) *Young People and Social Change: New Perspectives*, 2nd edn, Maidenhead: Open University Press.

Gabbidon, S.L. and Greene, H.T. (eds) (2005) *Race, Crime and Justice: A Reader*, Routledge: New York.

Gans, H.J. (1980 [1968]) 'Urbanism and suburbanism as ways of life', in Bocock, R., Hamilton, P., Thompson, K. and Waton, A. (eds) *An Introduction to Sociology*, London: Fontana.

Garfinkel, H. (1956) 'Conditions of successful degradation ceremonies', *American Journal of Sociology* 61 (2): 420–4.

—— (1967) *Studies in Ethnomethodology*, Englewood Cliffs, NJ: Prentice Hall.

Garland, D. (1997) 'Of crimes and criminals: the development of criminology in Britain', in Maguire, M., Morgan, R. and Reiner, R. (eds) *The Oxford Handbook of Criminology*, 2nd edn, Oxford: Clarendon Press.

Garratt, D. (2004) 'Youth cultures and sub-cultures', in Roche, J., Tucker, S., Thomson, R. and Flynn, R. (eds) *Youth in Society: Contemporary Theory, Policy and Practice*, 2nd edn, London: Sage.

Gavron, D. (2000) *The Kibbutz: Awakening from Utopia*, Lanham, MD: Rowman & Littlefield.

Geertz, C. (1973) *The Interpretation of Cultures*, New York: Basic Books.

Gelles, R.J. (1979) *Family Violence*, London: Sage.

General Assembly of the United Nations (1989) *The Convention on the Rights of the Child*, Adopted by the General Assembly of the United Nations on 20 November 1989. [UN Convention] www.unicef.org/crc/

Giddens, A. (1989) *Sociology*, Cambridge: Polity Press.

—— (1991) *Modernity and Self-identity: Self and Society in the Late Modern Age*, Oxford: Polity Press.

—— (1993) *The Transformation of Intimacy: Love, Sexuality and Eroticism in Modern Societies*, Cambridge: Polity Press.

—— (2006) *Sociology*, 5th edn, Cambridge: Polity Press.

Gilchrist, R., Phillips, P. and Ross, A. (2003) 'Participation and potential participation in UK higher education', in Archer, L., Hutchings, M. and Ross, A. (2003) *Higher Education and Social Class: issues of exclusion and inclusion*, London: Routledge Falmer.

Gilligan, C. (1982) *In a Different Voice: Psychological Theory and Women's Development*, Cambridge, MA: Harvard University Press.

Gillis, J.R. (1981) *Youth and History: Tradition and Change in European Age Relations, 1770–Present*, New York: Academic Press.

—— (1997) *A World of Their Own Making: Myth, Ritual, and the Quest for Family Values*, Cambridge, MA: Harvard University Press.

Gilroy, P. (1992) 'The end of anti-racism', in Donald, J. and Rattansi, A. (eds) *'Race', Culture and Difference*, London: Sage.

Gittins, D. (1993) *The Family in Question: Changing Households and Familiar Ideologies*, 2nd edn, Basingstoke: Macmillan.

—— (1998) *The Child in Question*, Basingstoke: Macmillan.

Glauser, B. (1997) 'Street children: deconstructing a construct', in James, A. and Prout, A. (eds) *Constructing and Reconstructing Childhood: Contemporary issues in the Sociological Study of Childhood*, 2nd edn, London: Routledge.

Glendinning, C. (1992) *The Costs of Informal Care*, London: HMSO.

Goffman, E. (1963) *Stigma: Notes on the Management of Spoiled Identity*, Englewood Cliffs, NJ: Prentice Hall.

—— (1968) *Asylums: Essays on the Social Situation of Mental Patients and Other Inmates*, London: Penguin.

—— (1969) *The Presentation of Self in Everyday Life*, Harmondsworth: Penguin.

Goodman, A., Johnson, P. and Webb, S. (1997) *Inequality in the UK*, Oxford: Oxford University Press.

Gordon, L. (1988) *Heroes of their own Lives: The Politics and History of Family Violence, Boston 1880–1960*, London: Virago.

Gorz, A. (1982) *Farewell to the Working Class*, London: Pluto.

Graham, H. (1983) 'Caring: a labour of love', in Finch, J. and Groves, D. (eds) *A Labour of Love: Women, Work and Caring*, London: Routledge & Kegan Paul.

—— (1991) 'The concept of caring in feminist research: the case of domestic service', *Sociology* 25 (1): 61–78.

—— (1997) 'Feminist perspectives on caring', in Bornat, J., Johnson, J., Pereira, C., Pilgrim, D. and Williams, F. (eds) *Community Care: A Reader*, 2nd edn, Basingstoke: Macmillan and Open University.

—— (1998) 'Promoting health against inequality', *Health Education Journal* 57: 292–302.

—— (2007) *Unequal Lives: Health and Social Inequalities*, Maidenhead: Open University Press.

Graham, M. (2002) *Social Work and African-Centred Worldviews*, Birmingham: The Venture Press.

—— (2007) *Black Issues in Social Work and Social Care*, Bristol: The Policy Press.

Gramsci, A. (1971) *Selections for the Prison Notebooks*, London: New Left Books.

Grbich, C. (1990) 'Socialisation and social change: a critique of three positions', *British Journal of Sociology* 41 (4): 517–30.

Green, E.C. (1999) 'Engaging indigenous African healers in the prevention of AIDS and STDs', in Hahn, R.A. (ed.) *Anthropology in Public Health*, Oxford: Oxford University Press.

Green, G. and Sobo, E.J. (2000) *The Engendered Self: Managing the Social Risks of HIV*, London: Routledge.

Green, H. (1988) *Informal Carers*, Series GHS No. 15, London: HMSO.

Green, J. (ed.) (2007) *Making Space for Indigenous Feminism*, Black Point, Nova Scotia: Fernwood Publishing.

Gregson, N. and Lowe, M. (1994) *Servicing the Middle Classes*, London: Routledge.

Griffiths, V. (1995) *Adolescent Girls and Their Friends: A Feminist Ethnography*, Aldershot: Avebury.

Gubrium, J.F. and Silverman, D. (1989) *The Politics of Field Research*, London: Sage.

Gunaratnam, Y. (1997) 'Breaking the silence: black and ethnic minority carers and service provision', in Bornat, J., Johnson, J., Pereira, C., Pilgrim, D. and Williams, F. (eds) *Community Care: A Reader*, 2nd edn, Basingstoke: Macmillan and Open University.

Habermas, J. (1981a) *The Theory of Communicative Action, i: Reason and the Rationalisation of Society*, London: Heinemann.

—— (1981b) *The Theory of Communicative Action, ii: The Critique of Functionalist Reason*, London: Heinemann.

Hahn, R.A. (ed.) (1999) *Anthropology in Public Health*, Oxford: Oxford University Press.

Hall, G.S. (1904) *Adolescence: Its Psychology and its Relations to Physiology, Anthropology, Sociology, Sex, Crime, Religion and Education*, New York: Appleton.

Hall, S. (1991) 'The local and the global: globalisation and ethnicity', in King, A. (ed.) *Culture, Globalisation and the World-System*, Basingstoke: Macmillan.

Hall, S., Critcher, C., Jefferson, T., Clarke, J. and Roberts, B. (1978) *Policing the Crisis: Mugging, the State and Law and Order*, Basingstoke: Macmillan.

Hall, S., and Jefferson, T. (eds) (1976) *Resistance through Rituals: Youth Sub-Cultures on Post-War Britain*, London: Hutchinson.

Hamilton, P. (1985) 'Editor's foreword', in Cohen, A.P. (1985) *The Symbolic Construction of Community*, London: Routledge.

Hanmer, J. and Statham, D. (1988) *Women and Social Work: Towards a Woman-Centred Practice*, Basingstoke: Macmillan.

Harding, S. (1987) *Feminism and Methodology*, Milton Keynes: Open University Press.

—— (1991) *Whose Science? Whose Knowledge? Thinking from Women's Lives*, Milton Keynes: Open University Press.

Hareven, T.K. (1996) 'Recent research on the history of the family', in Drake, M. (ed.) *Time, Family and Community: Perspectives on Family and Community History*, Oxford: Blackwell.

Harris, J. (2003) *The Social Work Business*, London: Routledge.

Harris, R. (1989) 'Child protection, child care and child welfare', in Wilson, K. and James, A. (eds) *The Child Protection Handbook*, Hemel Hempstead: Harvester Wheatsheaf.

Hartmann, H. (1981) 'The family as the locus of gender, class and political struggle', *Signs* 6: 366–94.

Harvey, D. (1973) *Social Justice and the City*, London: Edward Arnold.

Harvey, L. (1990) *Critical Social Research*, London: Unwin Hyman.

Hasler, F. (2004) 'Direct payments', in Swain, J., French, S., Barnes, C. and Thomas, C. (eds) *Disabling Barriers – Enabling Environments*, 2nd edn, London: Sage.

Haugen, G.M.D. (2007) 'Caring children: exploring care in post-divorce families', *The Sociological Review* 55 (4): 653–70.

Heathcote, F. (1981) 'Social disorganisation theories', in FitzGerald, M., McLennan, G. and Pawson, J. (eds) *Crime and Society: Readings in History and Theory*, Milton Keynes: Open University Press.

HEFCE (2003) *Schooling Effects on Higher Education Achievement*, Issues paper July 2003/32, Bristol: HEFCE.

Heidensohn, H. and Gelsthorpe, L. (2007) 'Gender and crime', in Maguire, M., Morgan, R. and Reiner, R. (eds) *The Oxford Handbook of Criminology*, 4th edn, Oxford: Oxford University Press.

Hekman, S. (1990) *Gender and Knowledge: Elements of a Postmodern Feminism*, Cambridge: Polity Press.

Heller, T., Reynolds, J., Gomm, R., Muston, R. and Pattison, S. (eds) (2000) *Mental Health Matters: A Reader*, Basingstoke: Macmillan in association with the Open University.

Henwood, M. (1990) *Community Care and Elderly People*, London: Family Policy Studies Centre.

Heraud, B.J. (1970) *Sociology and Social Work: Perspectives and Problems*, Oxford: Pergamon Press.

Herbert, M. (1997) 'Adolescence', in Davies, M. (ed.) *The Blackwell Companion to Social Work*, Oxford: Blackwell.

Hertz, R. (ed.) (1997) *Reflexivity and Voice*, London: Sage.

Hester, S. and Eglin, P. (1992) *A Sociology of Crime*, London: Routledge.

Hill, M. (1987) *Sharing Child Care in Early Parenthood*, London: Routledge & Kegan Paul.

Hill, M. and Aldgate, J. (eds) (1996) *Child Welfare Services: Developments in Law, Policy, Practice and Research*, London: Jessica Kingsley.

Hill, M. and Tisdall, K. (1997) *Children and Society*, Harlow, Essex: Addison Wesley Longman Ltd.

Hill Collins, P. (1990) *Black Feminist Thought*, London: Harper Collins.

—— (2005) *Black Sexual Politics: African Americans, Gender and the New Racism*, New York: Routledge.

Hillery, G.A. (1955) 'Definitions of community: areas of agreement', *Rural Sociology* 20 (2): 111–23.

Hirschi, T. (1969) *Causes of Delinquency*, Berkeley: University of California Press.

Hochschild, A. (1990) *The Second Shift: Working Parents and the Revolution at Home*, New York: Viking Press.

Hockey, J. and James, A. (1993) *Growing Up and Growing Old: Ageing and Dependency in the Life Course*, London: Sage.

Holman, B. (1988) *Putting Families First: Prevention and Child Care*, Basingstoke: Macmillan.

—— (1997) *FARE Dealing: Neighbourhood Involvement in a Housing Scheme*, London: Community Development Foundation.

Horgan, P. (2009) 'Interrogating the ethics of telecare services: a conceptual framework for dementia home care professionals', unpublished MPhil. thesis, Edinburgh: University of Edinburgh.

Howe, D. (1987) *An Introduction to Social Work Theory: Making Sense in Practice*, Aldershot: Gower.

—— (1991) 'The family and the therapist: towards a sociology of social work method', in Davies, M. (ed.) *The Sociology of Social Work*, London: Routledge.

—— (1994) 'Modernity, postmodernity and social work', *British Journal of Social Work* 24: 513–32.

Hudson, A. (1989) '"Troublesome girls": towards alternative definitions and policies', in Cain, M. (ed.) *Growing up Good: Policing the Behaviour of Girls in Europe*, London: Sage.

Hudson, B. (1984) 'Femininity and adolescence', in McRobbie, A. and Nava, M. (eds) *Gender and Generation*, Basingstoke: Macmillan.

Hudson, J. (2002) 'Community care in the information age', in Bytheway, B., Bacigalupo, V., Bornat, J., Johnson, J. and Spurr, S. (eds) *Understanding Care, Welfare and Community: A Reader*, London: Routledge and Open University.

Huff, D. (1973) *How to Lie with Statistics*, Harmondsworth: Penguin.

Humphries, S. (1995) *Hooligans or Rebels? Oral History of Working Class Childhood and Youth, 1889–1939*, 2nd edn, Oxford: Blackwell.

Hunter, S. and Ritchie, P. (eds) (2007) *Co-Production and Personalisation in Social Care*, London: Jessica Kingsley.

Ife, J. (2002) *Community Development, Creating Community Alternatives – Vision, Analysis and Practice*, Melbourne, Australia: Nelson.

Illich, I. (1975) *Medical Nemesis: The Expropriation of Health*, London: Calder and Boyars.

James, A. and Prout, A. (1997) 'Introduction', in James, A. and Prout, A. (eds) *Constructing and Reconstructing Childhood: Contemporary issues in the Sociological Study of Childhood*, 2nd edn, London: Routledge.

Jamieson, L. (1987) 'Theories of family development and the experience of being brought up', *Sociology* 21: 591–607.

—— (1998) *Intimacy: Personal Relationships in Modern Societies*, Cambridge: Polity Press.

Jamieson, L. and Toynbee, C. (1990) 'Shifting patterns of parental control', in Corr, H. and Jamieson, L. (eds) *The Politics of Everyday Life*, Basingstoke: Macmillan.

—— (1992) *Country Bairns: Growing Up 1900–1930*, Edinburgh: Edinburgh University Press.

Jefferson, T. (1992) 'Wheelin' and stealin'', *Achilles Heel* 13: 10–12.

Jeffery, R. (1979) 'Normal rubbish: deviant patients in casualty departments', *Sociology of Health and Illness* 1 (1); 90–107.

Jenks, C. (2005) *Childhood*, 2nd edn, London: Routledge.

Johnson, J. (1998) 'The emergence of care as a policy', in Brechin, A., Walmsley, J., Katz, J. and Peace, S. (eds) *Care Matters: Concepts, Practice and Research in Health and Social Care*, London: Sage.

Johnson, N. (1995) 'Domestic violence: an overview', in Kingston, P. and Penhale, B. (eds) *Family Violence and the Caring Professions*, Basingstoke: Macmillan.

Jones, C. (1997) 'British social work and the classless society: the failure of a profession', in Jones, H. (ed.) *Towards a Classless Society?* London: Routledge.

—— (2009) 'What makes adoptive family life work? Adoptive parents' narratives of the making and remaking of adoptive kinship', unpublished PhD thesis, Durham: University of Durham.

Jones, D.W. (2002) *Myths, Madness and the Family: The Impact of Mental Illness on Families*, Basingstoke: Palgrave.

Jones, G. and Wallace, C. (1992) *Youth, Family and Citizenship*, Buckingham: Open University Press.

Jones, H. (1997) *Towards a Classless Society?* London: Routledge.

Jones, K., Brown, J., and Bradshaw, J. (1978) *Issues in Social Policy*, London: Routledge & Kegan Paul.

Jordan, B. (1996) *A Theory of Poverty and Social Exclusion*, Cambridge: Polity Press.

Karn, J. (2007) *Narratives of Neglect: Community, Regeneration and the Governance of Security*, Cullompton, Devon: Willan Publishing.

Kelly, L. (1988) *Surviving Sexual Violence*, Cambridge: Polity Press.

Kelly, L., Burton, S. and Regan, L. (1994) 'Researching women's lives or studying women's oppression? Reflections on what constitutes feminist research', in Maynard, M. and Purvis, J. (eds) *Researching Women's Lives from a Feminist Perspective*, London: Taylor & Francis.

Kemshall, H. (1995) 'Feminist criminology and probation practice: the implications for teaching DipSW probation courses', *Social Work Education* 14 (3): 79–93.

Khan, M.S. (2009) *Domestic Workers and Socialisation in South Africa: The Socialisation Process Of The Black African Girl Child That Arrives in the Occupational Role Of Domestic Worker*, Johannesburg: VDM Verlag.

Kitzinger, J. (1990) 'Who are you kidding? Children and sociology in the UK', in Chisholm, L., Buchner, P., Kruger, H. and Brown, P. (eds) *Childhood, Youth and Social Change: A Comparative Perspective*, London: Falmer Press.

Klein, D.M. and White, J.M. (1996) *Family Theories: An Introduction*, London and California: Sage.

Kleinman, A. (1988) *The Illness Narratives: Suffering, Healing and the Human Condition*, New York: Basic Books.

Knuttila, M. (2005) *Introducing Sociology: A Critical Approach*, Oxford: Oxford University Press.

Kohlberg, L. (1981) *Essays on Moral Development, Vol. 1: The Philosophy of Moral Development: Moral Stages and the Idea of Justice*, Cambridge: Harper & Row.

Kumar, K. (1995) *From Post-Industrial to Post-Modern Society: New Theories of the Contemporary World*, Oxford: Basil Blackwell.

Laing, R.D. (1971) *The Politics of the Family and Other Essays*, London: Tavistock Publications.

Langan, M. and Day, L. (eds) (1992) *Women, Oppression and Social Work: Issues in Anti-discriminatory Practice*, London: Routledge.

Lasch, C. (1977) *Haven in a Heartless World*, New York: Basic Books.

Laslett, T.P. (1972) 'Mean household size in England since the 16th century', in Laslett, T.P. and Wall, R. (eds) *Household and the Family in Past Time*, Cambridge: Cambridge University Press.

Lavalette, M. and Cunningham, S. (2002) 'The sociology of childhood', in Goldson, B., Lavalette, M. and McKechnie, J. (eds) *Children, Welfare and the State*, London: Sage.

Leach, E. (1967) *A Runaway World*, London: BBC Publications.

Leat, D. and Gay, P. (1987) *Paying for Care*, Report 661, London: Policy Studies Institute.

Lee, N. (2001) *Childhood and Society: Growing up in an Age of Uncertainty*, Buckingham: Open University Press.

Lees, S. (1986) *Sexuality and Adolescent Girls*, London: Hutchinson.

Lemert, E.M. (1951) *Social Pathology*, New York: McGraw-Hill.

Leonard, P. (1966) *Sociology in Social Work*, London: Routledge & Kegan Paul.

Levin, I. (2004) 'Living apart together: a new family form', *Current Sociology*, 52 (2): 223–40.

Levitt, I. (1988) *Poverty and Welfare in Scotland 1890–1948*, Edinburgh: Edinburgh University Press.

Lewis, J. and Meredith, B. (1988) *Daughters Who Care Alone*, London: Routledge.

Lewis, O. (1949) *Life in a Mexican Village*, Urbana, IL: University of Illinois Press.

Lind, A. (2004) 'Legislating the family: heterosexist bias in social welfare policy frameworks', *Journal of Sociology and Social Welfare* 31 (4): 19–34.

Llewellyn, A., Agu, L. and Mercer, D. (2008) *Sociology for Social Workers*, Cambridge: Polity Press.

Lupton, D. (1995) *Medicine as Culture: Illness, Disease and the Body in Western Societies*, London: Sage.

—— (1997) 'Foucault and the medicalisation critique', in Peterson, A. and Bunton, R. (eds) *Foucault, Health and Medicine*, London: Routledge.

MacDonald, R. (ed.) (1997) *Youth, the 'Underclass' and Social Exclusion*, London: Routledge.

Macfarlane, A. (1996) 'Aspects of intervention: consultation, care, help and support', in Hales, G. (ed.) *Beyond Disability: Towards and Enabling Environment*, London: Sage in association with the Open University.

Macionis, J.J. and Plummer, K. (2008*) Sociology: A Global Introduction*, 4th edn, New Jersey: Prentice Hall.

Mackenbach, J.P., Bakker, M.J., Kunst, A.E. and Diderichsen, F. (2002) 'Socioeconomic inequalities in health in Europe', in Mackenbach, J.P. and Bakker, M.J. (eds) *Reducing Inequalities in Health: A European Perspective*, London: Routledge.

Maguire, M., Morgan, R. and Reiner, R. (eds) (2007) *The Oxford Handbook of Criminology*, 4th edn, Oxford: Oxford University Press.

Mahood, L. (1995) *Policing Gender, Class and Family: Britain, 1850–1940*, London: UCL Press.

MacPherson of Cluny, Sir William (1999) *The Stephen Lawrence Inquiry: Report of an Inquiry*, Cm 4262-I, London: The Stationery Office.

Marriott, H. (2003) *The Selfish Pig's Guide to Caring*, Clifton-Upon-Teme, Worcestershire: Polperro Heritage Press.

Marsh, I., Keating, M., Punch, S. and Harden, J. (2009) *Sociology: Making Sense of Society*, 4th edn, Harlow, Essex: Pearson.

Marsland, D. (1987) *Education and Youth*, London: The Falmer Press.

Martin, J. and Roberts, C. (1984) *Women and Employment: A Lifetime Perspective*, London: HMSO.

Marx, K. and Engels, F. (1976) *Collected Works*, London: Lawrence and Wishart.

Mason, D. (ed.) (2003) *Explaining Ethnic Differences: Changing Patterns of Disadvantage in Britain*, Bristol: The Policy Press.

Mason, J., May, V. and Clarke, L. (2007) 'Ambivalences and the paradoxes of grandparenting', *The Sociological Review* 55 (4): 687–706.

Matza, D. and Sykes, G. (1961) 'Juvenile delinquency and subterranean values', *American Sociological Review* 26: 712–19.

Mayall, B. (ed.) (1994) *Children's Childhoods: Observed and Experienced*, London: The Falmer Press.

—— (2002) *Towards a Sociology for Childhood: Thinking from Children's Lives*, Buckingham: Open University Press.

Maynard, M. (1985) 'The response of social workers to domestic violence', in Pahl, J. (ed.) *Private Violence and Public Policy*, London: Routledge & Kegan Paul.

—— (1990) 'The re-shaping of sociology? Trends in the study of gender', *Sociology* 24 (2): 269–90.

—— (2002) 'Studying age, race and gender: translating a research proposal into a project', *International Journal of Social Research Methodology*, 5(1): 31–40.

Mayo, M. (2000) *Cultures, Communities and Identities: Cultural Strategies for Participation and Empowerment*, Basingstoke: Palgrave Macmillan.

McBrewster, J., Miller, F.P. and Vandome, A.F. (2009) *Societal Attitudes Toward Homosexuality*, Beau Bassin, Mauritius: Alphascript Publishing.

McCrone, D. (2001 [1992]) *Understanding Scotland: The Sociology of a Nation*, 2nd edn, London: Routledege.

McIntosh, M. (1979) 'The welfare state and the needs of the dependent family', in Burnam, S. (ed.) *Fit Work for Women*, London: Croom Helm.

—— (1996) 'Social anxieties about lone motherhood and ideologies of the family: two sides of the same coin', in Silva, E.B. (ed.) *Good Enough Mothering? Feminist Perspectives on Lone Motherhood*, London: Routledge.

McKie, L. and Cunningham-Burley, S. (eds) (2005) *Families in Society: Boundaries and Relationships*, Bristol: The Policy Press.

McLaughlin, E., Muncie, J. and Hughes, G. (eds) (2003) *Criminological Perspectives: Essential Readings*, 2nd edn, London: Sage and Open University.

McLeod, E. and Bywaters, P. (2000) *Social Work, Health and Equality*, London: Routledge.

McMillan, D.W. and Chavis, D.M. (1986) 'Sense of community: a definition and theory', *Journal of Community Psychology* 14: 6–23.

McRobbie, A. and Garber, J. (1976) 'Girls and subcultures', in Hall, S. and Jefferson, T. (eds) *Resistance through Rituals: Youth Subcultures in Post-War Britain*, London: Hutchinson and CCCS, University of Birmingham.

Mead, G.H. (1934) *Mind, Self and Society*, Chicago: Chicago University Press.

Mead, M. (1928) *Coming of Age in Samoa*, London: Penguin.

Merton, R. (1957) *Social Theory and Social Structure*, New York: Free Press.

Mesch, G.S. and Talmud, I. (2010) *Wired Youth: The Social World of Adolescence in the Information Age*, London: Routledge.

Miller, D.L. (1997) *City of the Century: The Epic of Chicago and the Making of America*, New York: Simon & Schuster.

Mills, C.W. (1959) *The Sociological Imagination*, Oxford: Oxford University Press.

Mills, D. (1996) 'Community and nation in the past: perception and reality', in Drake, M. (ed.) *Time, Family and Community: Perspectives on Family and Community History*, Oxford: Blackwell.

Mirza, H. (1992) *Young, Female and Black*, London: Routledge.

Mooney, G. (1998) '"Remoralizing" the poor?: gender, class and philanthropy in Victorian Britain', in Lewis, G. (ed.) *Forming Nation, Framing Welfare*, London: Routledge.

Mooney, G. and Neal, S. (2009) 'Community: themes and debates', in Mooney, G. and Neal, S. (eds) *Community: Welfare, Crime and Society*, Maidenhead: Open University Press.

—— (eds) (2009) *Community: Welfare, Crime and Society*, Maidenhead: Open University Press.

Moore, L. (1993) 'Educating for the woman's sphere', in Breitenbach, E. and Gordon, E. (eds) *Out of Bounds*, Edinburgh: Edinburgh University Press.

Moore, S. (1988) *Investigating Deviance*, London: Unwin Hyman.

Morgan, D.H.J. (1975) *Social Theory and the Family*, London: Routledge & Kegan Paul.

—— (1996) *Family Connections: An Introduction to Family Studies*, Cambridge: Polity Press.

—— (2002) 'Sociological perspectives on the family', in Carling, A., Duncan, S. and Edwards, R. (eds) *Analysing Families: Morality and Rationality in Policy and Practice*, London: Routledge.

Morgan, M. (1996) 'The meanings of high blood pressure among Afro-Caribbean and white patients', in Kelleher, D. and Hillier, S. (eds) *Researching Cultural Differences in Health*, London: Routledege.

Morgan, P. (1995) *Farewell to the Family? Public Policy and Breakdown in Britain and the USA*, London: Institute of Economic Affairs.

Morris, J. (1991) *Pride against Prejudice: Transforming Attitudes to Disability*, London: Women's Press.

—— (1995) 'Creating a space for absent voices: disabled women's experience of receiving assistance with daily living activities', *Feminist Review* 51: 68–93.

—— (1997) '"Us" and "them"? Feminist research and community care', in Bornat, J., Johnson, J., Pereira, C., Pilgrim, D. and Williams, F. (eds) *Community Care: A Reader*, 2nd edn, Basingstoke: Macmillan and Open University.

Morris, K. (2008) *Social Work and Multi-Agency Working: Making a Difference*, Bristol: The Policy Press /BASW.

Morrow, V. (2003) 'Moving out of childhood', in Maybin, J. and Woodhead, M. (eds) *Childhoods in Context*, Milton Keynes: Open University.

Mouzelis, N. (1995) *Sociological Theory: What Went Wrong? Diagnosis and Remedies*, London: Routledge.

Mulhall, A. (2001) 'Epidemiology', in Naidoo, J. and Wills, J. (eds) *Health Studies: An Introduction*, Basingstoke: Palgrave.

Mullender, A. (1996) *Rethinking Domestic Violence: The Social Work and Probation Response*, London: Routledge.

—— (2008) 'Gendering the social work agenda', in Davies, M. (ed.) *Blackwell Companion to Social Work*, 3rd edn, Oxford: Blackwell.

Muncie, J. (1999) *Youth and Crime*, London: Sage.

—— (2009) *Youth and Crime*, 3rd edn, London: Sage.

Muncie, J. and FitzGerald, M. (1981) 'Humanising the deviant: affinity and affiliation theories', in FitzGerald, M., McLennan, G., and Pawson, J. (eds) *Crime and Society: Readings in History and Theory*, Milton Keynes: Open University Press.

Muncie, J., McLaughlin, E. and Langan, M. (1996) *Criminological Perspectives: A Reader*, London: Sage and Open University.

Muncie, J. and Sapsford, R. (1999) 'Issues in the study of "the family"', in Muncie, J., Wetherell, M., Dallos, R. and Cochrane, A. (eds) *Understanding the Family*, 2nd edn, London: Open University and Sage.

Muncie, J. and Wetherell, M. (1995) 'Family policy and political discourse', in Muncie, J., Wetherell, M., Dallos, R. and Cochrane, A. (eds) *Understanding the Family*, London: Open University and Sage.

Murdock, G.P. (1965) *Social Structure*, 2nd edn, New York: Free Press.

Murray, C. (1990) *The Emerging British Underclass*, London: Institute of Economic Affairs, Health and Welfare Unit.

—— (1993) 'The time has come to put a stigma back on illegitimacy', *Wall Street Journal*, 14 November.

—— (1994) With commentaries by Alcock, P., David, M., Phillips M. and Slipman, S., *Underclass: The Crisis Deepens*, Choice in Welfare Series No. 20, London: IEA.

Musgrove, F. (1968) *Youth and the Social Order*, London: Routledge & Kegan Paul.

Musgrave, P. (1972) *The Sociology of Education*, 2nd edn, London: Methuen.

Naffine, N. (1987) *Female Crime: The Construction of Women in Criminology*, London: Allen & Unwin.

Nava, M. (1983) 'From utopianism to scientific feminism', in Segal, L. (ed.) *What Is To Be Done about the Family?* Harmondsworth: Penguin.

—— (1984) 'Youth service provision, social order and the question of girls', in McRobbie, A. and Nava, M. (eds) *Gender and Generation*, Basingstoke: Macmillan.

Nazroo, J. (1999) 'Uncovering gender differences in the use of marital violence: the effect of methodology', in Allan, G. (ed.) *The Sociology of the Family: A Reader*, Oxford: Blackwell.

Nettleton, S. and Watson, J. (1998) *The Body in Everyday Life*, London: Routledge.

Nettleton, S. (2006) *The Sociology of Health and Illness*, 2nd edn, Cambridge: Polity Press.

Newman, T. (1996) 'Rights, rites and responsibilities', in Roberts, H. and Sachdev, D. (eds) *Young People's Social Attitudes: Having their Say: the Views of 12–19 Year Olds*, London: Barnardo's.

Newburn, T. and Stanko, E.A. (1994) 'When men are victims: the failure of victimology', in Newburn, T. and Stanko, E.A. (eds) *Just Boys Doing Business: Men, Masculinities and Crime*, London: Routledge.

Nissel, M. and Bonnerjea, L. (1982) *Family Care of the Handicapped Elderly: Who Pays?* London: Policy Studies Institute.

Nsamenang, A.B. (2002) 'Adolescence in sub-Saharan Africa: an image constructed from Africa's triple inheritance', in Brown, B.B., Larson, R.W. and Saraswathi, T.S. (eds) *The World's Youth: Adolescence in Eight Regions of the Globe*, Cambridge: Cambridge University Press.

Oakley, A. (1972) *Sex, Gender and Society*, London: Temple Smith.

—— (1974) *The Sociology of Housework*, London: Martin Robertson.

—— (1974) *Housewife*, London: Allen Lane.

—— (1980) *Women Confined: Towards a Sociology of Childbirth*, Oxford: Martin Robertson.

—— (1984) *The Captured Womb: A History of the Medical Care of Pregnant Women*, Oxford: Blackwell.

—— (1993) *Women, Medicine and Health*, Edinburgh: Edinburgh University Press.

—— (2005) *The Ann Oakley Reader: Gender, Women and Social Science*, Bristol: The Policy Press.

Office of National Statistics (ONS) (2009) *Social Trends* 39, Basingstoke: Palgrave Macmillan. Available at: www.statistics.gov.uk/socialtrends/

Ogbar, J.O.G. (2005) *Black Power: Radical Politics and African American Identity*, Baltimore, MD: Johns Hopkins University Press.

Okoli, R. (2009) 'Children's work: experiences of street vending children and young people in Enugu, Nigeria', unpublished PhD thesis, University of Edinburgh.

Oldman, D. (1994) 'Childhood as a mode of production', in Mayall, B. (ed.) *Children's Childhoods: Observed and Experienced*, London: The Falmer Press.

Oliver, M. (1990) *The Politics of Disablement*, Basingstoke: Macmillan.

Oni, J.B. (1995) 'Fostered children's perception of their health care and illness treatment in Ekiti Yoruba households, Nigeria', *Health Transition Review* 5: 21–34.

Opie, I. (1993) *The People in the Playground*, Oxford: Oxford University Press.

Osgerby, B. (1998) *Youth in Britain since 1945*, Oxford: Blackwell.

Oyemade, A. (1980) 'Child care practices in Nigeria: an urgent plea for social workers', *Child Abuse and Neglect* 4 (2): 101–3.

Palmer, G., Carr, J. and Kenway, P. (2005) *Monitoring Poverty and Social Exclusion*, York: Joseph Rowntree Foundation.

Palmer, S. (2006) *Toxic Childhood: How The Modern World Is Damaging Our Children And What We Can Do About It*, London: Orion.

Pantazis, C., Gordon, D. and Levitas, R. (2006) *Poverty and Social Exclusion in Britain: The Millennium Survey*, Bristol: The Policy Press.

Park, R.E. (1936) 'Human ecology', *American Journal of Sociology* 42 (1): 15.

—— (1950) *Race and Culture*, Glencoe, IL: Free Press.

—— (1967 [1915]) 'The city: suggestions for the investigation of human behavior in the city', *American Journal of Sociology* 20 (5): 577–612.

Park, R.E., Burgess, E. and McKenzie, R. (1925) *The City*, Chicago, IL: University of Chicago Press.

Parker, G. (1990) *With Due Care and Attention: A Review of Research on Informal Care*, 2nd edn, London: Family Policy Studies Centre.

Parker, G. and Lawton, D. (1994) *Different Types of Care, Different Types of Carer*, London: HMSO.

Parker, R. (1981) 'Tending and social policy', in Goldberg, E.M. and Hatch, S. (eds) *A New Look at the Personal Social Services*, Discussion Paper 4, London: Policy Studies Institute.

Parker, R., Ward, H., Jackson, S., Aldgate, J. and Wedge, P. (1991) *Assessing Outcomes in Child Care: Looking after Children*, London: HMSO.

Parsons, T. (1955) 'The American family: its relation to personality and the social structure', in Parsons, T. and Bales, R.F. (eds) *Family Socialisation and Interaction Process*, New York: Free Press.

—— (1964 [1951]) *The Social System*, New York: Free Press.

—— (1983 [1949]) 'The social structure of the family', in Anshen, R.N. (ed.) *The Family, Its Functions and Destiny*, New York: Harper.

Parton, N. (1985) *The Politics of Child Abuse*, Basingstoke: Macmillan.

—— (1991) *Governing the Family: Child Care, Child Protection and the State*, Basingstoke: Macmillan.

—— (1994) 'Problematics of government, (post) modernity and social work', *British Journal of Social Work* 24: 9–32.

—— (ed.) (1996) *Social Theory, Social Change and Social Work*, London: Routledge.

—— (2004) 'Post theories for practice: challenging the dogmas', in Davies, L. and Leonard, P. (eds) *Social Work in the Corporate Era: Practices of Power and Resistance*, Aldershot: Ashgate.

—— (2006) *Safeguarding Children: Early Intervention and Surveillance in a Late Modern Society*, London: Palgrave Macmillan.

Parton, N., Thorpe, D. and Wattam, C. (eds) (1997) *Child Protection: Risk and Moral Order*, Basingstoke: Macmillan.

Patel, N. (1990) *'Race' against Time: Social Services Provision to Black Elders*, London: Runnymede Trust.

Payne, C. (1994) 'The systems approach', in Hanvey, C. and Philpot, T. (eds) *Practising Social Work*, London: Routledge.

Payne, M. (1995) *Social Work and Community Care*, Basingstoke: Macmillan.

Pearson, G. (1983) *Hooligan: A History of Respectable Fears*, Basingstoke: Macmillan.

Phillips, A. (1993) *The Trouble with Boys*, London: Pandora.

Phillipson, C. and Biggs, S. (1995) 'Elder abuse: a critical overview', in Kingston, P. and Penhale, B. (eds) *Family Violence and the Caring Professions*, Basingstoke: Macmillan.

Pierson, J. (2008) *Going Local: Working in Communities and Neighbourhoods*, London: Routledge.

Pilcher, J. (1995) *Age and Generation in Modern Britain*, Oxford: Oxford University Press.

Pilkington, A. (2003) *Racial Disadvantage and Ethnic Diversity in Britain*, Basingstoke: Palgrave Macmillan.

Pollock, L. (1987) *A Lasting Relationship: Parents and Children over Three Centuries*, London: Fourth Estate.

Popay, J., Hearn, J. and Edwards, J. (1998) *Men, Gender Divisions and Welfare*, London: Routledge.

Postman, N. (1983) *The Disappearance of Childhood*, London: W.H. Allen.

Preston-Shoot, M. (2005) 'Editorial', *Social Work Education* 24 (6): 601–2.

Pringle, K. (1996) *Men, Masculinities and Social Welfare*, London: UCL Press.

—— (1998) *Children and Social Welfare in Europe*, Buckingham: Open University Press.

Prout, A. (2005) *The Future of Childhood*, London: Routledge/Falmer.

Pryke, S. (2002) 'The origins of classic social theory', in Marsh, I. (ed.) *Theory and Practice in Sociology*, Harlow, Essex: Pearson Education Ltd.

Pullar, A. (2009) 'Violent and non-violent convicted women offenders in Fife: an analysis of offending patterns, criminogenic need and effective service provision', unpublished PhD dissertation, Edinburgh: University of Edinburgh.

Purdy, M. and Banks, D. (2000) *The Sociology and Politics of Health*, London: Routledge.

Qureshi, H. and Walker, A. (1989) *The Caring Relationship*, Basingstoke: Macmillan.

Qvortrup, J. (1994) 'Childhood matters: an introduction', in Qvortrup, J., Bardy, M., Sgritta, G. and Wintersberger, H. (eds) *Childhood Matters: Social Theory, Practice and Politics*, Aldershot: Avebury.

—— (1995) 'Childhood and modern society: a paradoxical relationship?', in Brannen, J. and O'Brien, M. (eds) *Childhood and Parenthood*, London: Institute of Education, University of London.

Qvortrup, J., Bardy, M., Sgritta, G. and Wintersberger, H. (eds) (1994) *Childhood Matters: Social Theory, Practice and Politics*, Aldershot: Avebury.

Rafferty, J. and Steyaert, J. (2007) 'Social work in a digital society', in Lymbery, M. and Postle, K. (eds) *Social Work: A Companion to Learning*, London: Sage.

Ramazanoglu, C. (1989) *Feminism and the Contradictions of Oppression*, London: Routledge.

Ramazanoglu, C. with Holland, J. (2002) *Feminist Methodology: Challenges and Choices*, London: Sage.

Rank, M.R. and Kain, E.L. (1995) *Diversity and Change in Families: Patterns, Prospects and Policies*, Englewood Cliffs, NJ: Prentice-Hall.

Rapoport, R. and Rapoport, R. (1965) 'Work and family in contemporary society', *American Sociological Review* 30 (3): 381–94.

Redfield, R. (1947) 'The folk society', *American Journal of Sociology* 52 (3): 293–308.

Redhead, S. (1990) *The End-of-the-Century-Party: Youth and Pop toward 2000*, Manchester: Manchester University Press.

Reiss, I.L. (1965) 'The universality of the family', *Journal of Marriage and the Family* 27 (November): 443–53.

Rex, J. and Moore, R. (1967) *Race, Community and Conflict: A Study of Sparkbrook*, Oxford: Oxford University Press.

Richmond, M. (1917) *Social Diagnosis*, New York: Russell Sage Foundation.

Riddell, S. (1998) 'The dynamic of transition to adulthood', in Robinson, C. and Stalker, K. (eds) *Growing up with Disability*, London: Jessica Kingsley.

Roberts, E. (1996) 'Women and the domestic economy 1890–1970: the oral evidence', in Drake, M. (ed.) *Time, Family and Community: Perspectives on Family and Community History*, Oxford: Blackwell.

Roberts, K. (1995) *Youth and Employment in Modern Britain*, Oxford: Oxford University Press.

—— (1997) 'Is there an emerging British "underclass"? The evidence from youth research', in MacDonald, R. (ed.) *Youth, the 'Underclass' and Social Exclusion*, London: Routledge.

Robertson, R. (1992) *Globalization: Social Theory and Global Culture*, London: Sage.

Robinson, L. (2004) 'Black adolescent identity', in Roche, J., Tucker, S., Thomson, R. and Flynn, R. (eds) *Youth in Society: Contemporary Theory, Policy and Practice*, 2nd edn, London: Sage.

—— *Psychology for Social Workers: Black Perspectives on Human Development and Behaviour*, 2nd edn, London: Routledge.

Roche, J., Tucker, S., Thomson, R. and Flynn, R. (eds) (2004) *Youth in Society: Contemporary Theory, Policy and Practice*, 2nd edn, London: Sage.

Rock, P. (2007) 'Sociological theories of crime', in Maguire, M., Morgan, R. and Reiner, R. (eds) (2007) *The Oxford Handbook of Criminology*, 4th edn, Oxford: Oxford University Press.

Rodger, J.J. (1996) *Family Life and Social Control: A Sociological Perspective*, Basingstoke: Macmillan.

Rogers, W.S. (1989) 'Effective co-operation in child protection work', in Morgan, S. and Righton, P. (eds) *Child Care: Concerns and Conflicts*, London: Hodder and Stoughton.

Rose, N. (1999) *Governing the Soul: The Shaping of the Private Self*, 2nd edn, London: Routledge.

Rosenfield, R.L., Bachrach, L.K., Chernausek, S.D., Gertner, J.M., Gottschalk, M., Hardin, D.S., Pescovitz, O.H., Saenger, P., Herman-Giddens, M.E., Slora, E. and Wasserman, R. (2000) 'Current age of onset of puberty', *Pediatrics* 106 (3): 622–3.

Rowbotham, S. (1973) *Women's Consciousness, Man's World*, Harmondsworth: Penguin.

Russell, G. (1983) *The Changing Role of Fathers*, Milton Keynes: Open University Press.

Rutter, M., Graham, P., Chadwick, O.F.D. and Yule, W. (1976) 'Adolescent turmoil: fact or fiction?', *Journal of Child Psychology and Psychiatry* 17: 35–56.

Said, E. (1993) *Culture and Imperialism*, London: Chatto Press.

Saporiti, A. (1994) 'A methodology for making children count', in Qvortrup, J., Bardy, M., Sgritta, G. and Wintersberger, H. (eds) *Childhood Matters: Social Theory, Practice and Politics*, Aldershot: Avebury.

Saraswathi, T.S. and Larson, R.W. (2002) 'Adolescence in global perspective: an agenda for social policy', in Brown, B.B., Larson, R.W. and Saraswathi, T.S. (eds) *The World's Youth: Adolescence in Eight Regions of the Globe*, Cambridge: Cambridge University Press.

Saul, J. (2003) *Feminism: Issues and Arguments*, Oxford: Oxford University Press.

Savage, M. and Warde, A. (2002) *Urban Sociology, Capitalism and Modernity*, 2nd edn, Basingstoke: Macmillan.

Schon, D.A. (1983) *The Reflective Practitioner: How Professionals Think in Action*, London: Temple Smith.

The Scottish Office Social Work Services Group (1991) *National Objectives and Standards for Social Work Services in the Criminal Justice System*, Edinburgh: The Scottish Office Social Work Services Group.

—— (1996) *National Guidelines on Diversion to Social Work and Other Service Agencies as an Alternative to Prosecution*, Edinburgh: The Scottish Office Social Work Services Group.

Scourfield, J.B. (1998) 'Probation officers working with men', *British Journal of Social Work* 28 (4): 581–600.

Scraton, P. (ed.) (1997) *'Childhood' in 'Crisis'?* London: UCL Press.

Scraton, P. and Chadwick, K. (1991) 'The theoretical and political priorities of critical criminology', in Stenson, K. and Cowell, D. (eds) *The Politics of Crime Control*, London: Sage.

Segal, L. (1983) *What Is To Be Done about the Family?*, Harmondsworth: Penguin.

—— (1990) *Slow Motion: Changing Masculinities*, London: Virago.

—— (1999) *Why Feminism?*, Cambridge: Polity Press.

Senior, M. with Viveash, B. (1998) *Health and Illness*, Basingstoke: Macmillan.

Sennett, R. (1973) *The Uses of Disorder*, Harmondsworth: Penguin.

—— (1992 [1977]) *The Fall of Public Man*, New York: W.W. Norton.

—— (1998) *The Corrosion of Character: The Personal Consequences of Work in the New Capitalism*, New York: W.W. Norton.

Shaw, M., Galobardes, B. and Lawlor, D. (2007) *The Handbook of Inequality and Socioeconomic Position*, Bristol: The Policy Press.

Shilling, C. (2003) *The Body and Social Theory*, 2nd edn, London: Sage.

Showalter, E. (1987) *The Female Malady*, London: Virago.

Sibeon, R. (1991) *Towards a New Sociology of Social Work*, Aldershot: Avebury.

Simmel, G. (1971 [1903]) 'The metropolis and mental life', in Thompson, K. and Tunstall, J. (eds) *Sociological Perspectives*, Penguin: Harmondsworth.

Skeggs, B. (1997) *Formations of Class and Gender*, London: Sage.

Slevin, J. (2000) *The Internet and Society*, Cambridge: Polity Press.

Smart, C. (1976) *Women, Crime and Criminology: A Feminist Critique*, London: Routledge & Kegan Paul.

—— (1990) 'Feminist approaches to criminology or postmodern woman meets atavistic man', in Gelsthorpe, L. and Morris, A. (eds) *Feminist Perspectives in Criminology*, Buckingham: Open University Press.

Smart, C. and Smart, B. (1978) *Women, Sexuality and Social Control*, London: Routledge & Kegan Paul.

Smith, A. (2006) *Crime Statistics: An Independent Review*, November, www.crimereduction.homeoffice.gov.uk/statistics/statistics057.htm

Smith, C. and White, S. (1997) 'Parton, Howe and postmodernity: a critical comment on mistaken identity', *British Journal of Social Work* 27: 275–95.

Smith, D. (1988) *The Everyday World as Problematic*, Milton Keynes: Open University Press.

Smith, D.J. (1995) *Criminology for Social Work*, Basingstoke: Macmillan.

—— (1997) 'Ethnic origins, crime and criminal justice', in Maguire, M., Morgan, R. and Reiner, R. (eds) *The Oxford Handbook of Criminology*, 2nd edn, Oxford: Clarendon Press.

Smith, D.M. (1987) 'Peers, subcultures and schools', in Marsland, D. (ed.) *Education and Youth*, London: The Falmer Press.

Smith, M. (1965) *Professional Education for Social Work in Britain*, London: Allen & Unwin.

Smith, M. (2009) *Rethinking Residential Child Care: Positive Perspectives*, Bristol: The Policy Press.

Smith, M.A. and Kollock, P. (1999) *Communities in Cyberspace*, London: Routledge.

Social Work Services Inspectorate (1995) *Social Work Services in the Criminal Justice System: Achieving National Standards*, Edinburgh: The Scottish Office.

Sontag, S. (2001) *Illness as Metaphor and AIDS and Its Metaphors*, New York: Picador.

Speight, S., Smith, R., La Valle, I., Schneider, V. and Perry, J. with Coshall, C. and Tipping, S. (2009) Childcare and Early Years Survey of Parents 2008, Department for Children, Schools and Families, Research Report DCSF-RR136, DCSF Publications: Nottingham. Available at www.natcen.ac.uk/

Springhall, J. (1986) *Coming of Age: Adolescence in Britain 1860–1960*, Dublin: Gill and Macmillan.

Stanley, L. (ed.) (1990) *Feminist Praxis: Research, Theory and Epistemology in Feminist Sociology*, London: Routledge.

Stewart, F. (1992) 'The adolescent as consumer', in Coleman, J.C. and Warren-Adamson, C. (eds) *Youth Policy in the 1990s: The Way Forward*, London: Routledge.

Straus, M.A. and Gelles, R.J. (1986) 'Societal change and change in family violence from 1975 to 1985 as revealed by two national surveys', *Journal of Marriage and the Family* 48: 465–79.

Sutherland, E.H. (1939) *Principles of Criminology*, 3rd edn, Philadelphia: Lippincott.

Sutherland, E.H. and Cressey, D.R. (1978) *Criminology*, 10th edn, New York: Columbia University Press.

Swain, J., French, S., Barnes, C. and Thomas, C. (2004) *Disabling Barriers – Enabling Environments*, 2nd edn, London: Sage.

Swingewood, A. (1984) *A Short History of Sociological Thought*, London: Macmillan.

Symonds, A. (1998) 'Social construction and the concept of "community"', in Symonds, A. and Kelly, A. (eds) *The Social Construction of Community Care*, Basingstoke: Macmillan.

Taylor, C. and White, S. (2006) 'Knowledge and reasoning in social work: educating for humane judgement', *British Journal of Social Work* 35: 937–54.

Taylor, I., Evans, K. and Fraser, P. (1996) *Tale of Two Cities: Global Change, Local Feeling and Everyday Life in the North of England – A Study in Manchester and Sheffield*, London: Routledge.

Taylor, I., Walton, P. and Young, J. (1975) *Critical Criminology*, London: Routledge & Kegan Paul.

Tester, S. (1996) 'Women and community care', in Hallett, C. (ed.) *Women and Social Policy: An Introduction*, London: Harvester Wheatsheaf.

Thane, P. (1981) 'Childhood in history', in King, M. (ed.) *Childhood, Welfare and Justice: A Critical Examination of Children in the Legal and Childcare Systems*, London: Batsford.

—— (1996) 'Gender, welfare and old age in Britain, 1870s–1940s', in Digby, A. and Stewart, J. (eds) *Gender, Welfare and Old Age in Britain*, London: Routledge.

Thomas, C. (1993) 'De-constructing concepts of care', *Sociology* 27 (4): 649–69.

Thomas, N. (2000) *Children, Family and the State: Decision-making and Child Participation*, Basingstoke: Macmillan.

Thomas, W.I. (1966) 'The relation of research to the social process', in Janowitz, M. (ed.) *W.I. Thomas on Social Disorganisation and Social Personality*, Chicago: The University of Chicago Press.

Thompson, P. (1981) 'Life histories and the analysis of social change', in Bertaux, D. (ed.) *Biography and Society*, Beverly Hills: Sage.

Thomson, N. (2006) *Anti-Discriminatory Practice*, 4th revised edn, Basingstoke: Palgrave Macmillan.

Tisdall, K. (1996) 'From the Social Work (Scotland) Act 1968 to the Children (Scotland) Act 1995: pressures for change', in Hill, M. and Aldgate, J. (eds) *Child Welfare Services: Developments in Law, Policy, Practice and Research*, London: Jessica Kingsley.

Tizard, A. and Phoenix, B. (2001) *Black, White or Mixed Race?: Race and Racism in the Lives of Young People of Mixed Parentage*, 2nd edn, London: Routledge.

Tönnies, F. (1955 [1877]) *Community and Association*, London: Routledge & Kegan Paul.

Townsend, P. (1962) *The Last Refuge: A Survey of Residential Institutions and Homes for the Aged in England and Wales*, London: Routledge & Kegan Paul.

Townsend, P. and Davidson, N. (1982) *Inequalities in Health: The Black Report*, Harmondsworth: Penguin Books Ltd.

Toynbee, P. and Walker, D. (2008) *Unjust Rewards: Ending the Greed that is Bankrupting Britain*, London: Granta.

Triseliotis, J. (1980) *New Developments in Adoption and Foster Care*, London: Routledge & Kegan Paul.

Tronto, J.C. (1993) *Moral Boundaries: A Political Argument for an Ethic of Care*, London: Routledge.

Tucker, S. and Liddiard, P. (1998) 'Young carers', in Brechin, A., Walmsley, J., Katz, J. and Peace, S. (eds) *Care Matters: Concepts, Practice and Research in Health and Social Care*, London: Sage.

Turner, B.S. (1996) *The Body and Society: Explorations in Social Theory*, 2nd edn, London: Sage.

—— (1997) 'From governmentality to risk: some reflections on Foucualt's contribution to medical sociology', in Peterson, A. and Bunton, R. (eds) *Foucault, Health and Medicine*, London: Routledge.

Ungerson, C. (1983) 'Why do women care?', in Finch, J. and Groves, D. (eds) *A Labour of Love: Women, Work and Caring*, London: Routledge & Kegan Paul.

Ussher, J. (ed.) (1997) *Body Talk*, London: Routledge.

Van Den Haag, E. (1975) *Punishing Criminals*, New York: Simon and Schuster.

Vernon, A. (2002) *User-defined Outcomes of Community Care for Asian Disabled People*, Bristol: The Policy Press.

Walby, S. (1990) *Theorising Patriarchy*, Oxford: Blackwell.

—— (1997) *Gender Transformations*, London: Routledge.

—— (2009) *Globalization and Inequalities: Complexity and Contested Modernities*, London: Sage.

Walklate, S. (1989) *Victimology*, London: Unwin Hyman.

Wall, D.S. and Williams, M. (2007) 'Policing diversity in the digital age: maintaining order in virtual communities', *Criminology and Criminal Justice* 7 (4): 391–415.

Wall, R. (1992) 'Relationships between generations in British families past and present', in Marsh, C. and Arber, S. (eds) *Families and Households: Divisions and Change*, Basingstoke: Macmillan.

Wallace, C. (1987) 'Between the family and the state: young people in transition', in White, M. (ed.) *The Social World of the Young Unemployed*, London: Policy Studies Institute.

Waterhouse, L. (2008) 'Child abuse', in Davies, M. (ed.) *Blackwell Companion to Social Work*, 3rd edn, Oxford: Blackwell.

Waterhouse, L., Dobash, R. and Carnie, J. (1994) *Child Sexual Abusers*, Edinburgh: The Scottish Office.

Waxler-Morrison, N., Anderson, J.M., Richardson, E. and Chambers, N.A. (2005) *Cross-Cultural Caring: A Handbook for Health Professionals*, 2nd edn, Vancouver: UBC Press.

Weber, M. (1970) 'Politics as a vocation' and 'Science as a vocation', in Gerth, H.H. and Mills, C.W. (eds) *From Max Weber*, London: Routledge & Kegan Paul.

Weber, M. (1974 [1902]) *The Protestant Ethic and the Spirit of Capitalism*, London: Unwin.

Weedon, C. (1987) *Feminist Practice and Post-structuralist Theory*, Oxford: Blackwell.

Weeks, J. (1986) *Sexuality*, London: Tavistock.

Weeks, J., Heaphy, B. and Donovan, C. (1999) 'Partners by choice: equality, power and commitment in non-heterosexual relationships', in Allan, G. (ed.) *The Sociology of the Family: A Reader*, Oxford: Blackwell.

Weeks, J., Heaphy, B. and Donovan, C. (2001) *Same Sex Intimacies: Families of Choice and Other Life Experiments*, London: Routledge.

Wells, K. (2009) *Childhood in a Global Perspective*, Cambridge: Polity Press.

White, M. (1988) *And Grandmother's Bed Went Too: Poor But Happy in Somers Town*, London: St Pancras Housing Association, Camden.

White, S., Fook, J. and Gardiner, F. (eds) (2006) *Critical Reflection in Health and Social Care*, Maidenhead: Open University Press.

White, S. and Stancombe, J. (2003) *Clinical Judgement in the Health and Welfare Professions: Extending the Evidence Base*, Maidenhead: Open University Press.

Whitehead, M. (1992) *The Health Divide*, Harmondsworth: Penguin.

Whyte, B. (1998) 'Rediscovering juvenile delinquency', in Lockyer, A. and Stone, F.H (eds) *Juvenile Justice in Scotland: Twenty-Five Years of the Welfare Approach*, Edinburgh: T&T Clark.

Widdowson, E. (2004) 'Retiring lives? Old age, work and welfare', in Mooney, G. (ed.) *Work: Personal Lives and Social Policy*, Bristol: The Policy Press in association with the Open University.

Wilczynski, A. (1995) 'Child-killing by parents: social, legal and gender issues', in Dobash, R.E., Dobash, R.P. and Noaks, L. (eds) *Gender and Crime*, Cardiff: University of Wales Press.

Wilkins, L.T. (1964) *Social Deviance: Social Action and Research*, London: Tavistock.

Wilkinson, R. (1984) *Health, Economic Structure and Social Indicators*, London: Centre for Economic Policy Research Discussion papers 17.

—— (1996) *Unequal Societies*, London: Routledge.

—— (2005) *The Impact of Inequality: How to Make Sick Societies Healthier*, London: Routledge.

Wilkinson, R. and Pickett, K. (2009) *The Spirit Level: Why More Equal Societies Almost Always Do Better*, London: Allen Lane.

Williams, F. (1997) 'Women and community', in Bornat, J., Johnson, J., Pereira, C., Pilgrim, D. and Williams, F. (eds) *Community Care: A Reader*, 2nd edn, Basingstoke: Macmillan and Open University.

Williams, G. (1984) 'The genesis of chronic illness: narrative reconstruction', in Bury, M. and Gabe, J. (eds) (2004) *The Sociology of Health and Illness: A Reader*, London: Routledge.

—— (2004) 'The genesis of chronic illness: narrative reconstruction', in Bury, M. and Gabe, J. (eds) *The Sociology of Health and Illness: A Reader*, London: Routledge.

Williams, S.J., Gabe, J. and Calnan, M. (2000) *Health, Medicine and Society: Key Theories, Future Agendas*, London: Routledge.

Willis, P. (1977) *Learning to Labour*, Farnborough: Saxon House.

Willmott, P. and Young, M. (1960) *Family and Class in a London Suburb*, London: Routledge & Kegan Paul.

—— (1990) *Common Culture: Symbolic Work at Play in the Everyday Cultures of the Young*, Milton Keynes: Open University Press.

Wilson, E. (1977) *Women and the Welfare State*, London: Tavistock.

—— (1982) 'Women, the "community" and the "family"', in Walker, A. (ed.) *Community Care: The Family, the State and Social Policy*, Oxford: Basil Blackwell/Martin Robertson.

—— (1995) 'The invisible flaneur', in Watson, S. and Gibson, K. (eds) *Postmodern Cities and Spaces*, Oxford: Blackwell.

Wilson, J. (1975) *Thinking about Crime*, New York: Basic Books.

Wilson, M. (1996) 'Working with the CHANGE men's programme', in Cavanagh, K. and Cree, V.E. (eds) *Working with Men: Feminism and Social Work*, London: Routledge.

Wilson, W.J. (1980) *The Declining Significance of Race*, 2nd edn, Chicago: The University of Chicago Press.

Wirth, L. (1938) 'Urbanism as a way of life', *American Journal of Sociology* 44 (1): 1–24.

World Health Organization (1946) *Constitution of the World Health Organization*, New York: World Health Organization Interim Commission.

Wright, F.D. (1986) *Left to Care Alone*, Aldershot: Gower.

Wrong, D.H. (1961) 'The over-socialised conception of man in modern sociology', *American Sociological Review* 26 (April): 183–93.

Wyness, M. (2006) *Childhood and Society: An Introduction to the Sociology of Childhood*, Basingstoke: Palgrave Macmillan.

Yelloly, M.A. (1980) *Social Work Theory and Psychoanalysis*, New York: Van Nostrand Reinhold.

Young, J. (1986) 'The failure of criminology: the need for a radical realism', in Matthews, R. and Young, J. (eds) *Confronting Crime*, London: Sage.

—— (1999) *The Exclusive Society: Social Exclusion, Crime and Difference in Late Modernity*, London: Sage.

Young, M. and Willmott, P. (1957) *Family and Kinship in East London*, London: Routledge & Kegan Paul.

—— (1973) *The Symmetrical Family: A Study Of Work And Leisure in the London Region*, London: Routledge & Kegan Paul.

Zaretsky E. (1976) *Capitalism, the Family and Personal Life*, London: Pluto Press.

Index